Intracranial Pressure

Experimental and Clinical Aspects

Edited by

M. Brock and H. Dietz

With 142 Figures

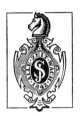

Springer-Verlag Berlin · Heidelberg · New York 1972

LRNN K

ISBN 3–540–06039–1 Springer-Verlag Berlin · Heidelberg · New York
ISBN 0–387–06039–1 Springer-Verlag New York · Heidelberg · Berlin

© by Springer-Verlag Berlin · Heidelberg 1972. Library of Congress Catalog Card Number 72–91885
Printed in Germany. Typesetting and printing: Universitätsdruckerei Mainz GmbH
Bookbinding: Karl Hanke, Düsseldorf

Preface

This volume contains the papers presented at the *First International Symposium on Intracranial Pressure*, held at the Neurosurgical Clinic of the Medizinische Hochschule Hannover (Hannover Medical School), July 27 to 29, 1972. The texts submitted have been included in their original form whenever possible. The editors have made only minor corrections and rearrangements, since rapid publication was considered to be more important than homogeneity in style. The sessions of this book correspond to the sessions of the symposium. At the end of each session the reader will find a summary of the topics presented and discussed, especially prepared by the chairman and co-chairman concerned.

Three main aspects of ICP were dealt with at the Symposium: *Methodology* (Sessions 1 and 2), *Pathophysiology* (Sessions 3 to 6), and *Clinical Aspects* (Sessions 7 to 10).

Following the symposium a special round table was held on the major topics covered by the meeting. The participants of this round table discussed drafts prepared by T. W. LANGFITT, B. JENNETT and N. LUNDBERG. These contributions have also been included as special chapters at the end of this book, and are believed to reflect the current attitudes as to the topics discussed.

The volume is closed by a *Glossary*, which was also discussed at the round table and constitutes an initial attempt to define some of the terms most commonly used in the field of ICP. Since this glossary was prepared for medical use, its authors have deliberately avoided going into details of pure physics. Obviously this glossary is incomplete and it is hoped that it will be enlarged and improved in the future.

The organizers of the symposium wish to express their deep appreciation to all who contributed to making this meeting so fruitful and interesting, especially the members of the Advisory Board, W. J. F. BEKS, W. GROTE, B. JENNETT, T. W. LANGFITT and N. LUNDBERG, who selected the papers presented.

We are grateful to Springer-Verlag for technical aid in the preparation of this book and for its prompt publication.

Hannover, November 1972   The Editors

Contents

Session 8 : Hydrocephalus (Clinical)

Session 9 : Drugs and Anesthetic Agents (Clinical)

List of Contributors

ADAMS, H., University Department of Neuropathology, Institute of Neurological Sciences, Southern General Hospital, Glasgow (Scotland)

ADAMS, R. W., Mayo Graduate School of Medicine, University of Minnesota, Rochester, MN (USA)

BAETHMANN, A., Institut für Chirurgische Forschung, Chirurgische Universitäts-Klinik, München (W. Germany)

BANNO, K., Department of Neurosurgery, Nagoya University, School of Medicine, Nagoya (Japan)

BARGE, M., Centre Hospitalier Universitaire de Grenoble, Grenoble (France)

BECKER, D. P., Division of Neurological Surgery, Medical College of Virginia, Richmond, VA (USA)

BEKS, J. W. F., Neurosurgical Clinic, Akademisch Ziekenhuis, Groningen (Netherlands)

BENABID, A. L., Centre Hospitalier Universitaire de Grenoble, Grenoble (France)

BETZ, E., Physiologisches Institut, Lehrstuhl I, Tübingen (W. Germany)

BOCK, W. J., Neurochirurgische Universitäts-Klinik, Essen-Holsterhausen (W. Germany)

BRENDEL, W., Institut für Chirurgische Forschung, Chirurgische Universitäts-Klinik, München (W. Germany)

BROCK, M., Neurochirgische Klinik, Medizinische Hochschule Hannover, Hannover-Kleefeld (W. Germany)

BRODERSEN, P., Department of Clinical Physiology, Bispebjerg Hospital, Copenhagen (Denmark)

BRUCE, D. A., Division of Neurosurgery, Hospital of the University of Pennsylvania, Philadelphia, PA (USA)

CAPRA, N. F., Division of Neurology, University of Alabama Medical Center, Birmingham, AL (USA)

CAVENESS, W. F., NINDS, National Institutes of Health, Bethesda, MD (USA)

COLLINS, C. C., Smith-Kettlewell Institute of Visual Sciences, Department of Visual Sciences, University of the Pacific, San Francisco, CA (USA)

COOPER, R., Burden Neurological Institute and Frenchay Hospital, Bristol (England)

CORONEOS, N. J., Department of Anesthesia, University of Leeds, Leeds (England)

DAHLMANN, W., Neurologische Universitätsklinik, Göttingen (W. Germany)

DIEFENTHÄLER, K., Fa. Voss und Stange, Hannover-Langenhagen (W. Germany)

DIETZ, H., Neurochirurgische Klinik, Medizinische Hochschule Hannover, Hannover-Kleefeld (W. Germany)

DORSCH, N. W. C., The National Hospital, Queen Square, London (England)

DONAGHY, R. M. P., University of Vermont, College of Medicine, Medical Center, Hospital of Vermont, Burlington, VT (USA)

EDVINSSON, L., Neurosurgical Clinic, University of Lund, Lund (Sweden)

ENZENBACH, R., Institut für Chirurgische Forschung, Chirurgische Universitäts-Klinik, München (W. Germany)

EVANS, J. P., Edificio El Dorado, Medellin (Colombia), South America

FURUSE, M., Department of Neurosurgery, Nagoya University, School of Medicine, Nagoya (Japan)

GARIBI, J., Institute of Neurological Sciences, The Southern General Hospital, Glasgow (Scotland)

GIBSON, R. M., Department of Anesthesia, University of Leeds, Leeds (England)

GOBIET, W., Neurochirgische Universitäts-Klinik, Essen-Holsterhausen (W. Germany)

GOSCH, H. H., Section of Neurosurgery, University of Michigan Medical Center, Ann Arbor, MI (USA)

GOURGAND, M., Centre de Calcul de l'Université de Clermont-Ferrand, Chamalieres (France)

GRAHAM, D. I., University Department of Neuropathology, Institute of Neurological Sciences, Southern General Hospital, Glasgow (Scotland)

GRANHOLM, L., Department of Neurosurgery, University Hospital, Lund (Sweden)

GRONERT, G. A., Mayo Clinic and Mayo Foundation, Department of Anesthesiology, Rochester, MN (USA)

GROTE, E., Neurochirurgische Universitätsklinik, Gießen (W. Germany)

GROTE, W., Neurochirurgische Klinik, Essen-Holsterhausen (W. Germany)

GUEIT, U. M., Centre de Calcul de de l'Université de Clermont-Ferrand, Chamalieres (France)

HALSEY, J. H., Division of Neurology University of Alabama Medical Center, Birmingham, AL (USA)

HARPER, A. M., Wellcome Surgical Research Institute, Glasgow (Scotland)

HARTUNG, C., Abteilung für Krankenhaustechnik, Medizinische Hochschule Hannover, Hannover-Kleefeld (W. Germany)

HASE, U., Neurochirurgische Klinik, Universität Mainz, Mainz (W. Germany)

HECK, A. F., Department of Neurology, University of Maryland, School of Medicine, Baltimore, MD (USA)

HEKMATPANAH, J. Division of Neurological Surgery, University of Chicago, IL (USA)

HEMMER, R., Neurochirurgische Klinik, Universität Freiburg, Freiburg (W. Germany)

HESS, K. H., NINDS, National Institutes of Health, Bethesda, MD (USA)

HEY, O., Neurochirurgische Klinik, Universität Mainz, Mainz (W. Germany)

HOFF, J. T., Department of Neurological Surgery, University of California, School of Medicine, San Francisco, CA (USA)

HØJGAARD, K., Department of Clinical Physiology, Bispebjerg Hospital, Copenhagen (Denmark)

HULME, A., Burden Neurological Institute and Frenchay Hospital, Bristol (England)

IKEYAMA, A., Department of Neurosurgery, Nagoya University, School of Medicine, Nagoya (Japan)

IWATA, K., Division of Neurosurgery, University of Texas, Galveston, TX (USA)

JANNY, L., Service de Neuro-Chirurgie de l'Université de Clermont-Ferrand, Chamalieres (France)

JANNY, P., Neuro-Chirurgien des Hôpitaux, Hôpital Fontmaure, Chamalieres (France)

JENNETT, B., Department of Neurosurgery, Institute of Neurological Sciences, Southern General Hospital, Glasgow (Scotland)

JOHNSTON, I. H., Division of Clinical Physics, Institute of Neurological Sciences, Southern General Hospital, Glasgow (Scotland)

JØRGENSEN, P. B., Department of Neurosurgery, Rigshospitalet, University of Copenhagen, Copenhagen (Denmark)

JOUAN, J. P., Service de Neuro-Chirurgie de l'Université de Clermont-Ferrand, Chamalieres (France)

KASTE, M., Department of Neurosurgery, University of Helsinki, Helsinki (Finland)

KATO, M., NINDS National Institutes of Health, Bethesda, MD (USA)

KEANEY, N. P., Department of Anaesthesia, University of Leeds, Leeds, Yorkshire (England)

KERCKHOFFS, H. P. M., Neurosurgical Clinic, Akademisch Ziekenhuis, Groningen (Netherlands)

KINDT, G. W., Section of Neurosurgery, University of Michigan Medical Center, Ann Arbor, MI (USA)

KJÄLLQUIST, Å., Department of Neurosurgery B, University Hospital, Lund (Sweden)

KUCHIWAKI, H., Department of Neurosurgery, Nagoya University, School of Medicine, Nagoya (Japan)

KULLBERG, G., Department of Neurosurgery B, University Hospital, Lund (Sweden)

KUTAS, V., National "Frederic Joliot Curie", Institute of Radiobiology and Radiohygiene, Budapest (Hungary)

KUURNE, T., Department of Neurosurgery, University of Helsinki, Helsinki (Finland)

LANGFITT, T. W., Division of Neurosurgery, Hospital of the University of Pennsylvania, Philadelphia, PA (USA)

LASSEN, N. A., Department of Clinical Physiology, Bispebjerg Hospital, Copenhagen (Denmark)

LEUTHEUSSER, J., Department of Mechanical Engineering, University of Toronto, Toronto (Canada)

LEWIS, H. P., Institute of Developmental Research, Children's Hospital, Cincinnati, OH (USA)

LICHTENSTEIN, S., Department of Neurosurgery, University of Toronto, Toronto (Canada)

LIESEGANG, J., Neurochirurgische Klinik, Essen-Holsterhausen (W. Germany)

LJUNGGREN, B., Brain Research Laboratory, University Hospital, Lund (Sweden)

LÖFGREN, J., Neurosurgical Department, University of Gothenburg, Sahlgren's Hospital, Gothenburg (Sweden)

LORENZ, R., Neurochirurgische Universitätsklinik, Gießen (W. Germany)

LUNDBERG, N., Department of Neurosurgery B, University Hospital, Lund (Sweden)

MAEDA, S., Department of Neurosurgery, Nagoya University, School of Medicine, Nagoya (Japan)

MAGAVLY, C., Neurochirurgische Klinik, Universität Mainz, Mainz (W. Germany)

MAHIG, J., University of Florida, College of Engineering, Gainsville, FL (USA)

MARGUTH, F., Neurochirurgische Universitäts-Klinik, München (W. Germany)

MARKAKIS, E., Neurochirurgische Klinik, Medizinische Hochschule Hannover, Hannover-Kleefeld (W. Germany)

MARMAROU, A., Drexel University, Philadelphia, PA (USA)

McDOWALL, D. G., Department of Anaesthesia, University of Leeds, Leeds, Yorkshire (England)

McGRAW, C. P., Division of Neurosurgery, University of Texas, Galveston, TX (USA)

McLAURIN, R. L., Institute of Developmental Research, Children's Hospital, Cincinnati, OH (USA)

MEINIG, G., Neurochirurgische Klinik, Universität Mainz, Mainz (W. Germany)

MELA, L., Division of Neurosurgery, Hospital of the University of Pennsylvania, Philadelphia, PA (USA)

MICHENFELDER, J. D., Mayo Clinic and Mayo Foundation, Department of Anesthesiology, Rochester, MN (USA)

MILLER, J.D., Institute of Neurological Sciences, The Southern General Hospital, Glasgow (Scotland)

MITCHELL, R. A., Department of Neurological Surgery, University of California, School of Medicine, San Francisco, CA (USA)

MORESHEAD, G., Veterans Administrations Hospital and University of Florida College of Medicine, Gainsville, FL (USA)

NAGAI, H., Department of Neurosurgery, Nagoya University, School of Medicine, Nagoya (Japan)

NAKATANI, S., Department of Surgery, Neurosurgery Division, Georgetown University, School of Medicine, WA (USA)

NIELSEN, K. C., Department of Neurosurgery, University Hospital, Lund (Sweden)

NORNES, H., Department of Neurosurgery, University Rikshospitalet, Oslo (Norway)

NUMOTO, M., University of Vermont, College of Medicine, Medical Center, Hospital of Vermont, Burlington, VT (USA)

O'BRIEN, M. D., Regional Neurological Centre, Newcastle General Hospital, Newcastle-upon-Tyne (England)

OLSEN, E. R., Department Neurological Surgery, University of California, Medical Center, San Francisco, CA (USA)

OMMAYA, A. K., National Institutes of Health, Bethesda, MD (USA)

PARAICZ, E., Institute of Neurosurgery, Budapest (Hungary)

PATERSON, A., Division of Clinical Physics, Institute of Neurological Sciences, Southern General Hospital, Glasgow (Scotland)

PICKERODT, V. W. A., University of Leeds, Department of Anaesthesia, Leeds (England)

PÖLL, W., Neurochirurgische Klinik, Medizinische Hochschule Hannover, Hannover-Kleefeld (W. Germany)

PONTÉN, U., Department of Neurosurgery B, University Hospital, Lund (Sweden)

PRILL, A., Neurologische Universitätsklinik, Göttingen (W. Germany)

REULEN, H. J., Neurochirurgische Klinik, Universität Mainz, Mainz (W. Germany)

RIISHEDE, J., Department of Neurosurgery, Rigshospitalet, University of Copenhagen, Copenhagen (Denmark)

RIVANO, C., Neurosurgical Clinic, University of Genova (Italy)

ROMODANOV, A. P., Institute of Neusurgery, Kiev (USSR)

ROOS, B.-E., Department of Neurosurgery, University Hospital, Umea (Sweden)

ROOS, W., Physiologisches Institut der Universität, Tübingen (W. Germany)

ROSSI, G. F., Neurosurgical Institute, Catholic University, Roma (Italy)

ROUGEMONT, J. DE, Centre Hospitalier Universitaire de Grenoble, Grenoble (France)

ROWAN, J. O., Division of Clinical Physics, Institute of Neurological Sciences, Southern General Hospital, Glasgow (Scotland)

SALMON, J. H., Division of Neurosurgery, University of Cincinnati, College of Medicine and Veterans Administration Hospital, Cincinnati, OH (USA)

SCHETTINI, A., Veterans Administration Hospital and University of Florida College of Medicine, Gainsville, FL (USA)

SCHMIEDECK, P., Institut für Chirurgische Forschung, Chirurgische Universitäts-Klinik, München (W. Germany)

SCHNEIDER, E., Institut für Chirurgische Forschung, Chirurgische Universitäts-Klinik, München (W. Germany)

SCHUTZ, H., Department of Neurosurgery, University of Toronto, Toronto (Canada)

SHALIT, M. N., Department of Neurosurgery, Hadassah University Hospital, Jerusalem (Israel)

SHULMAN, K., Department of Neurological Surgery, Albert Einstein College of Medicine, Bronx, NY (USA)

SIANI, C., Anesthesiology and Intensive Care Institute, University of Genova, Genova (Italy)

SIESJÖ, B. K., Department of Clinical Research, University of Lund (Sweden)

SILVERSTEIN, P. R., Division of Neurosurgery, Hospital of the University of Pennsylvania, Philadelphia, PA (USA)

SIMKOVICS, M., Institute of Neurosurgery, Budapest (Hungary)

STEPHENS, R. J., The Department of Neurosurgical Studies, Institute of Neurology, The National Hospitals, London (England)

SUNDBÄRG, G., Department of Neurosurgery, University Hospital, Lund (Sweden)

SUNDT, T. M., Mayo Clinic and Mayo Foundation, Department of Neurologic Surgery, Rochester, MN (USA)

SYMON, L., The Department of Neurosurgical Studies, Institute of Neurology, The National Hospitals, London (England)

TANAKA, A., NINDS, National Institutes of Health, Bethesda, MD (USA)

TINDALL, G. T., Division of Neurosurgery, University of Texas, Galveston, TX (USA)

TROUPP, H., Department of Neurosurgery, University of Helsinki, Helsinki (Finland)

TSO, M. O. M., Armed Forces Institute of Pathology, Washington, DC (USA)

TURNER, J. M., Department of Anaesthesia, Universtity of Leeds, Leeds, Yorkshire (England)

TYM, R., Maylyns, Bledington, Oxford (England)

VALTONEN, S., Department of Neurosurgery, University of Helsinki, Helsinki (Finland)

VAMOSI, B., Physiologisches Institut der Universität, Tübingen (W. Germany)

VANDERVEER, R. W., Division of Neurosurgery, University of Texas, Galveston, TX (USA)

VAPALAHTI, M., Helsinki University, Central Hospital, Helsinki (Finland)

VOLLES, E., Neurologische Universitätsklinik, Göttingen (W. Germany)

VRIES, J. K., Resident in Neurological Surgery, Medical College of Virginia, Richmond, VA (USA)

WALTZ, A. G., Department of Neurology, University of Minnesota Hospitals, Rochester, MN (USA)

WEIDLER, R., Physiologisches Institut der Universität, Tübingen (W. Germany)

WEST, K. A., Department of Neurosurgery, University Hospital, Umea (Sweden)

WILLIAMS, B., Hull Royal Infirmary, Hull (England)

WINKELMÜLLER, W., Neurochirurgische Klinik, Medizinische Hochschule Hannover, Hannover-Kleefeld (W. Germany)

WÜLLENWEBER, R., Neurochirurgische Klinik, Universität Bonn, Bonn (W. Germany)

ZATTONI, J., Anesthesiology and Intensive Care Institute, University of Genova (Italy)

ZIMMERMAN, L. E., Armed Forces Institute of Pathology, Washington, DC (USA)

ZOZULIA, Y. A., Institute of Neurosurgery, Kiev (USSR)

ZWETNOW, N., Neurosurgical Department, University of Gothenburg, Sahlgren's Hospital, Gothenburg (Sweden)

Introduction

Historical View of the Interest in Intracranial Pressure

J. P. Evans

Those of us who are old enough to have lived several decades of our lives before the onset of the Second World War, and whose training period therefore demanded much less of us bibliographically than is the case today, tend to be concerned over our younger colleagues. As we observe those working in the field of intracranial pressure, elaborately equipped with multiple strain gauges, amplifiers, radioisotopic tracers and other implements – and then see them faced with the inordinate demands of a burgeoning literature – we are concerned lest they fail to look back over their shoulder, and thus fail to employ that most useful scientific instrument, the *retrospectroscope*. Through such failure they risk repeating the errors of history. To be quite honest with you, my original intent as I began the preparation of this paper, was to preserve my listeners from that same risk. Thus I quite diligently and with no little personal profit reviewed a considerable portion of the literature on the cerebrospinal fluid. But my serious and pedantic interest was quickly dispelled when I faced compressing into a few pages the field that has already been so amply covered. Outstanding among reviews is the excellent historical section in Nils Lundberg's monograph in the 1960 Acta [1], which is a model of bibliographic reporting. In 1962 there appeared the succinct and very readable and well illustrated "historical introduction" to the small text entitled *The Anatomy of the Cerebrospinal Fluid* by Millen and Woolam of Cambridge Univ [2]. Pearce Bailey has a charming historical introduction to the Lups and Haan *The Cerebrospinal Fluid* [3]. And more recently, there has appeared a second edition of the well known work of Davson [4], with many historical references. Hence, I abandoned my original approach, believing that the purpose of this conference might be equally well served by a focusing on the three quarters of a century from 1875. First, however, since the subject of intracranial pressure is so intricately related to the form and function of the cerebrospinal fluid system, one should draw attention to the fact that as early as 1764 the first clear description of the fluid bathing the human brain and spinal cord, with recognition moreover of its communication with the ventricles, was given by the Neapolitan anatomist, Domenico Cotugno. Viets includes a direct translation from the 1775 edition of Cotugno's Latin treatise. The names of Munro Secundus, of Magendie, of Kellie and of Key and Retzius readily come to mind as contributors to the anatomical basis for our present understanding of CSF pressures [5].

If one accepts the monumental two-volume 1876 contribution of Key and Retzius [6] as a starting point of our modern understanding of the cerebrospinal fluid system, one may then think of later developments in terms of quarter centuries. I should like to make two comments about the first period, extract from Harvey Cushing's Cameron lectures of 1925 much of the story of the second, that from 1900 to 1925, then make some personal comments concerning the 1925 to 1950 period and neglect entirely the fourth quarter since this last is the time very familiar to all of us here.

The first clear reference that I have found suggestive of current concepts of the mechanism supportive of CSF pressure is in an obscure and rather speculative paper by James Cappie which appeared in 1880 in the second volume of Brain [7]. I quote, "... the second and, so far as the present enquiry is concerned, a more important source of pressure is the movement of fluids ... The greater the bulk and the more rapid the movement, the stronger will be the pressure ... From this restricted point of view as to the origin of intracranial pressure, its balance will depend simply on local alterations in the distribution of blood through the vessels. Every change in its circulation will be accompanied by change of pressure in or on the brain."

I have been unable to lay my hands on the account of Corning who in 1855, according to Cushing [8] "first pricked the spinal meninges for the purpose of introducing drugs", but I have been able to review Quincke's 1891 paper entitled "Über Hydrocephalus" [9], read in Wiesbaden at the 10th Congress for Internal Medicine. On page 334 he recounts that on 21 March, 1891 he, dealing with a "großer und sehr kräftig gebauter Mann ..." attempted to needle the lumbar subarachnoid space. He failed. Imagine how he must have felt on the second try, done on April 3rd under cloroform anesthesia, "Als die Nadel 6 cm tief eingesenkt war, tropfte Cerebrospinalflüssigkeit ab; der Druck über der Punktionsöffnung betrug 50 cm Wasser = 37 mmHg. In einer Stunde wurden 80 ccm einer vollkommen klaren Flüssigkeit entleert, die bei einem spec. Gew. von 1.015 ziemlich reichlich Eiweiß enthielt."

What an exciting moment it must have been when that fluid began to appear! And suppose that his needle had gone astray and instead of obtaining clear fluid it had proven bloody, or that foraminal herniation and death had occurred? In that event, his discouragement might have meant long delay in further CSF studies.

The second period, that from 1900 to 1925 can fairly and without undue provincialism be said to have been dominated by the work of Harvey Cushing and his colleagues, notably Weed, Reford, Dandy and Blackfan, and Ayer, whose studies were so ably summarized by Cushing in one of his three Cameron lectures of 1925, delivered at Edinburgh [8]. Cushing wrote

"It was quite evident that MAGENDIE, who believed the fluid was secreted by the pia, much, for example, as pericardial fluid is secreted, had no idea of this movement as other than an ebb and flow and this truly Galenic conception of a cerebrospinal fluid circulation still holds in most modern text-books of physiology, even though KEY and RETZIUS gave a hint of the actual state of affairs by demonstrating the continuity of the fluid-holding leptomeninges as distinct from the subdural space, by suggesting (without satisfactory proof, to be sure) that the granulations of PACCHIONI represent portals through which the fluid passes from the arachnoidea into the large meningeal sinuses.

"This is about as far as the modern text-books of physiology with which I am familiar go on the subject – if they actually go so far; and though it is hinted in one of them that the fluid 'is believed to undergo a slow circulation', it is said to 'pass from the foramen Magendie into the subarachnoid spaces of the spinal cord, down which it travels on the posterior aspect and then ascends on the anterior aspect, where the greater part of its absorption occurs' . . ."

"This curious neglect of a vascular system which teems with bio-physical problems can only be explained on the grounds that the subject of intracranial dynamics is one of the few on which CARL LUDWIG, the father of modern physiology, did not focus his fertile mind, and his pupils unto the third generation have followed suit."

CUSHING then goes on to say that following his return from a Wanderjahr in Europe he returned to Baltimore with a specific program in mind, ". . . I had only the vaguest possible ideas of the cerebrospinal pathway; and if LEONARD HILL's statement, made in the course of his admirable Hunterian lectures in 1896, were true – 'that no pathological increase of cerebral tension can be transmitted to the cerebrospinal fluid, because the fluid can never be retained in the meningeal spaces at a tension higher than the cerebral veins' – I could not understand how it was that a fluid which acted chiefly as a water bed for the brain could give surgeons so much trouble, and so determined to find out something more about it if that were possible."

The 1925 Cameron lecture summarized admirably what he and his colleagues learned in the course of the $2^1/_2$ decades. In that lecture the term "dynamic" is used on several occasions. I trust I may be excused for injecting at this point a personal note for it relates to that very term. I entered medical school the year the Cameron lecture was delivered and HARVEY Cushing was my Professor of Surgery. Among my teachers were many men closely associated with him – STANLEY COBB, PERCIVAL BAILEY, TRACY PUTNAM, HARRY FORBES, and FRANK FREMONT-SMITH. In my second year in the school, STANLEY COBB demonstrated before our class in Neuropathology the classic CUSHING experiment of cerebral compression. Never was I aware among my teachers of a truly dynamic conception, other than that akin to a flow of water whose volume and pressure were increased should an obstruction occur anywhere along the course of fluid flow. Perhaps had I been other than an observer in FORBES' experimental laboratory, where he was working on cerebral circulation, I might have been alerted to the importance of the vascular bed. In any event, in my 4th and final year as a medical student, while serving as a clinical clerk on Dr. COBB's service at the Boston City Hospital I was asked by my Chief Resident, Dr. H. HOUSTON MERRITT, to perform a lumbar puncture on a moribund patient who was proven at autopsy some days later to be harboring a large glioblastoma multiforme. The initial pressure was high so that I waited for a period for the elevated pressure to subside. This it did not do and as I watched I observed slow wide swings in the fluid level in the manometer. Puzzled, I went to my seniors in search of an explanation but none was forthcoming. Through the retrospectroscope it is now evident enough that I was seeing what have since come to be known as the plateau waves of LUNDBERG.

It would be idle for me to attempt to summarize the Cameron lecture and it must in any event be known to all of you. I shall therefore move on to a very hurried consideration of the third quarter century (1925–1950), which was distinguished chiefly by a world wide interest in the composition of the cerebrospinal fluid both cellular and chemical. In the American area there was the 1937 appearance of MERRITT's and FREMONT SMITH's *The Cerebrospinal Fluid*, in the English literature GREENFIELD's book had appeared in 1925 and in other languages there were other publications. Meanwhile both physiologists and clinicians had begun detailed studies of the cerebral vascular system, in man and in animals, and efforts were made sporadically to obtain long-term readings of intracranial pressure using water manometers and modifications of earlier physiological apparatus [1].

Thus it was that the stage came to be set toward the end of the period for the electronic recording of intracranial pressure and a variety of accompanying physiological parameters. During the course of a sabbatical period in 1948 in JOHN FULTON's laboratories at Yale where I was engaged in the study of cerebral edema my attention was drawn by a co-worker, FRANK ESPEY, to the development by JOHN LILLIE of the Johnson Foundation at the University of Pennsylvania of a new device called a strain gauge, an instrument now familiar to all of us. On our return to Cincinnati FRANK ESPEY and I prevailed upon HENRY RYDER, a local internist, to join our team. RYDER spear-headed a series of studies carried out by our neurosurgical co-workers over a 4 year term, beginning cautiously in the monkey and then extending the work to humans [10]. These were days of considerable concern and anxiety, for it must be remembered that the antibiotics had just been introduced and the limits of reasonable and morally justifiable patient involvement were far less clear than today. This constant concern no doubt partially explains the paucity of long-term observations and our failure to observe many of the changes which have been subsequently recorded.

It is interesting to note how often investigators in other lands, and not infrequently other languages, are working concurrently on the same subject.

Thus GUILLAUME and JANNY [11], using similar techniques, reported on their clinical studies, and GOLDENSOHN and his co-workers published their experimental results [12], all the group's papers appearing in 1951, utilizing the new techniques for documentation. Should there be other reports of that period which I have inadvertently overlooked, I apologize for the oversight.

I shall not, however, further transgress my self-imposed limit of 1950 and I shall omit reference to the many brilliant observations of those of you who form the working base of this conference. I count it a privilege to be included as a participant and I share with you younger investigators the thrill of having had a part to play in this gradually evolving understanding, so important to the health and welfare of our fellow beings.

References

1. LUNDBERG, N.: Continuous recording and control of ventricular fluid pressure in neuro-surgical practice. Acta. psychiat. scand. (Suppl. 149) **36**, 1–193 (1960).
2. MILLEN, J. W., WOOLLAM, D. H. M.: The Anatomy of the Cerebrospinal Fluid, pp. 151. London: Oxford University Press 1962.
3. LUPS, S., HAAN, A. M. G. H.: The Cerebrospinal Fluid, pp. 350. Amsterdam: Elsevier 1954.
4. DAVSON, H.: Physiology of the Cerebrospinal Fluid, Chapter 10, p. 337–383. Boston: Little Brown and Co. 1967.
5. VIETS, H. R.: Domenico Cotugno: His description of the cerebrospinal fluid, with a translation of his Des Ischiade Nervosa Commentarias (1764) and a bibliography of his important works. Bull. Hist. Med. **3**, 701–738 (1935).
6. KEY, A., RETZIUS, G.: Studien in der Anatomie des Nervensystems und des Binde-gewebes, 2 vols. Stockholm 1876.
7. CAPPIE, JAMES: Brain **2**, p. 373–385 (1879–1880).
8. CUSHING, H. C.: Studies in Intracranial Physiology. London: Oxford University Press 1926. Lecture I. The Third Circulation and its Channels, pp. 1–51.
9. QUINCKE, H.: Über Hydrocephalus. Verhandl. des Cong. für Inn. Med. **10**, 321–340 (1891).
10. RYDER, H. W., ESPEY, F. F., KRISTOFF, F. V., EVANS, J. P.: Observations on the inter-relationships of intracranial pressure and cerebral blood flow. J. Neurosurg. **8**, 46–58 (1951).
11. GUILLAUME, J., JANNY, P.: Monométrie intracranienne continue. Intérêt de la méthode et premiers résultats. Rev. neurol. (Paris) **84**, 131–142 (1951).
12. GOLDENSOHN, E. S., WHITEHEAD, W. R., PARRY, T. M., SPENCER, J. N., GROVER, R. F., DRAPER, W. B.: Effect of diffusion respiration and high concentrations of CO_2 on cerebrospinal fluid pressure of anesthetized dogs. Amer. J. Physiol. **135**, 334–340 (1951).

Session 1

Methodology I

Subdural Pressure Monitoring in Head-Injured Patients[1]

G. T. TINDALL, C. P. McGRAW, and K. IWATA

Introduction

Accurate, continuous measurement of intracranial pressure (ICP) is of clinical importance in patients with elevated ICP. It indicates the appropriate time to initiate therapy, monitors the effectiveness of that therapy, and is a useful guide to the clinical state and prognosis of patients with head injury. ICP recordings can be correlated with other physiological parameters such as blood pressure, heart rate and respiratory rate. In this report we will describe a simple and practical method for continuous monitoring of ICP which we have developed and used in head-injured patients.

Material and Methods

The pressure transducer used is a diaphragm-type (titanium), full-bridge, absolute pressure gauge[2]. Its sensing diaphragm is recessed 2 mm behind a nylon screen, preventing protrusion of brain tissue into the transducer assembly. The transducer is sealed within a stainless steel housing (Fig. 1) 14 mm in diameter and 12 mm in length. A hexagonal head on the housing facilitates screwing the threaded assembly into a threaded trephine opening to achieve a watertight seal.

An excitation voltage (approximately 3 volts) is used, and the electrical output is directly proportional to the absolute pressure to which the diaphragm is exposed. A transducer is used only after *in vitro* calibration studies have shown that the drift of the transducer is less than 0.7 mmHg/day. Calibration requires measurement of the sensitivity (number of millivolts output/mmHg pressure) and the degree of drift (changes with time in millivolts output for the same absolute pressure). Calibration is carried out at 37° C in an airtight container. The pressure is increased in 10 mmHg increments and plotted against millivolt output. Calibration of the pressure transducer is carried out prior to sterilization (ethylene oxide) and immediately after removal from the patient.

A trephine opening is made and threaded in a clockwise direction. The dura mater is opened. After filling the space between the face of the transducer and the protective screen with sterile saline, the assembly is screwed into the burr

1 This study was supported by the National Institutes of Health Research Grant NS073770 5.
2 Model P-22, Konigsberg Instruments, 2010 E. Foothill, Pasadena, California 91107, U.S.A.

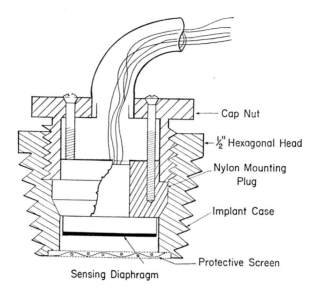

Fig. 1. Diagram of self-threading housing containing the transducer. The sensing diaphragm is mounted on a nylon plug that is compressed with the cap nut to make a watertight seal. The sensing diaphragm is recessed 2 mm behind the protective screen on the self-threading outer case. Reproduced with permission from Journal of Neurosurgery **37**, 117–121 (1972)

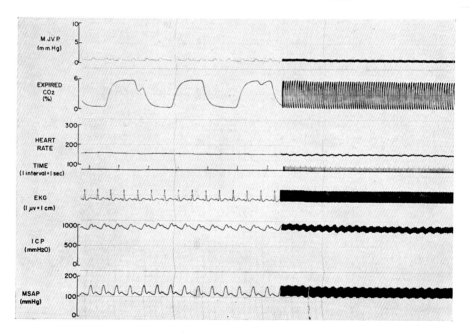

Fig. 2. Typical recording on a comatose head-injured patient. From top down: mean jugular venous pressure, per cent expired CO_2, time, EKG, subdural ICP, and systemic arterial pressure

hole and firmly seated using a $^5/_8$-inch wrench. The incision is closed, and the transducer lead wire is brought out through the skin incision. Continuous ICP recordings are made using a Grass amplifier and polygraph recorder[3] (Fig. 2).

Results

We have used the subdural pressure transducer in 36 patients with acute head injury for periods of time ranging from 1 to 20 days (average 6 days). Our experience now totals 5246 h of ICP recording. The average drift of the transducer while in patients has been less than 0.7 mmHg/day. Eleven patients regained consciousness while the transducer was in place and had no complaints referable to the device. Autopsies on 4 patients with fatal head injuries in whom the transducer had been used showed no significant pathological changes in the brain adjacent to the transducer.

Subdural ICP monitoring has proven to be an important adjunct in managing head-injured patients. Elevated ICP (> 22 mmHg) was observed in 23 of the 36 patients and was controlled by the administration of mannitol[4] (Fig. 3).

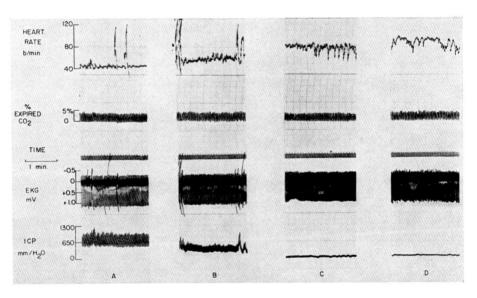

Fig. 3. Reduction of ICP by 20% mannitol administration. From top down: heart rate, per cent expired CO_2, time, EKG, subdural ICP. *A* shows ICP before administration of mannitol; *B*, *C*, and *D* show ICP at 30 min, 1 and 2 h respectively, after mannitol infusion was begun

---

3 Grass Polygraph, Model 8, Grass Instrument Co., Quincy, Mass. 02169, U.S.A.
4 A 20% mannitol solution was infused intravenously over a 2-h period at a dosage of 1 mg/kg.

Plateau pressure waves as described by LUNDBERG [1] were observed in 17 of the 36 patients. Although the administration of 20% mannitol was generally ineffective in preventing plateau waves, its use did decrease the magnitude of the ICP increase with each plateau wave. 4 of the 17 patients with plateau waves and 5 of the 19 without plateau waves subsequently died.

Discussion

Previous investigators have used numerous methods for determining ICP. Most have measured cerebrospinal fluid pressure in the lateral ventricle by means of a tube connected to an external pressure transducer or manometer [1]. Others [2] have measured ICP by inserting fluid-filled tambours into the subdural space and connecting them to an external pressure transducer. Intracranial implanting of miniature strain gauges with external connections to a recorder was proposed in 1966 [3, 4, 5]. Other types of pressure transducers were also proposed, such as a passive resonant circuit [6, 7]. However, these methods lacked reliability, and there was a need to determine the reliability of the transducer *in situ*.

The subdural pressure transducer is one of the most satisfactory methods presently available. An undesirable feature of this technique is the necessity for external wire connection to an amplifying and recording system, a disadvantage that may be obviated by the perfection of telemetry techniques. Several intracranial pressure transducers have been used [3, 4, 5] but have often proved unsatisfactory for prolonged implantation largely because of technical problems, the principal one being drift. We have found the transducer described in this report to be reliable for long periods of time and the degree of drift has been relatively small.

Summary

A simple and practical method for monitoring ICP based on a stable diaphragm-type, full-bridge, absolute pressure gauge has been developed. The transducer is contained in a self-threading case that will fit a 14 mm trephine. It is calibrated to absolute pressure at body temperature, sterilized and then placed in a trephine opening where it is in contact with the subdural space. Our experience with this transducer in 36 patients with acute head injury has been of considerable value in the clinical management of these patients. We believe that a stable, driftfree subdural pressure transducer is the most practical method available for continuous ICP measurement at the present time.

Key Words: Transducer, intracranial pressure, head injuries, mannitol.

References

1. LUNDBERG, N.: Continuous recording and control of ventricular fluid pressure in neurosurgical practice. Acta phsychiat. scand. (Suppl. 149) **36**, 1–193 (1960).

2. GUILLAUME, J., JANNY, P.: Manométrie intracranienne continue. Intérêt de la méthode et premiers résultats. Rev. Neurol. (Paris) **84**, 131–142 (1951).
3. HULME, A., COOPER, R.: A technique for the investigation of intracranial pressure in man. J. Neurol. Neurosurg. Psychiat. **29**, 154–156 (1966).
4. JACOBSON, S. A., ROTHBALLER, A. B.: Prolonged measurement of experimental intracranial pressure using a subminiature absolute pressure transducer. J. Neurosurg. **26**, 603–608 (1967).
5. COE, J. E., NELSON, W. J., RUDENBERG, F. H., GARZA, R.: Technique for continuous intracranial pressure reading. Technical note. J. Neurosurg. **27**, 370–375 (1967).
6. ATKINSON, J. R., SHURTLEFF, D. B., FOLTZ, E. L.: Radiotelemetry for the measurement of intracranial pressure. J. Neurosurg. **27**, 428–432 (1967).
7. BROCK, M., DIEFENTHÄLER, K., HUTTEN, H.: Continuous telemetric monitoring of intracranial pressure. Excerpta med. (congress series), **217**, 28 (1970).

Long-Time Monitoring of Epidural Pressure in Man

W. GOBIET, W. J. BOCK, J. LIESEGANG, and W. GROTE

Monitoring CSF pressure through a ventricular catheter has proven efficient in keeping intracranial pressure under control and has been applied by many authors [1–3]. In clinical use, however, a number of disadvantages have become apparent, such as uncontrolled loss of cerebrospinal fluid, blockage of the system, wrong measurement due to shifting of the external transducer, and danger of infection [4–5]. The development of miniature pressure transducers has made it possible to avoid these difficulties. The present paper reports our experience in measuring the pressure in the epidural space.

Material and Methods

We used the Sensotec BW 7 miniature pressure transducer which is very small: the sensitive element is only 6 mm in diameter and 2 mm thick. For protection against body liquids it is covered with modified Silastic rubber. Recordings were made with a Siemens electromanometer with automatic zero balance. In preliminary tests we found a zero-point drift of approx. 15 mmHg after 72 h under a test pressure of 30 mmHg.

The insertion was made through a special burr hole on the side contralateral to the intracranial lesion. The dura is stripped off from the bone for a distance of about 4 cm, so that the transducer can be placed between dura and bone.

Results

Epidural and ventricular fluid pressures were measured simultaneously in 11 patients. These measurements were performed on the second postoperative day, and lasted for 6 to 12 h. Both transducers were calibrated in accordance with the body temperature prior to insertion. Epidural pressures were always higher than ventricular fluid pressure, and this deviation was more marked at increasing pressures.

Figure 1 shows the values measured. With an epidural pressure of 100 mmHg the ventricular fluid pressure was approximately 15 mmHg lower. However, the form of the pressure waves was similar in both recordings. So far we have applied this method in 45 patients following several types of intracranial operations. The measurements extended for 3 to 5 days. After 3 days of implantation we found (even in vivo) a zero-point drift of about 15 mmHg.

With regard to epidural pressure levels three stages could be distinguished. In awake patients without signs of brain swelling, epidural pressure did not exceed 25 mmHg. With pressures up to 50 mmHg most patients presented slight disturbances. Above this level increasing unconsciousness, abnormal breathing and circulation patterns as well as other pathological signs were observed.

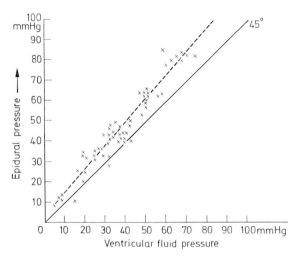

Fig. 1

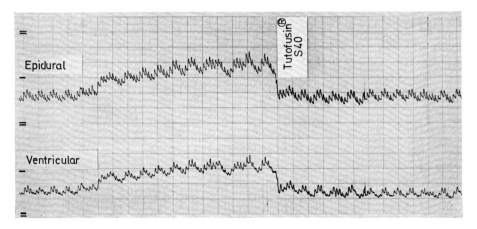

Fig. 2

Figure 2 shows the therapeutic effect of a hyperosmotic solution on increasing epidural pressure. The agreement between epidural and ventricular fluid pressures is apparent in this case. In another patient epidural pressure and EEG were recorded during a seizure (Fig. 3).

Plateau waves were recorded in 4 patients during increasing pressure and worsening of the clinical condition. With rising epidural pressure the amplitudes of the pressure waves increased. With a pressure rise of 50 mmHg, amplitude increased by 2–3 times.

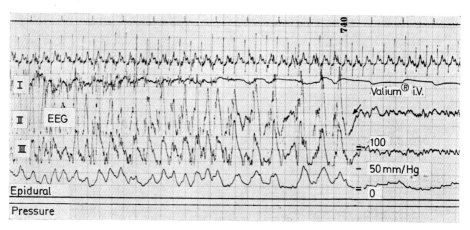

Fig. 3

No local disturbances attributable to the insertion of the transducer were observed. Due to its small dimensions the removal of the transducer does not present any difficulties. Only two incidents were observed: on one occasion the covering of the transducer was torn by an exceedingly high intracranial pressure, and in another case there was leakage of fluid through the coating. In both instances the transducer was restored by means of a new Silastic coating.

The problems of the method here described originate from the fact that at present it is impossible to build transducers without zero-point drift, and that the drift differs from one transducer to another. Drifting was less when the transducer was tested prior to implantation for about 12 h at a test pressure of 25 mmHg. It is not possible to check the zero point after implantation.

At present we are testing a new transducer, which can be mechanically calibrated following implantation. For this purpose the same pressure is applied to both sides of the membrane by means of two venting tubes. However, we have no data from long-time experiments since we have implanted the instrument only in a few instances.

Discussion

On the basis of our own experience and the data of others [4–8] it may be concluded that monitoring of epidural pressure with a miniature transducer provides reliable data for intracranial pressure control. The method is easy and offers no risk to the patient since measurements can be obtained without opening the CSF spaces. Its clinical use can be simplified by elimination of the external transducer and the ventricular catheter, thus avoiding misrepresentations due to specific effects of the measuring system. The method appears to be suitable for monitoring in neurosurgical intensive-care units.

Summary

Epidural pressure was measured with a miniature pressure transducer in 45 patients in a neurosurgical intensive-care unit. Epidural and ventricular fluid pressures were checked simultaneously and analogous data were found. Normal and pathological values, as determined in the epidural space, are discussed. A method for zero-point calibration during the recordings is described.

Key Words : Epidural pressure, ventricular fluid pressure, postoperative control, miniature pressure transducer.

References

1. Troupp, H., Valtonen, S., Vapalahti, M.: Intraventricular Pressure after Administration of Dehydrating Agents to Severely Brain-Injured Patients. Acta neurochir. 24, 89–95 (1971).
2. Lundberg, N., Troupp, H., Lorin, H.: Continuous Recording of the Ventricular Fluid Pressure in Patients with Severe Acute Traumatic Brain Injury. J. Neurosurg. 25, 581–590 (1965).
3. Kaufmann, G. E., Clark, K.: Continuous simultaneous monitoring of intraventricular and cervical subarachnoid cerebrospinal fluid pressure to indicate development of cerebral or tonsilar herniation. J. Neurosurg. 33, 145–150 (1970).
4. Nornes, H., Serck-Hanssen, F.: Miniature Transducer For Intracranial Pressure Monitoring In Man. Acta neurol. scand. 46, 203–214 (1970).
5. Jacobson, S. A., Rothballer, A. B.: Prolonged Measurement of Experimental Intracranial Pressure Using a Subminiature Absolute Pressure Transducer. J. Neurosurg. 26, 603–608 (1967).
6. Grote, W.: Gehirnpulsationen und Liquordynamik. Wien-New York: Springer 1964.
7. Nornes, H., Magnaes, B.: Supratentorial epidural pressure recorded during posterior fossa surgery. J. Neurosurg. 35, 541–549 (1971).
8. Schettini, A., McKay, L., Majors, R., Mahig, J., Nevis, A. H.: Experimental approach for monitoring surface brain pressure. J. Neurosurg. 34, 38–47 (1971).

Passive Radio Telemetry for the Measurement of Intracranial Pressure

E. R. OLSEN and C. C. COLLINS

The need for a technique that would permit the continuous measurement of physiologic pressure variations while being free of external leads led to the development of radiofrequency endoradiosondes [1]. Although many measurements can be made with internally powered active endoradiosondes, the measurement of intracranial pressure requires a minute passive device.

Transensors are passive telemetering devices without batteries or external wires and require one electronic part to perform the functions of a transducer, a modulator and a transmitter. They permit the ultimate in miniaturization of telemetering sensors and, requiring no batteries, theoretically possess unlimited life. Briefly, a transensor consists of a tuned circuit sensitized to the quantity being measured [2]. A transensor transduces a physiological pressure and transmits it by means of its absorption of electromagnetic energy from an external oscillator at a frequency related to the force acting on the transensor.

The original devices for passive telemetry operated in the low radiofrequency region (ca. 1 MHz) and utilized the pulsed echo ringing method for detection. The telemetering devices small enough to be implanted in the subdural space generally operate most efficiently at very high radiofrequencies (ca. 100 MHz). Such high frequency does not allow the use of pulsed echo ringing techniques since the ringing duration would be only a few nanoseconds (10^{-9} sec).

The initial transensors achieved resonant coupling between crossed transmitter and receiver coils to effect telemetering, a system that allowed full mechanical frequency response. However, measurement of subdural pressure did not require the use of a full kilocycle pressure band width. The transensor described here employs a simple panoramic absorption analyzer consisting of a repetitively swept grid-dip meter to follow the resonant absorption of the transensor [2]. This device is practical and more economical than other devices as it has fewer parts, but is it limited in frequency response by the scanning or sweeping rate of the active circuitry.

The pressure transensor, based on the principle of an aeroid barometer, consists of an air-filled pill-box with flexible pressure-distensible diaphragms. A flat spiral coil is mounted on each diaphragm; these coils constitute a high Q distributed resonant circuit whose frequency varies sensitively with relative coil spacing. As pressure acting on the diaphragms forces these coils together, both the stray capacity between the spirals and their mutual inductance increase. This lowers the resonant frequency of the configuration and the change is sensed through the intervening tissue by virtue of its absorption of electromagnetic energy. An external inductively coupled grid-dip oscillator rapidly sweeps the frequency of the detecting oscillator, and the absorption characteristics of the transensor are displayed on a synchronized oscilloscope. For automatic transensor frequency tracking, a tunnel diode switch detects the zero crossing of the differentiated absorption curve. The time to this zero crossing from the beginning of the sweep is demodulated to yield an analogue signal representing the transensor resonant frequency. Calibration is linear [2].

The implantable transensor presently used is encased in a 2-mm long, thin-walled glass tube whose ends are closed with thin glass [3] diaphragms 6-mm in diameter. Dielectric studs space each spiral coil approximately 0.5 mm from the outside of the diaphragm in order to maintain the Q of the transensor at above 30. This provides the detector with an adequate signal-to-noise ratio that is proportional to the Q of the transensor.

To obtain a continuous measurement of intracranial pressure, the transensor is placed in the subdural space through a burr hole and fixed to the dura to prevent migration. The dura is closed and the burr hole sealed with acrylic molded under the inner table of the skull to prevent loss of fluid or pressure [4]. Intracranial pressure is converted to a voltage sufficient to drive the pen of a chart recorder.

The size of a passive transensor is determined by how far it must be from the detector after it is implanted, the present output being detectable at 5 to 10 times the diameter of the coil. Transensors have been built with diameters of 2 to 16-mm and thicknesses of 1 to 2-mm [2, 5].

Early transensors transmitted pressure variations through Mylar diaphragms but these had the major disadvantage of long-term pressure drift due to the semipermeability and creep of the diaphragms. Other anticipated disadvantages were: 1. ionization of the copper coils through rupture of the diaphragms, resulting in excessive tissue reaction and formation of copper chlorides in the spinal fluid [6] and 2. meningeal scarring around the transensor leading to dampening of the diaphragm's response to pressure variations [7].

In the present transensor, the copper coil is bonded to the glass by firesealing with powdered glass frit and annealing of the coil sandwich. This burns out all organic material in the copper and oxidizes the outer surface of the wire. Long-term pressure drift does not occur since glass is relatively free of elastic anomalies and exhibits no creep or changes of spring constant over many decades [3]. Glass is also inert and non-irritating to tissues.

The 1 000 cycles-per-second mechanical resonant frequency of the capsule is more than adequate for measurement of intracranial pressure variations. The system is sensitive enough for variations of 0.5 mm H_2O to be recorded. The resonant radiofrequency is in the region of 100 MHz; pressure sensitivity is 100 KHz. The very small dynamic displacement of the capsule (10^{-6} cc per mm H_2O) does not significantly alter the intracranial compliance.

Summary

Continuous recording of pressure variations in the subdural space can be measured by means of a surgically implanted, glass, passive transensor. This transensor causes no tissue reaction and is not subject to long-term pressure drift. Since it acts passively, it is not limited to the life of one or more batteries. The cranial vault is sealed after implantation and no external connections are necessary. The transensor can be monitored immediately after implantation and has millisecond response.

Key Words: Transensor, implanted monitors, telemetry, pressure.

References

1. MacKay, R. S.: Bio-Medical Telemetry: Sensing and Transmitting Biological Information from Animal and Man. New York: John Wiley and Sons, Inc. 1968.
2. Collins, C. C.: Miniature passive pressure transensor for implanting in the eye. IEEE Transactions Bio.-Med. Engineering 14, 74–83 (1967).
3. Collins, C. C.: Passive telemetry with glass transensors. Proc. nat. Telemetry Cong. 146–151 (1967).
4. Olsen, E. R., Collins, C. C., Loughborough, W. F., Richards, V., Adams, J. E., Pinto, D. W.: Intracranial pressure measurement with a miniature passive implanted transensor. Amer. J. Surg. 113, 727–729 (1967).
5. Collins, C. C.: Biomedical transensors: A review. J. Bio. Sys. 1, 23–29 (1971).
6. Atkinson, J. R., Shurtleff, D. B., Foltz, E. L.: Radio telemetry for the measurement of intracranial pressure. J. Neurosurg. 27, 428 (1967).
7. Olsen, E. R., Collins, C. C., Altenhofen, T. R., Adams, J. E., Richards, V.: Intracranial tissue studies relating to glass transensors. Amer. J. Surg. 116, 3–7 (1968).

A Modified Equipment for the Continuous Telemetric Monitoring of Epidural or Subdural Pressure

M. Brock and K. Diefenthäler

Continuous pre and/or postoperative monitoring of intracranial pressure has long ceased to be a matter of merely academic interest in Neurosurgery [1, 2]. Telemetry appears to offer definite advantages as compared to monitoring with catheters and wires. Nevertheless, the application of telemetry to the continuous measurement of pressures within the skull has met with serious obstacles, among which the most important are:

1) problems caused by miniaturization,
2) difficulty in obtaining suitable energy sources and sufficiently wide transmission ranges,
3) stability of the pressure sensor (zero-line, temperature, hysteresis),
4) difficulty in obtaining quantitative measurements, and
5) possibility of repeated, reliable, in-vivo calibration.

The attempts to record biological pressures telemetrically [3, 4, 5] have provided only qualitative measurements by means of strongly temperature-dependent and drifting devices.

1969, while still working at the University of Mainz, together with Hutten, we developed an equipment for the continuous telemetric monitoring of epidural or subdural pressure in man [6, 7]. The unit consists of an implantable transmitter (Fig. 1) and an external receiver (Fig. 2). Its radius of action is 2 to 3 m. The transmitter fits into a conventional 16 mm burr hole and is held in place by 2 bone screws. It contains a capacitance sensor (copper-beryllium membrane), coated with silastic, an electronic circuit (with an astable multivibrator and a high-frequency oscillator, about 240 MHz), a 4 V mercury battery and an antenna. The frequency-modulated signals emitted by the transmitter are demodulated in the receiving unit and reproduced by means of a conventional pen-recorder.

Temperature sensitivity of the transmitter described originally was approximately 0.125 mmHg/$^\circ$ C and non-linearity was less than $\pm$ 2 mmHg for the range from —10 to +100 mmHg, so that overall precision was $\pm$ 3 mmHg for the above range, all sources of error being taken into account [7]. To permit quantitative measurements, the chamber of the pressure-sensor remains in communication with the atmosphere by means of a thin pressure-equalizing snorkel (polyethylene tube with an outer diameter of 1 mm) passed through the skin.

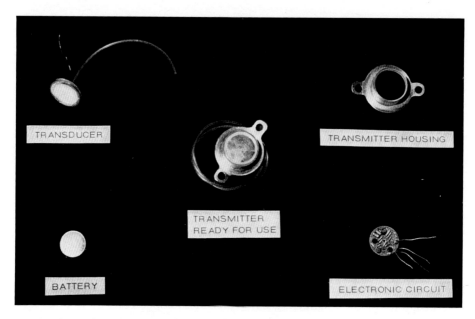

Fig. 1. The implantable transmitter (seen from its pressure-sensitive side) surrounded by its constituent parts

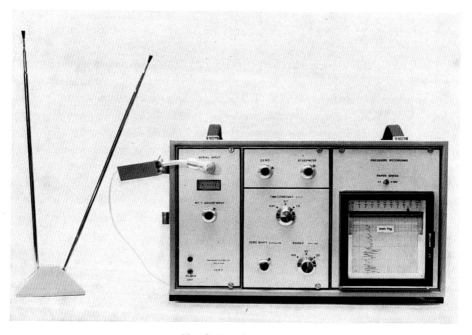

,Fig. 2. Receiver unit

While highly reliable, the original transmitter did not permit calibration in-vivo and still presented some zero-line instability since the silastic coating of the membrane appeared to swell in contact with tissue fluids. These draw-backs have been overcome in the latest model of transmitter currently in use.

Zero-line Stability

The diffusion of molecules of tissue fluid into the silastic coating causes it to swell and to compress the copper-beryllium membrane, leading to a humidity-dependent zero-line shifting. This can be prevented by shielding the silastic from direct contact with tissue fluids by means of a thin (20 μ) golden

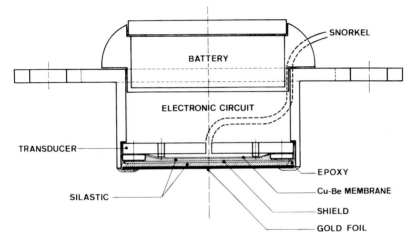

Fig. 3. Schematic section through the implantable transmitter, showing the arrangement of the Cu—Be membrane and its coatings

foil (Fig. 3). A foil of this type does not alter the physical properties of the pressure sensor. In-vitro experiments have shown a zero-line change inferior to 1% for periods of up to 15 days in contact with humidity.

In-vivo Calibration

In the latest model of pressure sensor, the pressure to be applied to the copper-beryllium membrane in order to cause it to establish contact with the opposite wall of the capacitance chamber (resulting in "collapsing" of the cham-ber) can be preestablished and is about 150 mmHg, the current upper limit of the measuring range. This "collapsing point" varies somewhat from one sensor to another but remains constant for each individual sensor at least for a period of several weeks. Furthermore, it is possible to recheck this "col-lapsing point" between one implantation of the sensor and the next.

When the copper-beryllium membrane touches the opposite wall of the capacitance chamber, pressure transmission ceases abruptly (by short-circuit) and the pen-recorder of the receiving unit drops to zero. This is a reversible situation; transmission is resumed as soon as the pressure is released.

In order to perform a zero-point calibration, the snorkel of the pressure chamber is connected, by means of a Y-tube, to a syringe and a mercury manometer. By suction with the syringe a negative pressure is applied to the chamber until it collapses and transmission ceases. The pressure at which this takes place, as indicated by the Hg-manometer, constitutes the "collapsing point". The collapsing point changes a few mmHg following implantation of the transmitter due to adhesion of the membrane to the dura mater. In practice, therefore, the measured epidural (or subdural) pressure and the negative pressure which must be applied through the snorkel to cause cessation of transmission are recorded shortly after implantation of the transmitter. The sum of both is the collapsing pressure and serves as a reference for repeated in-vivo calibration.

Example : In a given patient an epidural pressure of 20 mmHg is recorded following implantation of the sensor. Negative pressure of 130 mmHg has to be applied through the snorkel to produce collapsing of the pressure chamber. In this case the collapsing pressure is 150 mmHg. Two days later the epidural pressure indicated by the equipment is 35 mmHg and negative pressure of

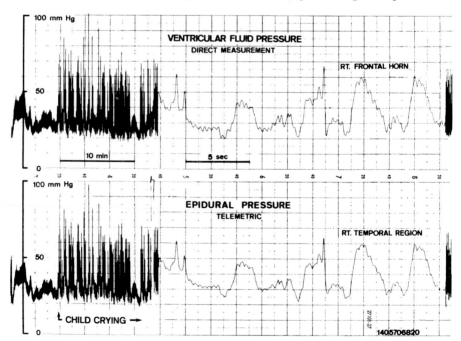

Fig. 4. Efficient recording of rapid dynamic pressure changes with the telemetric equipment as compared to direct ventricular fluid pressure measurement by means of a catheter connected to a pressure transducer. Two-year-old child with hydrocephalus

120 mmHg has to be applied through the snorkel to produce collapsing of the pressure chamber. Since the epidural pressure (35 mmHg) plus the negative pressure applied until the collapsing of the membrane occurred (120 mmHg) make 155 mmHg, which is 5 mmHg higher than the real collapsing point, the epidural pressure being recorded is 5 mmHg too high, being, in fact, 30 mmHg, and the zero-point must be corrected by 5 mmHg.

Simultaneous long-term recordings of ventricular fluid pressure with a catheter and of epidural pressure with the sensor described have demonstrated the high precision and reliability of the latter for the recording of rapid dynamic pressure changes (Fig. 4) as well as for long-term pressure monitoring (Fig. 5). The epidural sensor obviates the considerable difficulties sometimes

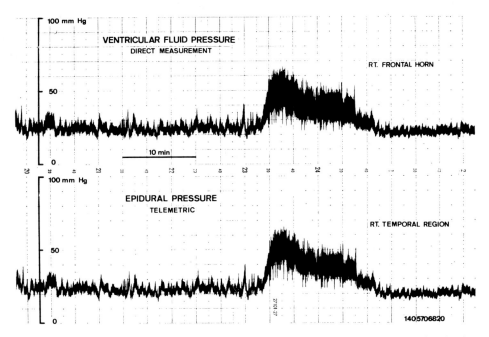

Fig. 5. Long-term monitoring (including a plateau-wave) in the same patient as in Fig. 4

posed by ventricular puncture in cases of a small or displaced ventricular system. Furthermore, reopening of the cutaneous incision to remove the transmitter after use seems to cause less potential harm than puncturing the brain tissue in order to place the tip of a catheter within the ventricular system.

References

1. GUILLAUME, J., JANNY, P.: Manométrie intracranienne continue. Intérêt de la methode et premiers resultats. Rev. Neurol. (Paris) 84, 131–142 (1951).
2. LUNDBERG, N.: Continuous recording and control of ventricular fluid pressure in neurosurgical practice. Acta psychiat. scand. (Suppl. 149) 1–193 (1960).

3. Atkinson, J. R., Shurtleff, D. B., Foltz, E. L.: Radio telemetry for the measurement of intracranial pressure. J. Neurosurg. **27**, 428–432 (1967).
4. Olsen, E. R., Collins, C. C., Loughborough, W. F., Richards, V., Adams, J. E., Pinto, D. W.: Intracranial pressure measurement with a miniature passive implanted pressure transensor. Amer. J. Surg. **113**, 727–729 (1967).
5. Fox, C. A., Wolff, H. S., Baker, J. A.: Measurement of intra-vaginal and intra-uterine pressures during human coitus by radio-telemetry. J. Reprod. Fertil. **22**, 243–251 (1970).
6. Brock, M., Diefenthäler, K., Hutten, H.: Continuous telemetric monitoring of intracranial pressure (ICP). Excerpta med. (congress series), **217**, 28 (1970).
7. Hutten, H., Diefenthäler, K., Brock, M.: Ein neues Gerät für die kontinuierliche telemetrische Messung des intrakraniellen Druckes beim Menschen. Biomed. Techn. **16**, 170–172 (1971).

Influence of Cerebral Vascular Factors on Brain-relative Stiffness

A. Schettini, J. Mahig, and G. Moreshead

Introduction

Dynamic intracranial pressure measurements epidurally[1] yield typical pressure response curves. The subarachnoid CSF compartment and subpial region are identified at two distinct inflection points. Beyond the subpial inflection point (surface brain pressure), the curve rises sharply [1]. Its slope resembles an elastic response and primarily represents the brain's resistance to deformation under moderate compression. The calculated slope (dP/dd) is then brain-relative stiffness. It is relative rather than absolute stiffness[2] because the entire force supported by the brain is not measured by the transducer head. However, pressure and displacement are known values at all times and the transducer surface area is fixed; therefore, the concept of stiffness in this case may be broadened by substituting pressure $\times$ area for the force (F).

We speculated that the slope of brain stiffness is determined by the interplay of the following factors: 1. brain visco-elastic properties; 2. kinematic influence of measurements through the intact dura; and 3. cerebral vascular tone and pressures. This reasoning prompted us to investigate, in a preliminary study, to what extent changes in brain stiffness reflected changes induced in the cerebral vascular compartment.

Materials and Methods

8 dogs (12–18 kg) were anesthetized with thiopental (30 mg/kg), intubated, and ventilated mechanically. Mean arterial pressure (MAP), cisternal CSF pressure and torcular sinus (in 4 dogs) pressure were monitored continuously. Arterial blood was analyzed for gas tensions and pH with a microelectrode system[3]. A coplanar transducer was inserted through a left parietal burr hole [1]. The transducer was calibrated prior to the experiment and when needed, during or after the experiment [1]. *In-vitro* calibrations at various dural displacements were also performed. Dynamic pressure measurements were made at 10–15 min intervals. The slope of brain stiffness was estimated from the pressure curve and was given by the ratio:

$$\frac{\Delta y \ (cm \ H_2O)}{\Delta x \ (displacement \ in \ mm)} .$$

---

1 By means of a specially designed coplanar transducer employed in our laboratories.
2 True stiffnes (e.g. of a spring) is the ratio of the applied force (F) to the displacement (d). The stiffness (k) is derived from the ratio F/d.
3 London Radiometer, Cleveland, Ohio, U.S.A.

The slope was then converted into dynes/cm (force/unit area) by the following formula:

$$\frac{Px\ (cm\ H_2O)}{displacement\ (cm)} \times \frac{H_2O\ density\ (grams)}{cm^3} \times (.223\ cm^2)^4 \times \frac{980\ dynes}{grams} = dynes/cm.$$

After control measurements, the animals were studied during hyposmotic edema, arterial hypertension, hypotension (both drug- and bleeding-induced), hypo- and hypercarbia, and venous occlusion. Hyposmotic edema was produced by infusing distilled water (50 ml/kg) at 9.89 ml/min; this was followed by 30% urea (3.5 ml/kg). Hypertension (200 mmHg) was induced with a 1% phenylephrine drip infusion. Hypotension (to 60 mmHg) was produced either by trimetaphan (Arphonad) drip infusion or by graded bleeding from the external jugular vein. In the hypocarbic experiment, the dog was hyperventilated after normocarbic control measurements. When control values were regained hypercarbia was induced with 10% CO_2 in oxygen, after which hyperventilation was reinstated. Bilateral external jugular occlusion at C4 was accomplished by clamping first the left jugular vein and then the right after 30 min. Both clamps were released 30 min later.

Results

Calibration *in vitro* through the dura demonstrated that the coplanar transducer was insensitive to membrane displacements ranging from 0.53 to 3.5 mm. Thus, the measurements reported in Table 1 are true submembrane pressure changes.

1. Hyposmotic Edema. Cisternal and surface brain pressures doubled, while brain-relative stiffness decreased to 60% of normal (a). Following urea administration, cisternal and surface brain pressures returned to normal, while brain-relative stiffness recovered by only 27% (b). Subsequently, stiffness began to decline as cisternal pressure increased (c) (Table 1).

2. Induced Hypotension. Trimetaphan-induced arterial hypotension (60 mmHg from 125 mmHg) raised surface brain and cisternal pressures by 50 and 100% above normal, respectively. Brain-relative stiffness, while exhibiting a small change at 15 min (a), decreased by 65,5% at 30 min (b). When trimetaphan was discontinued surface brain pressure and brain stiffness returned to normal; cisternal pressure, however, fell to 50% below normal, thus increasing the brain-cisternal pressure gradient, indicating persistent vasodilatation (c). When hypotension was reinstated the intracranial pressure gradient increased further, while stiffness decreased by only 23% (d, e) (Table 1).

3. Bleeding-Induced Hypotension. Initial bleeding (30 ml/kg) raised surface brain pressure (100%), cisternal pressure (100%), and stiffness (175%) (a). Further bleeding (15 ml/kg) to a MAP of 60 mmHg (50% of normal) reduced brain stiffness to 50% of normal and increased the surface brain-cisternal pressure gradient (b). Interruption of bleeding increased MAP (70 mmHg), intracranial pressure gradient and brain-relative stiffness (112% of normal).

In dog No. 1G36, subjected to the same graded bleeding, MAP pressure was maintained with phenylephrine infusion. Surface brain pressure nearly

---

4 Transducer-effective area.

Table 1. Results from 8 dogs included in the study. The experiments are presented in chronological order. For each animal, the series of measurements is indicated by lower case letters

Experiment		Time min	MAP mmHg	P_B mmHg	P_CSF mmHg	P_T mmHg	Brain R. Stiffness dynes/cm×10⁴	pH	PaCO₂ mmHg	PaO₂ mmHg
1. 1R135 (18 kg)	C		110	17	8		89.4	7.36	35.6	95
H. Edema	a)	90	155	29.5	22		12.7	7.49	28	210
Urea	b)	60	150	13	9		37.2			
	c)	90	150	14	15		29.8	7.52	25	190
2. 1R66 (12 kg)	C		125	17	9		38.8	7.36	34	260
	a)	15	60	22	16.5		37.2			
Trimetaphan	b)	30	60	24.5	16.5		13.4	7.41	30	260
Hypotension	c)	C	100	15.5	4.5		38.8			
	d)	15	80	19.5	6.5		35.8			
	e)	30	60	24.5	7.5		29.8	7.48	25	240
	f)	C	120	18.5	6.5		38.8			
I										
3. 1G36 (11.7 kg)	C		120	16	7.5		29.8	7.41	32.9	110
ᵃ30 ml/kg	a)	30	90	28	13.5		82.0			
ᵃ15 ml/kg	b)	45	60	29.5	7.5		14.9	7.33	25	160
	c)	120	70	25	3		63.3			
ᵃ30 ml/kg	d)	180	50	29.5	3		13.4	7.29	29	225
II										
1R56 (12 kg)	C		120	11.5	7		41	7.36	33	165
Bleeding	e)	30	100	22.5	8		55.9			
& Phenyl-	f)	45	100	20	8		58.1	7.50	25	160
ephrine	g)	120	80	20.5	9.5		59.6			
	h)	180	100	20	5		55.9	7.55	23	160
4. 1G3 (11 kg)	C		120	13	5		18.6	7.45	34.5	95
Phenyl-	a)	10	200	18	10.5		31.3			
ephrine	b)	30	200	26.5	9.5		127	7.44	25	160
Hyper-	c)	40	120	18.5	10.5		58.2	7.56	22	225
tension	d)	60	100	17	11		44.7			
I										
5. 109 (14.4 kg)	C		105	16.5	9.5	4	13.4	7.36	35.5	160
Hyper-	a)	30	120	14.5	7.5	3	11.2	7.39	25	140
ventilation	b)	60	126	16.5	7	3	12.7	7.55	22	140
II										
	c)	C	115	16	11	4	13.5	7.35	36	200
Hypercarbia	d)	20	140	41	27	13	60.3	7.18	80	285
	e)	40	165	48	38	21	70.8	6.94	110	310
Hyper-	f)	20	110	18	0	2	21.1	7.29	25	190
ventilation	g)	40	110	12	0	3	20.1			
	h)	60	115	14	1	3	16.4	7.39	22	160
I										
6. 1B1kWt106 (16 kg)	C		110	15	7	3.5	21.5	7.36	40	150
	a)	30	115	33.5	13.5	26	104	7.35	40	200
	b)	60	120	18.5	11	20	37.2	7.34	43	240
	c)	90	115	17.5	9	13.5	44.7	7.38	37	195
II										
1GrWt107 (15.4 kg)	C		120	13	5	4	14.9	7.38	30	160
	a)	30	120	18	9	13	22.4	7.44	32	240
	b)	60	125	22.5	14	17	11.2	7.41	30	190
	c)	90	120	16	7	9	13.9	7.39	30	190

ᵃ Rate of bleeding; MAP – Mean arterial pressure; P_B – Surface brain pressure; P_CSF – Cisternal CSF pressure; P_T – Torcular (confluens sinus) pressure; C – Control

doubled, while cisternal pressure rose by less than 15%. These pressure rises were sustained with (e, f) or without vasopressor (g). Stiffness was in direct proportion to surface brain pressure (r = .698) and increased by only 36%; this rise tended, however, to increase as the vasopressor was discontinued and bleeding progressed (g).

4. *Induced Hypertension.* Phenylephrine-induced hypertension (MAP to 200 from 120 mmHg) raised surface brain and cisternal pressures by 100% above normal (a, b). Brain-relative stiffness was in direct proportion to surface brain pressure (r = .969; p < 0.01); at 30 min, however, it had increased by 583% (b). When vasopressor was discontinued, after 60 min, stiffness was still 140% of normal (c, d).

5. *Acute Changes in Arterial Carbon Dioxide Tension.* In the normocarbic dog ($PaCO_2$ = 35.5 mmHg), hyperventilation effected only transient reductions in intracranial pressures and stiffness (a, b). In contrast, acute hypercarbia produced marked increases in stiffness (428%) and in torcular pressure (425%). These were out of proportion to the rises in surface brain (200%) and cisternal (250%) pressures (d, e). After 60 min of hyperventilation ($PaCO_2$ = 22 mmHg), brain-relative stiffness was still 20% above normal even though intracranial pressures had fallen to less than normal (g, h).

6. *Temporary Occlusion of the External Jugular Veins.* With jugular occlusion, brain-relative stiffness changed directly as a function of surface brain pressure (r = .987; p < 0.01) and torcular pressure (r = .825; p < 0.05). Certain differences, however, were noted. In dog No. 1 Blk/Wht 106, unilateral occlusion produced greater increases in stiffness (400%) and torcular pressure (600%) than in surface brain (100%) and cisternal (90%) pressures (a). These measurements remained high following bilateral occlusion even 30 min after release of the occlusion (b, c).

In dog No. 1Gr 107, however, stiffness fell to 25% below normal when torcular, surface brain, and cisternal pressures attained their maximum level (a, b, c). This suggests an increase in brain water.

Comments

Two major patterns of stiffness changes can be tentatively differentiated from our data: 1. stiffness changes in the opposite direction to surface brain pressure (Fig. 1); and 2. stiffness changes as a function of surface brain pressure (Fig. 2).

In hyposmotic edema, the increased water uptake (CSF and brain) enhances intracranial viscous forces and stiffness is reduced [2]. In trimetaphan-induced and in severe hypovolemic hypotension, the reduction in stiffness may be considered as a "vasodilating response" to a critically low perfusion pressure. The resulting cerebral blood pooling, however, damps any further reduction in stiffness.

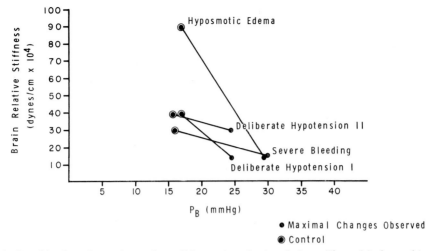

Fig. 1. Graphic plot of experimental conditions where brain-relative stiffness (y) changed in the opposite direction to surface brain pressure (x). Note that slope for the second bout of trimetaphan hypotension parallels that of severe bleeding, which suggests a common underlying mechanism of decreased flow and blood pooling. The slopes primarily indicate the general trend

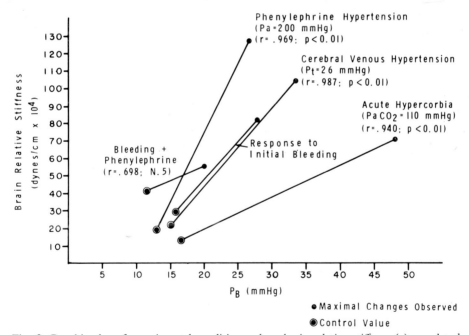

Fig. 2. Graphic plot of experimental conditions where brain-relative stiffness (y) correlated directly with surface brain pressure (x). Correlation coefficients are based upon an average of eight observations for each experiment. Note that slope of bleeding and phenylephrine-maintained arterial pressure parallels that of acute hypercarbia (vasodilator response with increased intracranial blood flow and volume). Each slope represents the general trend without telling rate of change in stiffness

In contrast, in phenylephrine hypertension the marked stiffness is predominantly a "vasoconstrictive response", *i. e.*, an increased perfusion pressure transmitted to the arterioles, making them stiffer. Presumably, this mechanism may also be invoked, to some extent, in jugular occlusion due to cerebral venous hypertension. At the other extreme, in acute hypercarbia, because of intense vasodilatation [3], stiffness increases due to increased intracranial vascular volume and flow. The fact that stiffness did not change during hyperventilation from normocarbia may imply that intracranial blood volume did not change.

Summary

A method for quantitating brain-relative stiffness *in vivo* is described. In a preliminary study, the influence of cerebral vascular factors on brain-relative stiffness was assessed in 8 dogs. The experimental data indicate that brain-relative stiffness is intimately related to brain water, cerebral vascular volume, and perfusion pressures[5].

Key Words: Brain stiffness, cerebral vascular factors.

References

1. Schettini, A., Mahig, J.: Intracranial pressure measurements and rheological behavior of the intracranial system. J. Neurosurg. **37**, 170–176 (1972).
2. Koeneman, J. B.: Viscoelastic properties of brain tissue. M. S. Thesis, Case Institute of Technology (1966).
3. Reivich, M.: Arterial pCO_2 and cerebral hemodynamics. Amer. J. Physiol. **206**, 25–35 (1964).

5 Supported by Clinical Investigatorship from the Veterans Administration. Acknowledgements to: Mrs. Cherie Cox for technical assistance and to Dr. J. Thornby for statistical analysis.

Some Pecularities of the Passage and Absorption in the Subarachnoid Space at Increased ICP Investigated by Radioisotope Methods

E. Paraicz, M. Simkovics, and V. Kutas

Isotope cisternography as introduced by di Chiro [1] and Dietz et al. [2] offers new possibilities for functional analysis of the CSF spaces and passage.

In many cases subarachnoid CSF blockage is the cause of hypertensive hydrocephalus [1, 3, 4, 5, 6]. Serial scintigrams also reveal markedly decreased absorption rates in communicating hydrocephalus [7, 8], and the tracer injected into the subarachnoid space fails to be resorbed or remains in the ventricular cavities [8, 9].

Material and Methods

We investigated 43 cases of increased intracranial pressure by radioscintigraphy of the CSF spaces. High specific activity ^{131}I-albumin was employed. Generally 100–200 mCi were introduced into the lumbar CSF spaces. The tracer flow in the CSF spaces was observed by means of a Picker Magnascanner 500. Scintigrams were performed 3–24 h after injection and occasionally after 48–72 h. The disappearance of the tracer from the CSF space was detected and its appearance in the plasma measured in a well-type crystal from blood samples collected over 24 h.

Results

The syndromes investigated can be divided into 2 groups:

1. Intracranial hypertension due to obstruction of CSF pathways or impaired absorption;

2. Space-occupying lesions.

Post-infectious adhesions may occlude the CSF spaces in patients of group 1. Hence, tracers injected into the lumbar spaces stop at the level of the blockage. After 24 h, however, 70% of the tracer has left the CSF spaces although no absorptive surface is present on the convexity. This proves the compensating absorptive functions of the infratentorial and spinal CSF spaces.

In some cases intracranial hypertension develops while free passage in the CSF spaces is maintained. Such patients have a markedly decreased absorption rate. RIHSA flow is substantially reduced, its absorption from the subarachnoid space is prolonged and it remains in the ventricles. This ventricular reflux is characteristic of communicating hydrocephalus. Similar differences were demonstrated in a case of Dandy-Walker syndrome presenting during infancy. The cyst was removed at the age of 16.5 months and the CSF passage was restored. Though the general condition of the infant improved, symptoms of intracranial hypertension persisted and skull growth was excessive. The tracer was still in the CSF spaces after 48 h (Fig. 1).

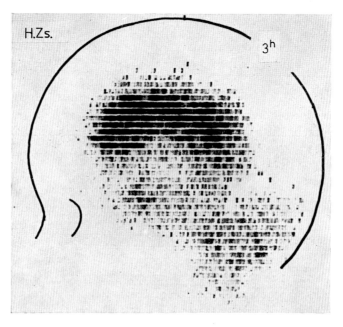

Fig. 1. Scintigram of a 3-year-old boy, $1^1/_2$ years after radical operation of a Dandy-Walker cyst. The picture was taken 4 h after intralumbal administration of 150 mCi RIHSA. The tracer occupies the ventricles and the cavity of the cyst in the posterior fossa, and remains there for 48 h. A typical communicating hydrocephalus was verified by this method, with a characteristic slow absorbtion rate

Scintigraphic studies in patients with hemispheric tumors have demonstrated that filling of the subarachnoid space is deficient or rare homolateral to the tumor. On the contralateral side, however, rapid subarachnoid circulation was demonstrated, most of the tracer disappearing within the first 24 h.

Tumors of the anterior or middle cranial fossa may decrease the passage of albumin injected into the lumbar space. This is apparently due to compression of the basal cisterns. In cases of posterior fossa tumors, normal spino-cranial passage and normal resorption are possible even when tonsillar herniation and cisternal compression takes place.

Data on Resorption

Plasma concentration of RIHSA increased rapidly during the first 3 h, even before any detectable amount of tracer reached the convexity (Fig. 2). It can

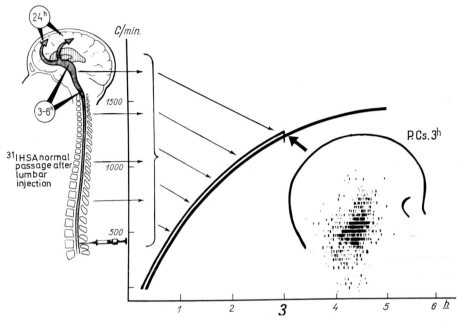

Fig. 2. Diagram of Absorption by the blood plasma of RIHSA introduced into the intralumbar spaces. The scan, 3 h after administration of the tracer shows that it reached only the basal cistern and CSF spaces. Tracer appearance in plasma is related to the spinal and subtentorial absorption surfaces

be demonstrated that this early absorption is related to the spinal and subtentorial absorptive surfaces. The role of these surfaces was increased in cases of incisural block and congenital aqueduct occlusion.

Summary

CSF circulation was investigated by means of isotope cysternography in various forms of intracranial hypertension. The importance of spinal and subtentorial absorption surfaces is emphasized. A compensatory subtentorial resorption of tracer is found in cases of incisural blockage accompanying congenital aqueduct obstruction. In cases of tumors occupying considerable space, tracer resorption is faster than in patients with hydrocephalus.

References

1. Di Chiro, G., Ashburn, W. L.: Isotope cisterno- and ventriculography. J. nucl. Med. 8, 266–267 (1967).

2. Dietz, H., Schürmann, K., Zeitler, E.: Beobachtungen der Liquordynamik auf Grund szintigraphischer Untersuchungen. In: Hydrodynamik, Elektrolyt- und Säure-Basen-Haushalt im Liquor und Nervensystem. Stuttgart: Thieme 1967.
3. Milhorat, T. H., Hamock, M. K., di Chiro, G.: The subrachnoid space in congenital obstructive hydrocephalus. Part. 1. J. Neurosurg. **35**, 1–6 (1971).
4. Pen-Tze Lin, J., Goddkin, R., Tong, E. C. K., Epstein, F. J., Vinciciguerra, E.: Radioiodinated serum albumin (RIHSA) cisternography in the diagnosis of incisural block and occult hydrocephalus. Radiology **90**, 36–41 (1967).
5. Tator, C. H., Fleming, J. F. R., Sheppard, R. H., Turner, V. M.: Radioisotopic test for communicating hydrocephalus. J. Neurosurg. **28**, 327–340 (1968).
6. Gaini, S. M., Paoletti, P., Villani, R., Frigani, G.: High specific activity I^{131} and Tc^{99m}-albumin for studying the cerebrospinal fluid circulation in infantile and childhood hydrocephalus. Acta neurochir. **23**, 31–46 (1970).
7. Abbott, M., Alksne, J. F.: Transport if intrathecal I^{125} RISA to circulating plasma. A test for communicating hydrocephalus. Neurology (Minneap.) **18**, 870–874 (1968).
8. Heinz, E. B., Davis, D. O., Karp, H. R.: Abnormal isotope cisternograph in symptomatic occult hydrocephalus. Radiology **95**, 109–120 (1970).
9. McCullough, D. C., Haerbert, J. C., di Chiro, G., Ommaya, A. K.: Prognostic criteria for cerebrospinal fluid shunting from isotope cisternography in communicating hydrocephalus. Neurology (Minneap.) **20**, 594–598 (1970).

Comments to Session 1

L. SYMON and J. O. ROWAN

Most of this session was concerned with technical problems of measurements of pressure in some portion of the cranial cavity. TINDALL's group reported their experience with subdural pressure recording which they had found satisfactory from the point of view of stability and temperature drift. It was of particular interest that they appeared to have solved the problem of fluid penetration in this transducer but several comments from the floor indicated that this happy experience had not been shared by other groups. GOBIET and the group in Essen reported the use of a commercially available epidural transducer, but SHULMAN and others questioned the temperature stability of this device and GOBIET admitted that it was necessary to refer all measurements to a calibration at 37° C and that the temperature characteristics were not very satisfactory.

The problem of very long term pressure recording was tackled by OLSEN and COLLINS using a non-commercial copper coil glass-mounted transensor. They had overcome the fluid penetration and plastic creep which have proved such a problem with this device. The small critical acceptance angle of the grid-dip external circuit was still something of a problem, and OLSEN admitted to having lost one transensor completely, although it had been in the animal for 3 years. He commented that X-ray localization diminished this hazard. ROWAN and several others questioned the quoted frequency response of this machine and it became clear that the figures quoted referred to components rather than to the system as a whole.

A further attempt to produce free-range monitoring capability was presented by the Hannover group, BROCK showing the development of the machine which he reported in Mainz two years ago.

In the discussion of all the transducers the necessity for external calibration capacity was repeatedly stressed. Only TINDALL appeared to be confident that the stability of this device was sufficient to dispense with external calibration completely. GOBIET had developed an external calibration system, and BROCK, despite telemetering the signal, had retained external connection to facilitate zero check by suction-apposition of the plates of his capacitance manometer.

GOBIET and BROCK appeared to have the only tranducers which could function in the negative range, the importance of negative recording capacity being stressed by PORTNOY and by SYMON, both of whom had recorded negative intracranial pressures of down to —33 mmHg at the foramen of Monro in shunted patients in the upright position.

Permanent implantation with telemetry, the ideal system, still seemed far away; only the device of Olsen and Collins held promise. Olsen admitted that he saw no way of accommodating zero reference in the transensor, but it seems possible that electromagnetic techniques may provide the means to do this, and for long term, particularly episodic, recording the transensor seems ideal. Most current clinical problems, however, are adequately studied by short-term implantation, for which a number of machines are now available. The differences experienced by various workers in the use of the same machine seems to render some form of external calibration essential at present. Eversden has shown that such zero reference potential can easily be attached to the majority of transducers. External connection is, therefore, necessary and we believe that with such an external connection the added cost and complexity of an implantable telemetering device is unjustified.

In the later part of the session Schettini's group presented their fascinating work on deformation stresses and provoked debate amongst the physicists about the appropriate mathematical analysis of such data. The novel and challenging approach, however, seemed to show cerebral blood content as the dominant factor in the resistance of the brain to deformation stress. The work, therefore, promised a new analytical approach to the fascinating relationships between intracranial pressure, brain tissue pressure, and cerebral blood flow.

Session 2

Methodology II

Comparative Clinical Studies of Epidural and Ventricular Pressure[1]

P. B. Jørgensen and J. Riishede

Introduction

Monitoring of ventricular pressure (VP) has been widely used in neuro-surgical practice. Because of certain disadvantages, other techniques of recording intracranial pressure (ICP) have been developed. Miniature transducers have been placed both subdurally and epidurally, and recordings made either directly or telemetrically. Since pressure gradients may exist within the intracranial space [1] and since elastic forces from the dura and the brain tissue act on a transducer placed on the brain surface [2], the correlation between ventricular pressure and pressure recorded by any such extracerebral device must be determined before the information can be useful to the clinician.

The purpose of the present investigation is to study this relationship in the case of the Nornes-Serck-Hanssen epidural transducer and to study its practical clinical applicability.

Material and Methods

Epidural pressure (EDP) was recorded in 20 patients for a total of 1356 h. Simultaneous recording of VP was performed in 7 of these patients over a total of 188 h. After sufficient of the dura had been stripped away from the bone, the pressure transducer described by Nornes and Serck-Hanssen [3] was placed epidurally 3 cm from the edge of a frontal burrhole with the pressure-sensitive membrane facing the dura. Care was taken that no bone chips were left around the transducer. Zero-point adjustment and calibration were performed before insertion and checked after removal.

VP was recorded as described by Lundberg [4]. Signals were recorded on a "Servogor" potentiometer strip recorder. Mean pressures were derived from the traces by adding one third of the systolic-diastolic difference to the diastolic pressure. Results are shown in Table 1.

Results

Function of the Epidural Transducer: Linearity and temperature-sensitivity were found in accordance with the manufacturer's specifications i.e. linearity:

1 Supported by a grant from Danish Medical Research Council.

0–300 mmHg: less than 1% full scale; temperature-sensitivity 0.01–0.03% full scale per °C. During continuous recordings from patients we found the zero-point drift was less than 5 mmHg per 24 h, and greatest during the first 24 h.

Table 1. Diagnoses and mean pressures

Diagnosis	Epidural			Ventricular		Difference EDP–VP	
	h	Range mmHg	Zero-drift mmHg	h	Range mmHg	mmHg	
1 Cerebral contusion	7	105–140	not known	4	85–125	15–20	Silicone rod broke during recording
2 Oligodendrogl.	23	20–115	−5	23	20–118	− 3	
3 Cerebral abscess	300	20–100	10	72	10– 90	2–15	
4 Aqueduct stenosis	170	5– 60	0	24	3– 55	3– 7	
5 Headache papiledema	72	15– 50	5	18	8– 40	4–10	
6 Headache papiledema	25	15– 40	3	25	10– 30	3–10	
7 Headache papiledema	22	5– 45	2	22	4– 40	0– 5	
8 Cerebral contusion	170	40– 70	20				Electrical instability; fluid in chamber
9 Cerebral contusion	12	40–130	−5				
10 Cerebral contusion	8	60–120	not known				Fluid in connection tube
11 Cerebral contusion	18	80–190	3				
12 Cerebral contusion	12	50–122	−1				
13 Epidural hematoma	110	20–115	2				
14 Epidural hematoma	100	10– 40	5				Electrical instability; cable broken
15 Epidural hematoma	72	15– 35	0				
16 Aneurysm	8	60– 80	0				
17 Aneurysm	36	35–300	3				
18 Malignant glioma	15	30– 70	3				
19 Benign glioma	150	5– 40	10				
20 Cerebral anoxia	26	70–140	3				
Total	1356			188			

Although decreasing, the total zero-point drift in long-term recordings could amount to 10 mmHg/150 h (case 19). The drift was usually positive but could be negative. Transducer break-down during recording occurred 4 times (cases 1, 8, 10, 14) and was immediately evident from the trace. The causes are shown in Table 1. In addition, 3 break-downs occurred at implantation. The causes were damage to the cable or fracture of the silicone rod from handling.

Pressure Relationship : Except in case 2 the recorded EDP always exeeded the VP. However, if zero-point drift is subtracted from the EDP-VP difference this is slightly positive in all cases. The EDP and VP curves were parallel except for zero-point drift, disturbances in the VP trace caused by movements of the connection tube and changes in the EDP due to turning of the head (Fig. 1).

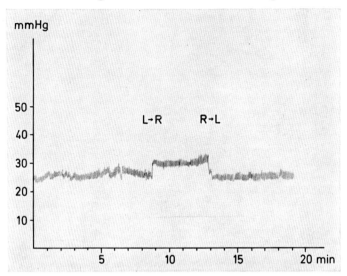

Fig. 1. Change in epidural pressure due to turning of the head, left-right and right-left. Expression of difference in hydrostatic pressure

Tapping of ventricular fluid (Fig. 2) and intravenous administration of mannitol caused similar changes. However, with increasing pressure, the EDP-VP difference increased slightly, but not more than 5 mmHg per 50 mmHg increase in EDP.

Discussion

In the system applied here the temperature sensitivity was satisfactorily low and easily corrected for. The zero-point drift was the main problem since it cannot be checked without removing the transducer. A drift of 5 mmHg/ 24 h, although low, does limit the transducer's usefulness to short-term recordings and to patients with high ICP, where the drift accounts for only a small fraction of the total pressure. For long-term recordings, in-situ zero-point control is mandatory, and epidural transducers meeting this requirement have been described [5]. We also found the fragility of the device a further limitation to its usefulness for routine clinical application.

LANGFITT et al. [1] found in experimental studies that pressure changes were freely transmitted within an open subarachnoid space. However, an increase in epidural pressure caused by an expanding epidural mass was not freely transmitted to the subarachnoid space due to the physical properties of the dura and its attachment to the skull. SUNDBÄRG and NORNES [6] compared

EDP and VP using the same technique and a similar transducer as in our study and found, as we did, that the EDP was always higher than the VP. SCHETTINI et al. [2] found a positive gradient between epidural and cisternal pressure in animals, but different slopes in the curves when the two pressures were reduced by hyperventilation. A similar discrepancy between EDP and VP during rapid pressure variations within the 10–70 mmHg range (Fig. 2) did not occur in our study.

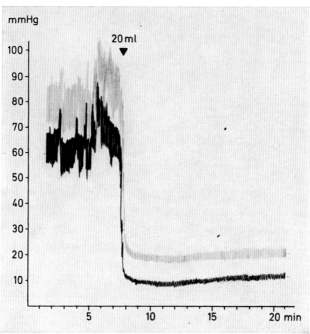

Fig. 2. Changes in pressures caused by withdrawal of ventricular fluid. The difference between EDP and VP is greater when the pressures are high than when they are low. Otherwise closely parallel curves

In the present study the forehead was used as reference level for the VP. When the patient is in the supine position the epidural transducer will be about 3 cm below this level, and the recorded difference in pressure must therefore be reduced accordingly. The importance of these hydrostatic factors becomes apparent from Fig. 1.

A clinically acceptable approximation for ventricular pressure can be derived from the epidural pressure recorded with the present technique as follows:

$$\text{VP} = \text{EDP} - \underset{\downarrow}{5} - \underbrace{\text{EDP}/50 \times 5}\ (\text{mmHg}).$$

estimated zero-point drift during first 24 h

dural wedge-pressure increasing by 5 mmHg per 50 mmHg increase in EDP.

This equation will correct approximately for the dural wedge pressure, which increases as EDP rises, and also for a zero-point drift of 5 mmHg, but only within the first 24 h. The accuracy of the calculated VP will be $\pm$ 5 mmHg if EDP is below 50 mmHg, $\pm$ 10 mmHg for EDP above 50 mmHg. This means that its accuracy is clinically acceptable only in short-term recordings of pressures in the higher range.

Recording of ventricular pressure via a catheter has definite advantages. Zero-point and calibration can be checked during recording, and it is possible to withdraw ventricular fluid for diagnostic and therapeutic purposes. However, in many patients, recording is not possible due to compression and dislocation of the ventricles. The risk of infection has often been considered a major disadvantage. In our opinion this risk is a point of concern, but in recordings over a few days it is very low if correct sterile procedures are applied.

Pressure recording from any single place will, theoretically, give information only about local pressure. For clinical purposes an estimation of the global ICP is necessary. Anatomically, the ventricular system seems ideal for measurement of the global ICP. An epidural recording will give reliable information if the relationship between EDP and VP for the applied system is known. To reduce possible local influence of a mass occupying a space the transducer should be placed over the hemisphere opposite the lesion.

Summary

The Nornes-Serck-Hanssen miniature transducer for recording of epidural pressure has been applied in 20 patients, in 7 of whom ventricular pressure was recorded at the same time. The epidural pressure was 5–10 mmHg higher than the ventricular pressure, the difference increasing slightly at higher pressures. Otherwise the pressure recordings were closely parallel. The method was found valuable only in short-term recordings in patients with high intracranial pressure since monitoring of zero-point drift is not possible during recording.

References

1. LANGFITT, T. W., WEINSTEIN, J. D., KASSELL, N. F., GAGLIARDI, L. J.: Transmission of increased intracranial pressure II. J. Neurosurg. **21**, 998–1005 (1964).
2. SCHETTINI, A., McKAY, L., MAJORS, R., MAHIG, J., NEVIS, A. H.: Experimental approach for monitoring surface brain pressure. J. Neurosurg. **34**, 38–47 (1971).
3. NORNES, H., SERCK-HANSSEN, F.: Miniature transducer for intracranial pressure monitoring in man. Acta neurol. scand. **46**, 203–214 (1970).
4. LUNDBERG, N.: Continuous recording of ventricular fluid pressure. Acta psychiat. scand. (Suppl. 149) **36**, (1960).
5. DORSCH, N. W. C., STEPHENS, R. J., SYMON, L.: An intracranial pressure transducer. Bio-med. Engng. **6**, 452–457 (1971).
6. SUNDBÄRG, G., NORNES, H.: Simultaneous recording of the ventricular fluid pressure and the epidural pressure. Acta neurol. scand. **46**, 634 (1970).

Simultaneous Recording of the Epidural and Ventricular Fluid Pressure

G. Sundbärg and H. Nornes

Continuous recording of the ventricular fluid pressure (VFP) is a reliable and clinically useful method of monitoring the intracranial pressure [1] but involves a potential risk of infection of the cerebrospinal fluid spaces. During recent years, small pressure transducers suitable for recording epidural or subdural pressure have become available. Nornes [2] has tested such a pressure-monitoring device in clinical practice, studying the epidural pressure (EDP). The method reveals even small alterations in intracranial pressure, but EDP values obtained are consistently higher than can be expected from the traditional VFP method. It therefore appeared necessary to compare simultaneous recordings of VFP and EDP systematically.

Material and Methods

VFP and EDP were recorded simultaneously for $2^1/_2$ h in one mongrel dog (12 kg) and for 3 h to 11 days in 7 human patients.

The epidural transducer was implanted according to the method described by Nornes and Serck-Hanssen [2]. The method for measuring VFP has been described in detail by Lundberg [1] and has since undergone only minor modifications.

The two pressure-sensitive systems were connected to a common two-channel potentiometer recorder. Owing to technical failures some of the simultaneous registrations had to be made with two separate recorders. Analysis of the data obtained by application of the *least squares* method gave the lines of regression presented in Fig. 1. Data concerning special measures such as inhalation of CO_2 or tapping of VF were not included in these analyses.

Brief Case Reports

Case no. 1: 19-year-old man with hydrocephalus after operation for glioma in the cervical medulla. Moderate intracranial hypertension relieved by Spitz-Holter shunt. Simultaneous recording for 24 h.

Case no. 2: 39-year-old man with persistent hydrocephalus after removal of cerebellar metastasis. Severe intracranial hypertension relieved by Spitz-Holter shunt. Simultaneous recording for 48 h.

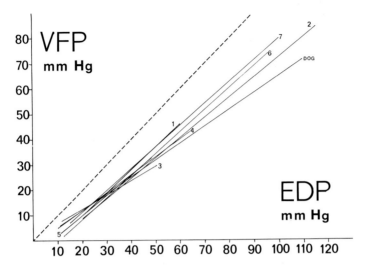

Fig. 1. Lines of regression showing the correlation between VFP and EDP in the dog and patients nos. 1–7 under standard conditions. Dotted line represents VFP = EDP

Case no. 3: 51-year-old woman with a considerable posttraumatic ventricular dilatation. Periodically slight elevation of the intracranial pressure. Simultaneous recording for 36 h.

Case no. 4: 18-year-old woman with severe traumatic brain injury and multiple cranial fractures. Intracranial pressure moderately raised. Simultaneous recording for 24 h.

Case no. 5: 37-year-old man with subarachnoid hemorrhage 7 days after rupture of aneurysm of middle cerebral artery. Moderate intracranial hypertension. Simultaneous recording for 3 h.

Case no. 6: 21-year-old woman with cerebellar tumor. Severe intracranial hypertension. Simultaneous recording for 3 days.

Case no. 7: 40-year-old woman, comatose after rupture of aneurysm from posterior communicating artery. Severely raised intracranial pressure. Simultaneous recording for 11 days.

Results

When the recordings were made under standard conditions, i.e. with no maneuvers interfering with the intracranial pressure, a linear correlation was invariably found between VFP and EDP ($r = 0.92$–0.99). (Fig. 1.). This linear correlation persisted during changes induced by injection of small amounts of fluid into the ventricles or the cisterna magna in the dog and during rise in pressure induced by inhalation of CO_2 as in the dog and patient no. 3.

Although the VFP/EDP ratio was linear under standard conditions and those mentioned above, the ratio varied from one patient to another (Fig. 1).

The EDP was invariably higher than the VFP and the difference increased with rising intracranial pressure.

At one point in the dog experiment it was necessary to drain CSF to control dangerous intracranial hypertension induced by inhalation of CO_2. After drainage, the tracings showed no correlation between the variations in the two pressures. The removal of about 1 ml of CSF had resulted in smaller decrease of the EDP value than would have been expected from the simul-

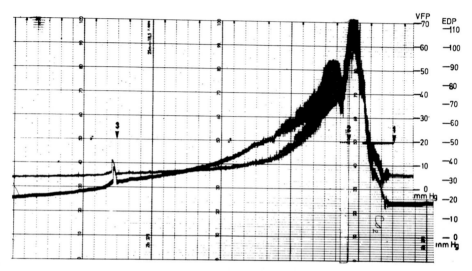

Fig. 2. Dog experiment. The effect of inhalation of CO_2, begun at (1), with subsequent tapping of CSF (2). Queckenstedt maneuver at (3), where the phase shifts between the pens can also be seen as graphically demonstrated in Fig. 3. The curve should be read from right to left

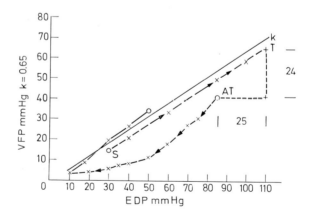

Fig. 3. Dog experiment. Graphic representation of the tracings in Fig. 2, i.e. the effect of CO_2 inhalation with subsequent tapping of CSF in relation to original regression line (k). T = tapping. AT = after tapping. S = inhalation of CO_2 begins

taneous fall in VFP. This discrepancy persisted until the intracranial pressure returned to normal (Fig. 2, 3). Similar observations were made in patients nos. 1 and 2. Changes in the VFP/EDP ratio were noted during and after repeated tapping and repeated periods of continuous drainage of CSF. These changes were of the same magnitude as in the dog.

Discussion

Two essentially different kinds of information may be gained by recording the intracranial pressure, viz. a "qualitative" evaluation of the trace, e.g. the occurrence of typical rapid-pressure variations of clinical significance [1], and a quantitative estimation of the pressure level during a certain period. Since the slopes of the lines of regression differ slightly, the VFP/EDP ratio varied somewhat from one patient to another, and since the ratio deviated from the standard, it appears that in certain circumstances recording of the EDP alone does not give such accurate quantitative information on the intracranial pressure as the VFP recording. At present, determination of the EDP is precise enough to distinguish between mild, moderate and severe intracranial hypertension.

The EDP was consistently higher than the VFP. COE et al. [3] found a similar constant difference between the VFP and the subdural pressure recorded by a small transducer on the brain surface. They ascribed this difference to the assumption that the tranducer membrane was permanently exposed to a "wedge pressure" which was added to the true intracranial pressure.

SCHETTINI et al. [4] discussed pressure differences between the epidural pressure measured with a device similar to the one we have used and the cisternal CSF pressure in experimental animals under different pressure conditions. They concluded that a consistent pressure gradient existed between cisternal CSF and brain surface pressure. They also found an increased discrepancy between the two pressures after hyperventilation. Certain sequences of our traces also disclosed true intercompartmental pressure gradients where severe intracranial hypertension was relieved by drainage of ventricular fluid.

Summary

Continuous simultaneous recordings of the epidural and the ventricular fluid pressures (EDP and VFP) lasting between $2^1/_2$ h to 11 days in 1 dog and 7 human patients were compared. Under standard conditions the correlation between the two pressures was linear. The slopes of the lines of regression varied moderately from patient to patient. The EDP was consistently higher than the VFP and this difference increased with the pressure. Deviations from the typical slopes were observed under certain conditions, e.g. lowering of high pressure by removal of fluid, which increased the pressure difference.

Key Words: Epidural pressure, ventricular fluid pressure, simultaneous pressure recording, intercompartmental pressure gradients.

References

1. LUNDBERG, N.: Continuous recording and control of ventricular fluid pressure in neurosurgical practice. Acta psychiat. scand. (Suppl. 149) 1–193 (1960).
2. NORNES, H., SERCK-HANSSEN, F.: Miniature transducers for intracranial pressure monitoring in man. Acta neurol. scand., **46**, 203–214 (1970).
3. COE, J. E., NELSON, J. W., RUDENBERG, F. H., GARZA, R.: Technique for continuous intracranial pressure recording. J. Neurosurg., **27**, 370–375 (1967).
4. SCHETTINI, A., McKAY, L., MAJORS, R., MAHIG, J., NEVIS, A. H.: Experimental approach for monitoring surface brain pressure. J. Neurosurg., **34**, 38–47 (1971).

Comparison of Extradural with Intraventricular Pressure in Patients after Head Injury

N. J. Coroneos, J. M. Turner, R. M. Gibson, D. G. McDowall,
V. W. A. Pickerodt, and N. P. Keaney

At the Cerebral Blood Flow Symposium last year in Rome, we described and presented some results obtained with a small, perforated metal capsule designed to measure pressure from the cephalic extradural space [1].

The extradural pressure recorded from the closed skull in the dog was compared with simultaneously measured cerebrospinal fluid pressure (CSFP) over a 6-h period (mean EDP $\pm$ SE). Excellent correlation was found.

We also described the results obtained from 20 postcraniotomy patients when EDP was compared with ventricular pressure. The capsule was linked to a small transducer mounted on the head bandage so as to allow frequent base-line and calibration checks.

In these patients the capsule was injected with 0.2 ml saline within 6 h of insertion, and again at 24 and 48 h after insertion. The extradural pressure readings obtained between 3 and 15 min after injection were compared with intraventricular pressure (IVP). Briefly, we found a disappointing correlation within 6 h of surgery, with EDP higher at low VP and lower than ventricular at pressure above 12 mmHg (160 mmH$_2$O). These observations were attributed to loss of CSF during surgery and to decompression of the extradural space from the mobile bone flap.

Good correlation was found at 24 h and 48 h after surgery, when the two factors mentioned were no longer thought to be exerting any significant effect. At 48 h the EDP was systematically higher than the IVP by approximately 7 mmHg or 90 mmH$_2$O, and an unanswered question at the time was whether this was a true physiological difference or whether it was due to excessive flushing of the system, possibly with an alteration in the characteristics of the dura.

As the measurement of intracranial pressure (ICP) can play an important role in the management of patients suffering a closed head injury, we now report a comparison of EDP recorded by this capsule with IVP in such patients after head injury. The effect of repeated flushing of the capsule on the EDP has been measured. In an attempt to determine whether EDP was different on the side of the injury, EDP was measured bilaterally in some of the patients and the readings compared with the more normal side.

There were 9 patients in the study, 3 with subdural haematomata, 1 with an extradural haematoma and 5 with cerebral contusions. 5 of the 9 had bilateral extradural capsules.

The technique was similar to that used in the earlier study, that is, after insertion the capsules were flushed with 0.2 ml of saline, and again at 24 and 48 h. Both the extradural capsule and the ventricular catheter were linked to an externally-mounted transducer. The results presented are those taken immediately before flushing and between 3 and 15 min after flushing, and are grouped according to the duration after insertion.

Figure 1 shows the relationship found between extradural and IVP up to 6 h after insertion of the capsule, although most readings were taken in the first hour. There is a tendency for the extradural capsule to under-read at high values of IVP; however, in the one patient with very high IVP, EDP values within 6 h gave a good indication that the ICP was elevated.

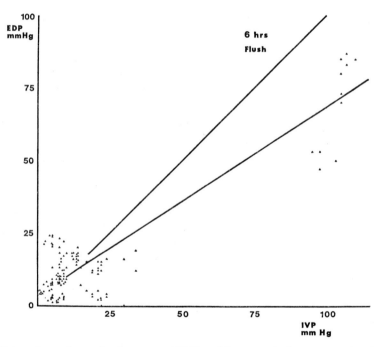

Fig. 1. Comparison of extradural pressure (EDP) and intraventricular pressure (IVP) within 6 h of insertion and after flushing the extradural capsule (EDC). Lines of identity and regression are shown. r = 0.92

At 24 h (Fig. 2) pre-flush correlation was good, except for 3 readings obtained in 2 patients when the EDP gave a zero reading. These values have not been included in the line of regression shown. After flushing, these abnormal readings came into line, presumably because flushing had cleared a blocked extradural capsule. At 24 h after flushing, then, there was excellent

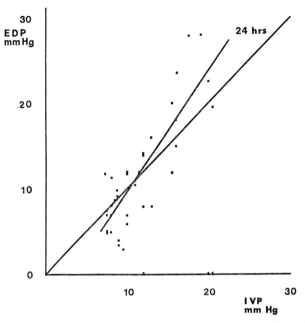

Fig. 2. Comparison of EDP and IVP at 24 h after insertion before flushing. Lines of identity and regression are shown. Calculated value for line of regression ignores the three points at zero EDP. r = 0.82

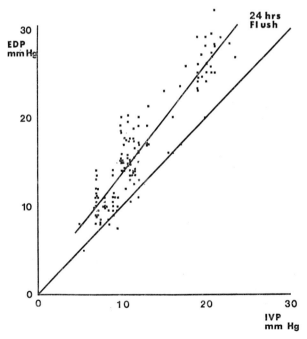

Fig. 3. Comparison of EDP and IVP at 24 h and after flushing EDC. Lines of identity and regression are shown. r = 0.92

linear correlation, (Fig. 3) r = 0.92, with the EDP slightly higher than IVP over the range studied. At 48 h the correlation is poor prior to flushing (Fig. 4) and is greatly improved by flushing (Fig. 5). However, flushing at this stage increases the measured EDP, especially at high ICP, so that the slope of the line of regression becomes 1.4. The effect of flushing is seen in Figure 6, which shows the extradural-intraventricular differences before and after flushing at the 48-h reading period. It will be seen that flushing elevated the EDP above IVP but, even so, after this effect had waned, EDP readings remained higher than the IVP, suggesting that pressure measured at this site by this technique genuinely is slightly above that measured in the ventricles.

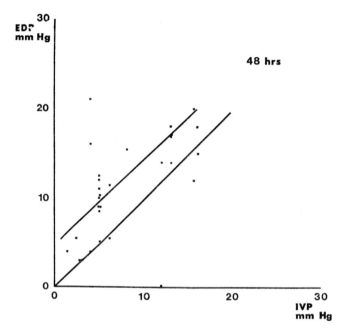

Fig. 4. Comparison of EDP and IVP at 48 h after insertion and before flushing. Lines of identity and regression are shown. r = 0.63

Figure 7 shows the relationship at 6 h in 5 patients in whom EDP was measured bilaterally. The capsule contralateral to the ventricular catheter and the space-occupying lesion when present is on the y axis. By chance all lesions were on the right, except in one case with bilateral subdural haematoma. There is no correlation between the two sides shortly after operation, and no consistent direction of difference between the two capsules. In particular, there is no evidence that the side of the lesion had a higher EDP than the more normal side. Whatever the origin of this pressure difference between the sides was at 6 h, it had disappeared by 24 h (Fig. 8), and was also absent at 48 h (Fig. 9).

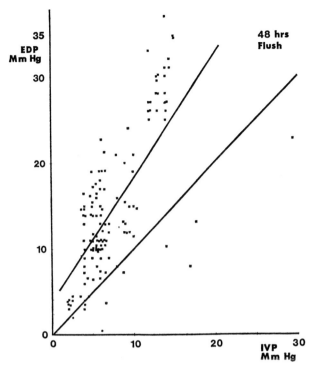

Fig. 5. Comparison of EDP and IVP at 48 h after insertion and after flushing. Lines of identity and regression are shown. r = 0.72

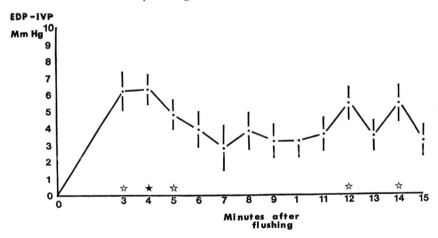

Fig. 6. Effect of flushing the extradural capsule at 48 h on the difference between EDP and IVP. Values are Means and Standard Errors. Stars indicate significant values: open stars = p ± 0.05; closed stars = p ± 0.01

We conclude, therefore, that this technique indicates the direction of change of pressure and also gives clinical warning of very high intracranial pressures

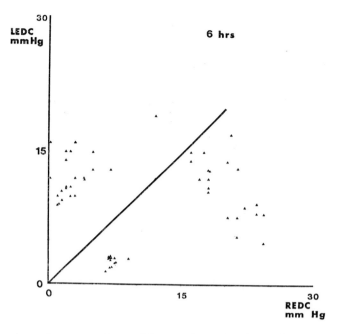

Fig. 7. Comparison of pressures observed from each extradural capsule at 6 h after insertion in patients with bilateral capsules. Line of identity only shown

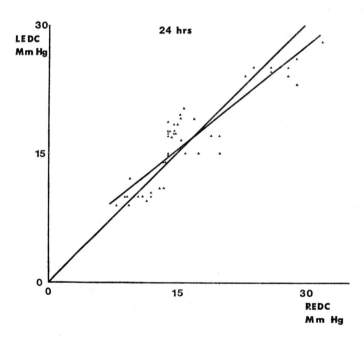

Fig. 8. Comparison of pressures observed from each extradural capsule at 24 h after insertion in patients with bilateral capsules. Lines of identity and regression are shown. r = 0.89

in the period up to 48 h after insertion. There is a tendency for the readings in the first 6 h to under-estimate the ventricular pressure, and for those at 48 h to overestimate. Flushing the capsule produces little change in EDP

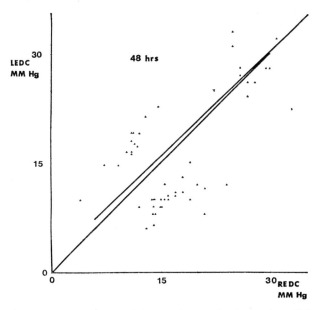

Fig. 9. Comparison of pressures observed from each extradural capsule at 48 h after insertion in patients with bilateral capsules. Lines of identity and regression are shown. r = 0.69

until the 48-h readings, but then there is an effect tending to increase the over-reading of EDP at this later time. In the 5 cases with bilateral capsules, a pressure differential was demonstrated within 6 h of insertion. This may have been due to the very abnormal intracranial situation existing immediately after surgical decompression. At 24 and 48 h there was no evidence of differences of pressure between the two sides. The pressures from the two extradural capsules, although equal at 24 and 48 h, were higher than ventricular pressure, and this observation suggests that there may be a true pathophysiological difference in pressure between the extradural space and the IVP in head-injured patients, EDP being greater than IVP.

Acknowledgements

During the course of this study NJC was in receipt of a Commonwealth Universities Medical Fellowship, sponsored by the British Council, and was latterly supported by a Grant from the Board of Governors of the United Leeds Hospitals. NPK was in receipt of a Grant from the Medical Research Council.

The authors wish to thank Messrs. M. STANDEN, B. GOUGH, A. RUSSELL and M. MAHER for technical assistance, and Mrs. M. ALBERS for secretarial help. They wish to acknowledge also the assistance of the medical and nursing staff at Leeds General Infirmary and at Chapel Allerton Hospital, Leeds.

Reference

1. Coroneos, N. J., McDowall, D. G., Gibson, R. M., Pickerodt, V. W. A., Keaney, N. P.: A Comparison of Intracranial Extradural Pressure with Subarachnoid Pressure. In: C. Fieschi (Ed.): Cerebral Blood Flow and Intracranial Pressure. Basel, S. Karger (1972), pp. 461–464.

A Statistical Approach to Long-Term Monitoring of Intracranial Pressure[1]

P. Janny, J. P. Jouan, L. Janny, M. Gourgand, and U. M. Gueit

Intracranial pressure (ICP) is, now, a familiar concept, its major variations being identifiable and admitting physiopathological interpretation.

However, this knowledge has as yet found little clinical application, probably for the following reasons: a) difficulty in picking up and transmitting pressures, which in most cases still requires a burr hole and a wire or plastic tubing connection; b) difficulty in selecting the useful data from the mass of information yielded by long-term monitoring.

The present work deals particularly with the latter aspect of the problem, and uses statistical methods; we saw two possible approaches, frequency analysis or amplitude analysis. We are convinced that both are equally valid, and have retained the second only for its apparently greater simplicity.

Material and Methods

13 patients with various diseases altering or not altering ICP were monitored over periods of 3 to 12 days. No complication of any kind was noted. Pressure was measured by a Philips electromanometer provided with a Statham P 23 Db gauge connected to a teflon catheter in the frontal horn of one ventricle. Patients were in the supine position, and the lateral projection of the foramen of Monro was taken as pressure reference level.

Continuous manometric signals were converted into numerical data by a galvanometric point-to-point recorder. Subsequently, a mechano-optical procedure[2] facilitated listing in mmHg of the pressure value of each point from the recording paper with $1/10$ to $4/10$ mmHg precision, depending on the scale of sensitivity.

A 2-min sampling period was chosen in conjunction with the recording apparatus described so as to exclude pulse and respiratory waves.

---

1 This work was supported by the U.E.R. de Médecine de l'Université de Clermont-Ferrand, with an aid of Massiot-Philips Society.

2 This procedure was developed by H. Joly, G.R.I.S., 135, rue Didot, 75014 – Paris, and M. Dubois, S.C.A.M., route de Lyon, 63000 – Clermont-Ferrand. We are also endebted to Mr. Bonnemoy, of the Centre de Calcul, for his critics, and contributions to statistical problems.

Numerical data acquired in this way were processed by different programs on a 7044-1401 IBM System.

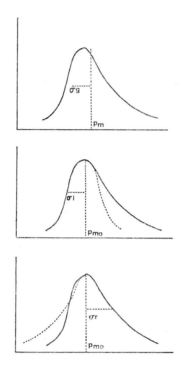

Fig. 1. Histograms are asymmetric, and their correct description requires not only mean pressure (Pm) and general standard deviation, but also Pmo = modal or most frequent pressure, σr and σl = standard deviation of right and left parts of the histograms

Pressure histograms were provided directly by the computer with pressure classes (0,5, 2 and 5 mmHg) along the abscissa, and the number of values on the ordinate. Each histogram was composed of pressure values collected over 24 h, with the assumption that any physiological variations would be included in this interval. In 6 patients the 24-h period was divided into 6-, 4- and 2-h periods, and corresponding histograms were obtained. Histograms were then analyzed with the usual parameters, i.e. mean pressure (Pm) and general standard deviation (σg). The histograms revealed an asymmetrical distribution and other parameters had to be introduced, namely modal and median pressure (Pmo and Pmd), left standard deviation (σl), or standard deviation of a theoretical population obtained by considering the data to the left of the modal pressure and matching them with hypothetical values to the right, and right standard deviation (σr) which is obtained in a similar way from the values to the right of the mode (Fig. 1). We also studied a dissymmetry coefficient (d)[3], and two flattening coefficients (al and ar)[4] calculated for both theoretical populations defined above.

These parameters were finally subjected to a correlation test, and the line of regression was calculated whenever the correlation was above the 95% confidence level.

Results

1. Sixteen 24-h histograms were obtained from 13 patients.

Their general appearance is that of a Gaussian curve but the distribution is not normal except in one case, as proven by the statistical study (Kolmogorof test) which definitely discards this hypothesis ($\alpha < {}^5/_{100}$).

The graphic aspect of the histograms depends greatly on the class interval; the 2 mmHg width appears to be the most convenient as it provides both a number of classes statistically sufficient, and a satisfactory physiological analysis.

Most of the histograms are skew, and consequently show a Pmo distinct from Pm and Pmd. Pm is generally greater than Pmo, so that the right side of the histogram is usually larger than the left side. This right-sided asymmetry is sometimes enhanced by the presence of second population of pressure values higher than those in the main bulk of sample but fewer in number.

There is a strong positive correlation between Pmo, Pm and Pmd in the 13 patients, as shown in Table 1. A slightly less marked correlation was found between these 3 parameters and standard deviations σr and σl, but the correlation with the general standard deviation σg is definitely weaker (Table 1).

Such a correlation, relating ICP to its fluctuation [$\sigma g = f$ (Pm)], was, however, statistically significant for each patient individually within each 30-min interval.

No correlation was found between the other pairs of parameters, both whether or not they were statistically obvious or had any physiological significance.

2. The 214 histograms obtained from 6-, 4- and 2-h observation periods are slightly different. Their general form is still that of a hump-shaped curve, even though some figures indicate a plurimodal distribution. Nonetheless, their numerical parameters may vary quite widely during the day. Furthermore, if Pmo, Pm and Pmd remain closely correlated in one patient, correlation between these pressure values and the standard deviation ($\sigma g, \sigma l$ and σr) becomes weaker and may even disappear.

3    $d = \dfrac{\sum \frac{(x - Pm)^3}{n}}{\sigma g^3}$

4    $ar = \dfrac{\sum \frac{(x - Pm)^4}{n}}{\sigma r^4}$ $al = \dfrac{\sum \frac{(x - Pm)^4}{n}}{\sigma l^4}$

Table 1. Correlations and regression lines between modal, mean, and median pressure – and general, left and right standard deviations

	Pmo	Pm	Pmd
Pmo		$r = 0.75$ $\alpha < 0.001$ $Pm = 0.936\ Pmo + 2.8$	
Pmd		$r = 0.96$ $\alpha < 0.001$ $Pm = 1.02\ Pmd - 0.07$	
σg	$r = 0.41$ $\alpha < 0.15$ $\sigma g = 0.20\ Pmo + 1.13$	$r = 0.77$ $\alpha < 0.001$ $\sigma g = 0.30\ Pm - 1.45$	$r = 0.78$ $\alpha < 0.001$ $\sigma g = 0.30\ Pmd - 1.55$
σl	$r = 0.55$ $\alpha < 0.05$ $\sigma l = 0.17\ Pmo + 0.45$	$r = 0.56$ $\alpha < 0.05$ $\sigma l = 0.14\ Pm + 1$	$r = 0.59$ $\alpha < 0.02$ $\sigma l = 0.15\ Pmd + 0.82$
σr	$r = 0.59$ $\alpha < 0.02$ $\sigma r = 0.40\ Pmo - 2.20$	$r = 0.65$ $\alpha < 0.01$ $\sigma r = 0.35\ Pm - 1.67$	$r = 0.67$ $\alpha < 0.01$ $\sigma r = 0.37\ Pmd - 1.96$

Discussion

1. These results provide judicious arguments for choosing a value likely to represent ICP. Since there is a strong correlation between Pmo, Pm and Pmd, any of these parameters might be used. We think, however, that Pm, although frequently referred to in the literature, is, in fact, like Pmd, less suitable than Pmo. While Pm and Pmd are theoretically calculated values, Pmo is an actual one, easily read on the histogram. Furthermore, Pm is by definition the most frequent pressure value, and is consequently perfectly consistent with a good definition of what one may call the basal ICP. It must, however, be noted that, in the case of the plurimodal histograms sometimes encountered when the recording time is short, Pmo may lack physiological meaning. It is then worth abiding by Pm.

2. Intracranial pressure fluctuates above and below Pmo, i.e. to the right and left of Pmo on the histograms. σr and σl provide a measure of these fluctuations. Pressure waves of any kind, and particularly the so-called plateau-waves, of course lie at the extreme right of the histogram where they may even "emerge" as a second peak, when they are frequent and elevated, as previously stated by KULLBERG [1] (Fig. 2).

Thus, on the whole σr depicts the pathological events tending to raise ICP, whereas σl provides information on the fluctuations by which ICP tends to return to physiological values.

The close correlations between Pmo and standard deviations σr and σl indicates that an increase in ICP is paralleled by an increase in the amplitude of its fluctuations. But it is essential to point out that the increment is not the same in both halves of the histograms, as is seen from a comparison of the lines of regression; high pressure waves increase as a function of Pmo about twice as fast as low pressure waves.

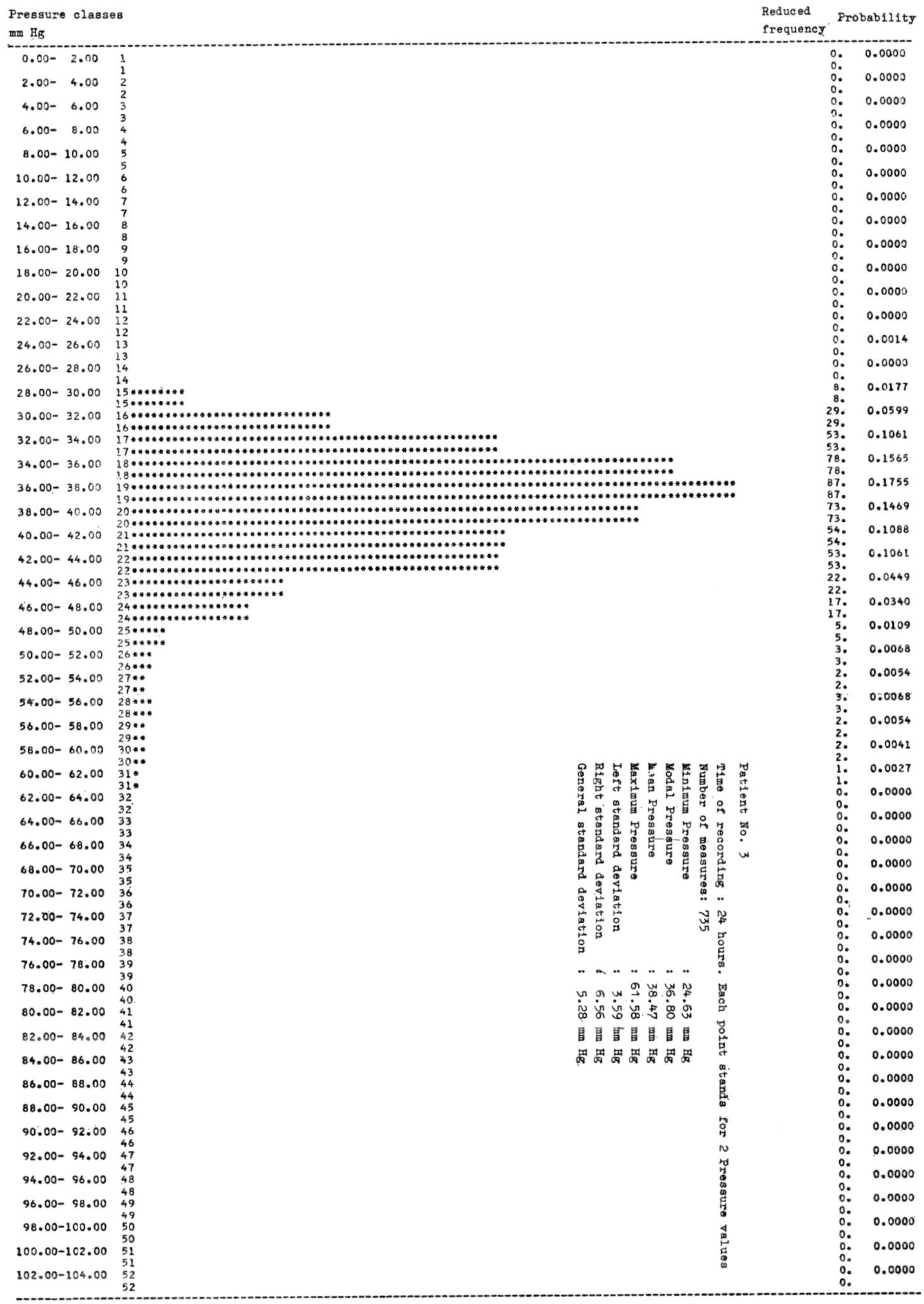

Pressure classes mm Hg		Reduced frequency	Probability
0.00- 2.00	1	0.	0.0000
2.00- 4.00	2	0.	0.0000
4.00- 6.00	3	0.	0.0000
6.00- 8.00	4	0.	0.0000
8.00- 10.00	5	0.	0.0000
10.00- 12.00	6	0.	0.0000
12.00- 14.00	7	0.	0.0000
14.00- 16.00	8	0.	0.0000
16.00- 18.00	9	0.	0.0000
18.00- 20.00	10	0.	0.0000
20.00- 22.00	11	0.	0.0000
22.00- 24.00	12	0.	0.0000
24.00- 26.00	13	0.	0.0014
26.00- 28.00	14	0.	0.0000
28.00- 30.00	15	8.	0.0177
30.00- 32.00	16	29.	0.0599
32.00- 34.00	17	53.	0.1061
34.00- 36.00	18	78.	0.1565
36.00- 38.00	19	87.	0.1755
38.00- 40.00	20	73.	0.1469
40.00- 42.00	21	54.	0.1088
42.00- 44.00	22	53.	0.1061
44.00- 46.00	23	22.	0.0449
46.00- 48.00	24	17.	0.0340
48.00- 50.00	25	5.	0.0109
50.00- 52.00	26	3.	0.0068
52.00- 54.00	27	2.	0.0054
54.00- 56.00	28	3.	0.0068
56.00- 58.00	29	2.	0.0054
58.00- 60.00	30	2.	0.0041
60.00- 62.00	31	1.	0.0027
62.00- 64.00	32	0.	0.0000
64.00- 66.00	33	0.	0.0000
66.00- 68.00	34	0.	0.0000
68.00- 70.00	35	0.	0.0000
70.00- 72.00	36	0.	0.0000
72.00- 74.00	37	0.	0.0000
74.00- 76.00	38	0.	0.0000
76.00- 78.00	39	0.	0.0000
78.00- 80.00	40	0.	0.0000
80.00- 82.00	41	0.	0.0000
82.00- 84.00	42	0.	0.0000
84.00- 86.00	43	0.	0.0000
86.00- 88.00	44	0.	0.0000
88.00- 90.00	45	0.	0.0000
90.00- 92.00	46	0.	0.0000
92.00- 94.00	47	0.	0.0000
94.00- 96.00	48	0.	0.0000
96.00- 98.00	49	0.	0.0000
98.00-100.00	50	0.	0.0000
100.00-102.00	51	0.	0.0000
102.00-104.00	52	0.	0.0000

Patient No. 3
Time of recording : 24 hours. Each point stands for 2 Pressure values
Number of measures: 735
Minimum Pressure : 24.63 mm Hg
Modal Pressure : 36.80 mm Hg
Mean Pressure : 38.47 mm Hg
Maximum Pressure : 61.58 mm Hg
Left standard deviation : 3.59 mm Hg
Right standard deviation : 6.56 mm Hg
General standard deviation : 5.28 mm Hg

Fig. 2. Typical 24-h histogram showing the right-sided asymmetry of the pressure distribution, and the presence of a second isolated hump corresponding to the plateau-waves

It is also apparent that at a Pmo of about 12 mmHg, the 2 parameters become equal and the histograms become symmetrical. Since this pressure value may be considered an upper physiological limit in a recumbent patient, it may be that under normal conditions ICP fluctuates symmetrically to each side of a mean value, and that asymmetry of the histograms reveals incipient pathological phenomena. These remarks show the advantage of using σr and σl rather than standard general deviation σg to describe fluctuations in intracranial pressure.

3. The above analysis is applicable in the case of 6-h histograms but seems less and less appropriate as observation periods become shorter and correlation weakens between Pmo and σr, σl. It is then probably better to describe fluctuations of such small pressure samples by the general standard deviation around the mean.

4. We hope, in conclusion, that these results may be useful in the development of an automatic analyzer capable of providing not only immediate records of ICP, but also its mean value and standard deviation over the last hour, and histograms of the fluctuations over the last 6 and/or 24 h, with indication of Pmo, σr and σl.

Summary

We have attempted to summarize the numerous data acquired during ICP recordings and to make them more intelligible.

The continuous signal supplied by an electromanometer was converted to numerical values every 2 min, and pressure histograms were obtained and described by appropriate parameters.

We have shown that such histograms and parameters contain the principal features of ICP during the recording period, i.e. 1. definition of a basal pressure, and 2. recording of the pressure fluctuations, and particularly of the high pressure waves. These results probably provide a valuable basis for an automatic continuous ICP analyzer.

Key Words: Intracranial pressure, monitoring, statistical analysis.

Reference

1. Kulberg, G.: Influence of corticosteroids on the ventricular fluid pressure. Act. neurol. scand. **41** (Suppl. 13), 445–452 (1965).

A Method for Statistical Analysis of Intracranial Pressure Recordings

G. KULLBERG

When the intracranial pressure is recorded for extended periods of time, the information contained in the record may be difficult to glean from mere inspection of the long, irregular tracing. Some sort of condensing and ordering procedure may be desirable to depict the characteristic features. We have chosen to analyze the quantitative representation of different pressure classes in the record, i.e. the pressure-class frequency distribution. In an earlier study [1] based on this method the data was extracted from the curves manually. Since then a special apparatus has been constructed which performs the analysis.

Methods

In curve sections of suitable length, for example 24-h periods of recording, the pressure is read at frequent, regular intervals. These pressure observations are grouped into pressure classes of 10 mmHg interval, i.e. 10–20, 20–30, 30–40 etc. mmHg. The number of observations in each class is noted. The data obtained constitutes the pressure-class frequency distribution. The distribution is conveniently represented as a histogram or frequency polygon by plotting the number of observations, expressed as percentages of the total, against the pressure classes.

The pressure data are provided by the analyzing apparatus[1] simultaneously with the pressure recording. The analyzer is equipped with 13 counters, each counter representing one pressure class. At present time intervals the analyzer senses the pressure level and identifies the pressure class, each time causing the corresponding counter to register one more digit. The time interval can be varied from 0.1 to 1 sec in several steps. The maximum counting capacity is 10000 counts. 10000 counts in 24 h will correspond to an interval of 8.64 sec. The counters are visible on the front panel of the analyzer and can be read at any time offering a practical bedside survey of the pressure pattern during the preceding period. If desired, a pressure diagram can easily be constructed from the data provided by the counters.

---

1 Constructed by Mr. TURE NILSSON at the Medical Engineering Department, University Hospital, Lund, Sweden.

Results

Examples of pressure-class frequency distribution of different types obtained by this method are shown in Figures 1 and 2. For comparison each distribution has been represented as a histogram, a frequency polygon and a hypothetical frequency curve obtained by simple freehand fitting. Pressure diagrams demonstrate the extent of the pressure variations and the presence of a more or less distinct "typical" pressure level, which is indicated by the high peak or hump. This "typical" or basal pressure is usually different from the mean pressure as the distributions are commonly skew, particularly when the basal pressure is high. Sometimes a double-humped distribution is obtained,

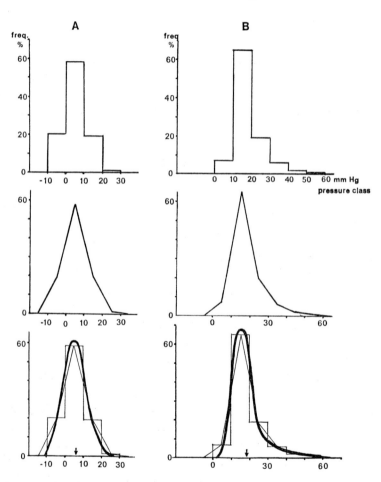

Fig. 1. Pressure-class frequency distributions, each represented as histogram (above), frequency polygon (centre), hypothetical frequency curve (below). Arrows indicate mean pressure. A) Essentially normal pressure and symmetrical distribution. B) Moderately raised pressure, skew distribution. (The examples represent 24-h periods of recording in a case of head injury: A in the recovery phase, B in the initial phase.)

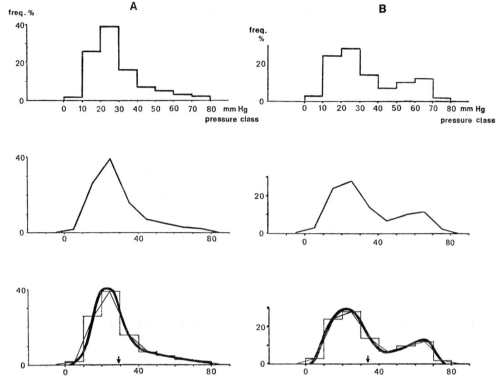

Fig. 2. Pressure-class frequency distributions, each represented as histogram (above), frequency polygon (centre), hypothetical frequency curve (below). Arrows indicate mean pressure. A) Raised basal pressure, skew distribution. B) Raised basal pressure, double-humped distribution, the hump to the right indicating plateau waves. (These distributions represent 48-h periods of recording in two patients with malignant glioma.)

the smaller hump reflecting the occurrence of plateau waves reaching equal height.

The diagrams also give an idea of the mean pressure (center of gravity of the frequency curve) and of the median pressure (vertical line dividing the curve area in equal parts).

Comparison of pressure diagrams representing consecutive periods of recording aid in the evaluation of slowly occurring changes in the pressure. Differences in the shape and the position of the distribution stand out clearly if a series of diagrams are superimposed in the same coordinate system.

Another way of representing a series of pressure-class data from a long period of recording in one single diagram is shown in Figure 3. In this chart days are indicated on the horizontal axis, cumulated pressure-class frequencies on the vertical axis. The pressure-class data for each day are marked by points in a vertical row. Points representing identical pressure levels on the different days

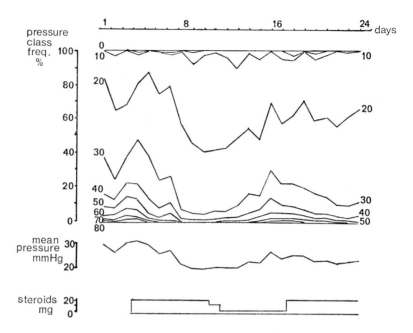

Fig. 3. "Isobar" chart. Cumulated pressure-class frequencies for each day marked by points in a vertical row. Points representing identical pressure-class limits on the different days joined by lines, "isobars". The area between two lines forms a band whose width is the frequency of the corresponding pressure-class. The dominating pressure-class(es) – the widest band (s) – indicate the level of the basal pressure. Calculated mean pressure values and treatment with steroids shown below. Note the decrease in frequency of the high-pressure classes and the downward shift of the basal pressure during steroid treatment

have been joined up by lines traversing the chart like isobars. The area between 2 adjacent lines forms a band whose width indicates the frequency of that particular pressure-class. Thus, the chart shows the changing representation of the different pressure-classes during the period recorded, in the example given the decrease of the high pressure-classes and the shift of the basal pressure to a lower class during steroid treatment.

Comments

The pressure data provided by the analyzer can also be used for calculation of mean pressure values and measures of dispersion, parameters of special statistical importance. However, the main value of the analyzing method lies in the pressure diagram. The diagram depicts natural properties and clinically important features of the pressure curve, such as the basal pressure level and the occurrence of high pressure episodes, which are poorly reflected by the mean and the standard deviation. Although giving less refined and elaborate information than may be obtained with a computer, the analyzer described seems to offer a good alternative suitable for routine clinical use.

Summary

It is suggested that tracings obtained during long-term recording of the intracranial pressure be analyzed by calculation of the pressure-class frequency distribution in order to obtain a condensed picture of the characteristic and clinically important features of the pressure curve. An apparatus for automatic analysis is described. Various forms of graphic representation of the data are presented.

Key Words: Intracranial pressure recording, statistical analysis, automatic analyzer.

Reference

1. KULLBERG, G., WEST, K. A.: Influence of corticosteroids on the ventricular fluid pressure. Acta neurol. scand. 41 (Suppl. 13), 445–452 (1964).

Comments to Session 2

R. Cooper and H. Nornes

In the determination of all clinical measurements there must be minimum interference with the patient consistent with obtaining a *sufficiently accurate* measure of the variable being investigated.

In the measurement of pressure inside the cranium this has led to the development of techniques of measuring pressure in the space between the skull and the dura. By these means incision of the dura can be avoided and the risk of infection reduced. Another advantage of the method is that at very high levels of ICP it may be dangerous to open the dura. In addition any loss of CSF through the dural incision will distort the measurement of the true conditions, especially at high pressures.

The main disadvantage of the epidural method of recording is that at low pressure levels an error of 5–10 mmHg may be interpreted as having clinical significance whereas the same error at high pressure is not important.

During the implantation of VFP transducers some CSF is bound to escape and several hours may elapse before a "steady state" is re-established. Thus any comparison of methods must be delayed until equilibrium is reached. There is discrepancy between the two techniques because the dura is relatively thick and measurement of the pressure through it will distort the true value.

Coe et al. (1969) suggested that transducers placed in the space between two semi-rigid bodies are subjected to a continuous "wedge pressure" and that the pressure recorded would be too high. Thus, epidural transducers can be expected to read too high.

Three studies comparing the VFP with the epidural pressure (EDP) have been described by the groups of Jørgensen, Sundbärg, and Coroneos.

Once having established equilibrium and with normocapnia, all measurements show that the EDP is higher than the VFP although both methods showed good linearity. The data presented showed that the proportional error increased at high mean pressure levels although there is a possibility that this might be due to minor leakage of CSF along the catheter at high pressure.

The VFP/EDP regression line does not pass through zero and shows an error up to 10 mmHg EDP when the VFP is zero. There is also evidence that during acute relative changes of cerebral constituents there are pressure gradients between ventricles and brain surface as measured by the epidural method.

In disturbed physiological conditions, such as in the presence of pathology or hypercarbia, the deviations of the two measures can be considerable (greater than 20 mmHg) and values of EDP must be treated with caution.

According to McDowall there can be great bilateral differences during the first 6 h after implantation that are not related to pathology, improving over the first 24 h but diverging again after 48 h. It is possible that these changes are consistent with changes taking place in the dura during this period.

The error introduced by the simpler and safer epidural technique might be insufficient to warrant incision of the dura but this now becomes a personal clinical decision in each patient.

Analysis of Intracranial Pressure Data

In any continuous monitoring of a rapidly changing variable such as ICP a voluminous amount of data can be collected over a period of days.

Even with slow-speed recorders the traces can be inconveniently long and some form of reduction of the data may be desirable. Additionally, analysis of the data may reveal characteristics that are clinically useful but not seen by scanning the raw data.

One transform of the data is to change the pressure/time record to a frequency histogram in which the length of time the pressure lies between certain limits is determined for various ranges of pressure. This time, usually expressed as a percentage of the total time of the recording, is plotted against the ranges, thus, from a 24-h recording a frequency histogram showing the time spent between limits 0–10, 10–20, 20–30, etc. mmHg can be constructed.

The shape of this histogram need not be, and only rarely is, symmetrical. This skewness can arise in many ways and can become bimodal if a large number of plateau waves occur in the record when the times spent at high and low pressures can be similar but with little time at levels between.

The analysis can be done by a digital computer or by specially constructed devices with counters for each pressure range (Kullberg). Since many histograms of 12 or 24-h periods can be plotted on one 3-dimensional graph the time course over periods of weeks can be seen.

The various statistical measures such as modal, mean or median pressure can be determined though it should always be remembered that it is unlikely that the original data is normally distributed and the validity of any statistical procedures should be carefully assessed.

Janny showed in his computer analysis that after the data has been filtered to remove cardiac and respiratory fluctuations there is a correlation between the mean pressure and the variability. This is probably due to the fact that more plateau waves occur when the mean pressure is high.

There is no doubt that new information can be obtained by computer analysis. Whether this will be of clinical value remains to be seen.

Reference

Coe, J. E., Nelson, J. W., Rudenberg, F. A., Yarza: Technique for continuous intracranial pressure recording. J. Neurosurg. **27**, 370–375 (1967).

Session 3

Cerebral Blood Flow and Metabolism
(Experimental)

Some Adjustment Mechanisms of Brain Metabolism during Increased Intracranial Pressure

H. Nagai, M. Furuse, K. Banno, A. Ikeyama, S. Maeda, and H. Kuchiwaki

In an earlier report [1] we described how the response of experimental animals progresses through the following four stages when the intracranial pressure was gradually raised: the compensation period (stage 1), the period of reduced CBF (stage 2), the period of the vasopressor response (stage 3) and the final stage (stage 4). In this classification, stage 3 was further divided into 2 parts based mainly on changes in EEG activity. In stage 3a, the EEG activity was maintained, whereas in stage 3b it became flat.

Material and Methods

Experiments were carried out on 22 adult mongrel dogs weighing 13 to 17 kg, under light Nembutal anesthesia (20–30 mg/kg body-weight). The animals were placed in a head-fixation apparatus. An endotracheal tube was inserted and respiration was spontaneous in all animals.

Continuous measurements of CBF by the heat clearance method, of systemic blood pressure, respiration, oxygen tension in the femoral artery and the confluence of sinuses, intracranial pressure in the frontal epidural space and EEG were recorded on a polygraph. In some cases, a Radiometer pH microelectrode was used to measure CSF and venous blood pH. Lactate levels in CSF were also determined by standard enzymatic methods. PCO_2 and HCO_3^- in CSF were calculated from the Siggaard-Andersen nomogram. The minute-ventilation was measured through a respiratory valve connected to a Wright spirometer. In most experiments intracranial pressure was increased in increments of 7.4 mmHg by injection of synthetic CSF into the cisterna magna at 1-min intervals until a level of approximately 110 to 147 mmHg was reached, but in experiments where chemical analysis of CSF was required the intracranial pressure was gradually increased by injection of water into a balloon inserted into the epidural space over one cerebral hemisphere.

Results

As the intracranial pressure rose, changes in the respiratory pattern occurred at stage 3a in many animals. The results recorded in 22 animals whose ventilation volumes were measured are shown in Fig. 1. As seen on the left of

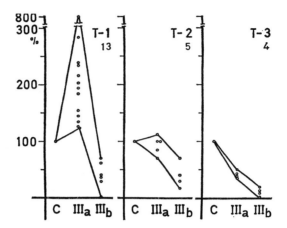

Fig. 1. Changes in respiratory minute-volume during increased ICP

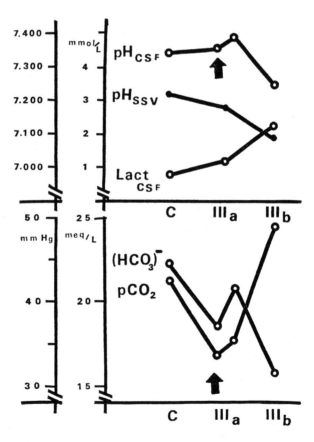

Fig. 2. Effect of increased ICP on acid-base and lactate metabolism of CSF

this figure, hyperventilation was observed in 13 out of the 22 experiments; the ventilation volumes had increased by 130 to 800% in each of these cases. As shown in the centre, there were 5 cases in which no changes in ventilation volumes were recorded, while in the other 4 animals a decrease in the ventilation volumes was noted at this time. Hyperventilation was also observed in cases of increased intracranial pressure produced by balloon inflation.

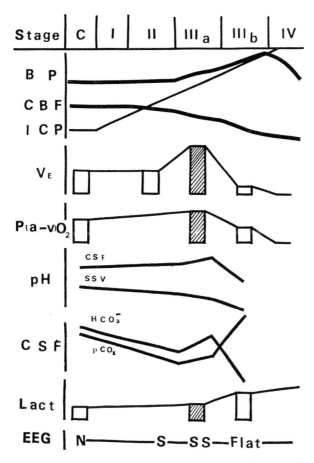

Fig. 3. Effect of increased intracranial pressure on cerebral metabolism

In order to investigate the part of ventilation in brain metabolism we measured PCO_2, HCO_3^- and pH in CSF as well as PO_2 in arterial and venous blood. All the cases where ventilation was increased showed a large discrepancy between the arterial and venous oxygen tensions, with increased PaO_2 and decreased PvO_2. It was considered that the increase in PaO_2 might be caused by hyperventilation and the decrease in PvO_2 by a fall in CBF. In any case, such an increase in arterio-venous oxygen difference may play a role in maintaining

$CMRO_2$ constant despite decreased CBF. On the other hand, PaO_2 decreased and PvO_2 increased when the ventilation volumes were reduced in stage 3 b. The increase in PvO_2 at this time means that brain tissue can no longer use oxygen and thus indicates loss of brain function. During these processes, although the venous blood pH fell gradually, the CSF pH was maintained within narrow limits at approximately 7.34 as shown in the upper part of Figure 2. At the beginning of stage 3 a, a considerable decrease in both HCO_3^- and PCO_2 in CSF was characteristic of the hyperventilated animals as shown on the lower part of Figure 2. If the buffer mechanism does not act in this situation, CSF pH becomes elevated because hyperventilation decreases PCO_2 in the CSF. However, although $HCO_3 -$ and PCO_2 fell by about the same amount there was no change in the CSF pH.

Late in stage 3 a, and after hyperventilation, the CSF HCO_3^- values increased in proportion to the PCO_2 accumulation in the CSF; again, there was no change in the CSF pH.

In brief, this ability to maintain the equilibrium between HCO_3^- and PCO_2 in CSF might play a role in keeping the CSF pH constant at stage 3 a. As shown in Figure 2, lactate concentration in CSF was 2.17 mM at stage 3 a, presenting no significant deviations from the control values. This might also be connected with the fact that CSF pH did not change so much in stage 3 a. In this stage, the vasoreactivity to changes in $PaCO_2$ persisted.

At stage 3 b the values of HCO_3^- in CSF decreased but there were striking increases in PCO_2 and lactate which resulted in a fall in CSF pH. At this time, the adjustment mechanisms of CSF pH and the vasoreactivity to changes in $PaCO_2$ were lost.

Comments

It is obvious from the experiments described above that the brain has some metabolic adjustment mechanisms during increased intracranial pressure. Initially, autoregulation acts to protect CBF against increased intracranial pressure. At stage 2 this mechanism is lost. At stage 3 the vasopressor response occurs and tends to maintain CBF. At stage 3 a hyperventilation is observed in many cases, and causes an increase in the arterio-venous oxygen difference. At this time CSF HCO_3^- decreases. This might play a role in keeping $CMRO_2$ constant and in adjusting CSF pH within a narrow range.

Reference

1. Nagai, H., Ikeyama, A., Furuse, M., et al.: Effect of increased intracranial pressure on cerebral hemodynamics. Observations of CBF, CBV and PO_2. In: Fieschi, C. (Ed.): Cerebral blood flow and intracranial pressure, p. 434–438. Stuttgart: S. Karger 1972.

Changes of Cerebral Hemodynamics and Energy Metabolism during Increased CSF Pressure and Brain Edema[1]

G. Meinig, H. J. Reulen, C. Magavly, U. Hase, and O. Hey

Introduction

Many studies have been performed in recent years on the influence of increased ICP on cerebral hemodynamics, and various mechanisms have been proposed for the explanation of the differing results. Many of these differences may be explained 1. by the technique used to produce increased ICP [3], 2. by the level of ICP, 3. by the definition of cerebral perfusion pressure, 4. by the state of vasomotor activity of the cerebral arterioles and 5. by the anatomical species differences of the cerebral venous outflow. Therefore, definition of the model and the parameters used is necessary in order that we may finally come to some common conclusions.

At the London CBF meeting we presented evidence that, in edematous tissue adjacent to a brain tumor, regional cerebral blood flow is closely related to the water content of the brain tissue, i.e., the amount of local edema [2]. These findings have since been substantiated by experimental studies in cold-injury edema [1]. It was concluded that local accumulation of edema fluid enlarges the volume of the affected tissue area and therefore increases the local tissue pressure. Rising extravascular pressure due to pathological accumulation of edema fluid in the extracellular space may approach the intravascular pressure in the downstream end of a capillary and tend to collapse this capillary. In order to maintain blood flow the intracapillary pressure must be as high – in fact a little higher. It has been shown that the "critical closing pressure", the arterial pressure at which flow stops, increases when extracapillary pressure is raised by accumulation of edema fluid. It may, therefore, be concluded from these data that increased *local tissue pressure* due to brain edema is a main factor responsible for the depression in flow observed in patients with brain tumors.

These studies, however, were performed with open skull or open dura and the ICP was normal or only slightly raised. The present study was undertaken to examine the additional influence of increased ICP on this relationship, i.e., the experiments being performed with closed skull. Water intoxication was used produce a *generalized* brain edema and a predictable increase in ICP.

1 Supported by a grant from the Deutsche Forschungsgemeinschaft.

Methods

Increasing amounts of generalized brain edema (BE) were produced in cats by intravenous infusion of distilled water equal to 5, 10, 15 or 20% of their body-weight. All animals were anesthetized with sodium pentobarbital (30 to 40 ml/kg), paralyzed with Flaxedil, normoventilated with a conventional Starling pump and functionally nephrectomized by ligation of both ureters, renal arteries and veins. Blood gases were analyzed intermittently using the Astrup microequipment and were kept within the normal range (pCO$_2$ 28–31 mmHg). Both temporal muscles were completely removed; the left lingual artery was cannulated for tracer injections. MABP, CSFP and, in some animals, intraventricular fluid pressure (IVP) were measured continuously.

rCBF (^{133}Xe-Clearance) was recorded before and immediately after the water load and again 60 and 120 min later. Following the last CBF measurement blood and CSF samples were withdrawn to determine pH, lactate and pyruvate. The brain was then frozen in situ with liquid nitrogen and brain tissue samples were removed to determine water content and metabolite concentrations (CrP, ATP, ADP, AMP, lactate, pyruvate).

Results

The effect of the water intoxication on CSFP and on rCBF is shown in Fig. 1. rCBF was found to remain unchanged following intravenous infusion of 50 ml of dest. water per kg body-weight and was decreased following infusion of 100, 150 and 200 ml/kg. Since the water load causes an increase in blood-volume and hemodilution, the same amount of saline was infused in control animals to examine whether these changes affect rCBF. Infusion of 0.9% saline resulted in a slight increase in the flow as compared to normal untreated animals. These slight increases in the different groups may by used to correct the rCBF values measured following water intoxication. The corrected values are indicated by the broken line. It must be mentioned that the clearance curves recorded in most animals of the 20% group, sometimes nearly plateau curves, probably represent external carotid blood flow.

In the lower panel the respective values of MABP, CSFP and CPP (difference between MABP and CSFP) are illustrated. Although an increase in CSFP occurred, the CPP was not significantly changed in the 10 and 15% groups. Therefore, the reduced blood flow recorded in both these groups cannot be explained by a decrease in CPP, and other factors must be responsible. In the 20% group CSFP often rose markedly within a few minutes and herniation occurred so that CSFP could no longer be measured. This group certainly has a reduced CPP, which was about 20 mmHg in the few animals where values for CSFP were obtained.

Water intoxication produces a significant degree of brain edema. The intensity of cerebral edema was directly proportional to the water load. The effect of cerebral edema on rCBF is shown in Figure 2. rCBF values are compared with the brain water-content as determined immediately after rCBF measurement. A close relationship exists between the increase in brain water-content and the decrease in cerebral blood flow. The respective values of the CPP are given at the top of the figure. Since a rise in MABP occurred concomitantly to the rise in CSFP, CPP is not significantly reduced and seems not to play an important role in the depression of flow.

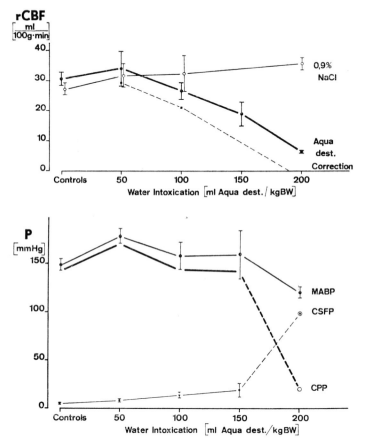

Fig. 1. rCBF, MABP, CSFP and CPP following water intoxication in cats equal to 5, 10, 15 or 20% of the body weight

The question arises as to whether the diminution of tissue perfusion leads to cellular hypoxia. A sensitive method for the assessment of tissue hypoxia is the measurement of the energy state or the oxidation/reduction state of the tissue. Brain lactate and brain lactate/pyruvate ratio increased and PCr and ATP decreased progressively with the amount of water injected. Significant changes of these metabolites were found in the 10, 15 or 20% groups. The fall in tissue perfusion in the 10 and 15% groups amounted to about 20 and 40%

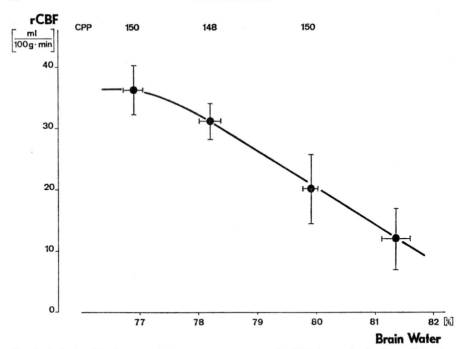

Fig. 2. Relationship between brain water content and rCBF in cerebral edema following water intoxication

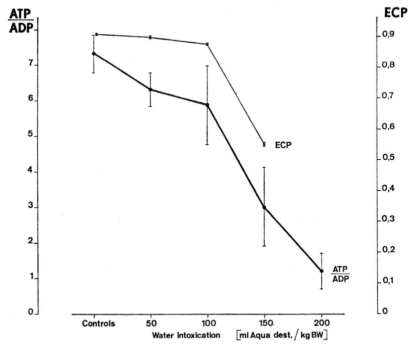

Fig. 3. Energy charge potential (ECP) and ATP/ADP ratio in brain tissue following a water intoxication equal to 5, 10, 15 or 20 % of the body weight

as compared with the control value. In the 20% group an almost complete breakdown of PCr and ATP occurred and the lactate concentration reached an extremely high value. Since cellular lactate and PCr concentrations may be influenced by changes in intracellular pH even if hypoxia is absent, the energy-charge potential of the adenine nucleotide pool was calculated to evaluate the presence of an imbalance between the production and utilization of high-energy compounds [5]. A definite decrease in ECP was found in the 15% as well as the 20% group, indicating inadequate oxygenation of brain tissue. It must be emphasized that CPP was about 150 mmHg in the 15% group (Fig. 3).

Discussion

In studies on the effects of increased ICP on CBF, ZWETNOW et al. [6], and recently MILLER et al. [3] showed that cerebral blood flow is upheld at normal values until the effective cerebral perfusion pressure is lowered to 30 to 50 mmHg. In addition they found only small changes in the brain lactate concentration and no changes in the PCr and ATP concentration at cerebral perfusion pressures within the autoregulatory range [4]. This is in contrast to the present findings. ZWETNOW and MILLER, however, have increased ICP by infusion of Ringer solution into the cisterna magna or the lumbar sub-arachnoid space. Obviously, this method, if performed precisely, does not alter the autoregulatory status of the cerebral arterioles. If autoregulation was defective, CBF followed CPP passively [3]. It must be emphasized that the reduction in flow rate occurred in the present study (10 and 15% groups) without any significant change in CPP. This must be due to brain edema and elevated tissue pressure, as indicated by the increased ICP. A reduction in CPP, as observed in the 20% group, caused an immediate further fall in CBF.

It may be concluded that the adaption of CBF to the CPP, which remains intact during ICP increase by enlarging the *CSF volume*, is lost in brain edema where ICP is increased due to enlargement of the *brain-tissue volume*. The underlying mechanisms may be an increased tissue pressure and a swelling of endothelial and/or perivascular glia cells with reduction of the diameter of the capillaries and the venules.

Summary

In brain edema induced by water intoxication, intracranial pressure (CSFP or IVP) was increased. Cerebral perfusion pressure (CPP) remained constant due to a concomitant rise in MABP. rCBF decreased in the presence of an unchanged CPP. The reduction in flow rate was closely related to the brain water content, i.e. the extent of cerebral edema.

Key Words: Water intoxication, brain edema, tissue pressure, rCBF.

References

1. Frei, H. J., Pöll, W., Reulen, H. J., Brock, M., Schürmann, K.: Regional energy metabolism, tissue lactate content and rCBF in cold injury edema. In: Russell, R. W. R. (Ed.): Brain and Blood Flow, pp. 125–129. London: Pitman 1972.

2. Hadjidimos, A., Reulen, H. J., Brock, M., Déruaz, J. P., Brost, F., Fischer, F., Samii, M., Schürmann, K.: rCBF, tissue water content and tissue lactate in brain tumors. In: Russel, R. W. R. (Ed.): Brain and Blood Flow, pp. 378–385. London: Pitman 1972.

3. Miller, J. D., Stanek, A., Langfitt, T. W.: Concepts of cerebral perfusion pressure and vascular compression during intracranial hypertension. Progr. Brain. Res. 35, 411–432 (1972).

4. Siesjö, B. K., Zwetnow, N. N.: Effects of increased cerebrospinal fluid pressure upon adenine nucleotides and upon lactate and pyruvate in rat brain tissue. Acta neurol. scand. 46, 187 (1970).

5. Siesjö, B. K., Messeter, K.: Factors determining intracellular pH. In: Siesjö, B. K., Sørensen, S. C. (Eds.): Homeostasis of the brain, pp. 244–263. Copenhagen: Munksgaard 1972.

6. Zwetnow, N. N.: Effects of increased cerebrospinal fluid pressure on the blood flow and on the energy metabolism of the brain. Acta physiol. scand. (suppl. 339), 1–31 (1970).

rCBF, CMRO$_2$ and Intracranial Pressures Following a Local Cold Injury of the Cortex[1]

D. A. Bruce, M. Vapalahti, H. Schutz, and T. W. Langfitt

We have previously reported [1] a group of head injured patients with diminished cerebral blood flow (rCBF) and cerebral metabolic rate for oxygen (CMRO$_2$) in whom intraventricular pressure was minimally elevated. Hypertonic mannitol produced a marked increase in rCBF in many of these patients, often without reduction of intraventricular pressure. The present experiments were designed to investigate the effects of a necrotic lesion of the brain simulating a contusion, on rCBF, CMRO$_2$ and intracranial pressures and to identify the mechanisms responsible for any changes in the measured parameters.

Methods and Procedure

Fifteen, 6–8 kg rhesus monkeys were anesthetized with Sernylan 0.01 mg/kg i.m., tracheostomized, paralyzed with gallamine and artificially ventilated to maintain a pCO$_2$ of 36–40 mmHg. Mean systemic arterial pressure (SAP), end-tidal CO$_2$, rectal temperature, sagittal sinus wedge pressure (SSWP), and cisterna magna pressure (CSFP) were continuously recorded. Retrograde cannulation of both common carotid arteries via the lingual arteries was performed and the external carotid arteries ligated. rCBF was determined by the ^{133}Xe injection method using three 5 mm probes positioned over each cerebral hemisphere and collimated such that the 95% isodose curves did not overlap. The collimator openings were 11 mm apart and frontal, precentral, and parietal locations were used. The left parietal probe was located 1.5 cm from the edge of a 1.5 cm occipital burr hole. A catheter was placed in the torcula and arterial and venous blood samples were drawn during each determination of rCBF for measurements of pO$_2$, pCO$_2$, pH, Hgb, Hct and oxygen saturation. The CMRO$_2$ was calculated as the a-v oxygen content × the mean CBF of all 6 probes. The EEG was recorded from 4 to 6 screws placed in the calvarium in the same vertical planes as the CBF probes.

Following 2 control flows autoregulation was tested by raising the SAP approximately 30 mmHg with i.v. angiotensin. Those monkeys in whom autoregulation was defective in more than one probe were discarded. Following these measurements a 1.5 cm copper tube filled with liquid nitrogen was

---

1 Supported by John A. Hartford Foundation, Inc.

placed on the intact dura of the left occipital burr hole and left in contact for 5 min. After completion of the lesion a rubber plug was placed in the burr hole. rCBF and $CMRO_2$ determinations were made each hour for 4 h.

4 of the 15 monkeys served as controls. In the experimental group 6 monkeys received mannitol, 1 g/kg i.v. 2 h after the lesion. 4 monkeys were given Evans blue prior to the lesion. A sample of brain under each probe was taken and dried over night in a heated vacuum desiccator in 5 monkeys. Water content was derived from the formula wet weight – dry weight/wet weight × 100. In 2 animals the brains were frozen in situ for measurements of metabolites. The metabolite data will not be included in this report.

Results

In the control group there was no change in rCBF or $CMRO_2$ over the 4 h. In the experimental group pO_2, pCO_2 and pH were constant except for a slight fall in pCO_2 at 2 h. In the control and experimental animals there was a slight all in Hgb over the 6 h of anesthesia, 12.9–10.9 g and 12.5–10 g respectively. In the control state the SSWP was 4–8 mmHg higher than the CSFP. In 3 animals the SSWP and CSFP rose rapidly over the first 2 h leading to a drop in CPP from 96.8 to 50.0 mmHg. In 1 animal the CSFP stopped recording and in the other 2, as intracranial pressures rose above 25–30 mmHg CSFP increased above SSWP and this relationship was maintained thereafter. Mean rCBF fell from 38.7 to 22.8 ml/100 g/min and the $CMRO_2$ fell, progressively from 2.6 to 1.92 ml/100 g/min at 2 h (Fig. 1). After 2 h there was a fall in CSFP, an increase in rCBF to 27.2 ml/100 g/min but a continued fall in $CMRO_2$ to 1.11 ml/100 g/min at 4 h.

In 8 monkeys the increases in SSWP (7–14 mmHg) and in CSFP (2 to 10 mmHg) were small. There was a decrease in $CMRO_2$ from 3.26 ± .27 to 2.61 ± .53 by the end of the second hour which was not statistically significant. Thereafter the $CMRO_2$ remained constant (Fig. 2). There was no change in rCBF in the 3 probes most distal from the lesion (Fig. 3). The left precentral probe next anterior to the perilesion probe showed a small but not significant change at 2 and 3 h returning to control values at 4 h. The perilesion probe fell significantly in the first hour 36.2 ± 2.2 to 29.4 ± 2.4 (p < .05), further by the second hour to 25.6 ± 2.3 (p < .005) and remained at this level (Fig. 3). The probe contralateral to the perilesion probe fell from 34.3 ± 3.2 to 28.1 ± 2.5 at 2 h (p < .05), to 27.1 ± 1.5 at 3 h (p < .02) then rose to 29.4 ± 2.5 at 4 h (N.S.). In none of these animals was there evidence of spread of Evans blue as far as the perilesion probe and there was no significant increase in water content under the perilesion probe (73.66 ± 1.2% control and 74.4 ± 1.9% perilesion). The EEG initially demonstrated slowing and decreased voltage in the perilesion lead, usually evident by 1 h and in several animals the lead contralateral to the perilesion lead showed similar changes by the second hour. Mannitol administered to 2 animals in the group with a large rise in intracranial pressure and to 4 animals in the group with little or no rise in intracranial pressures had no effect on rCBF despite lowering CSFP and SSWP.

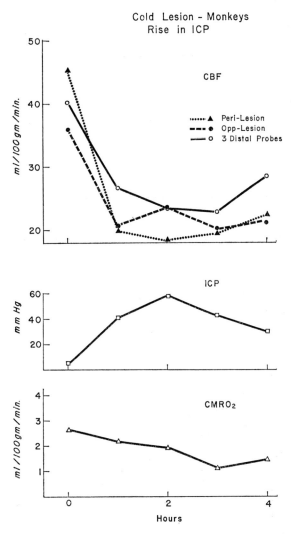

Fig. 1. rCBF, SSWP and CMRO₂ in 3 experimental monkeys who exhibited large increase in CSFP

Discussion

Diminished rCBF and diminished tissue energy levels have been shown to correlate well with changes in tissue water content [2, 3]. We have found a decrease in rCBF in the area proximal to a local intracerebral lesion and in the corresponding area in the contralateral hemisphere. A small drop in

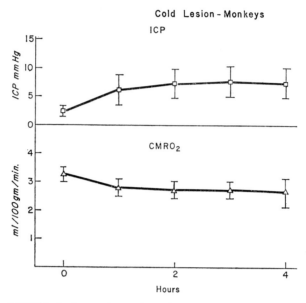

Fig. 2. CSFP and CMRO$_2$ in 8 experimental monkeys with minimal elevation of CSFP (bars represent S.E. of the mean)

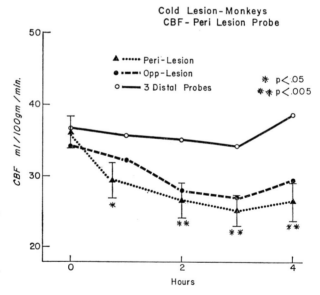

Fig. 3. rCBF of perilesion probe, contralateral probe and the mean of the 3 distal probes in 8 monkeys with minimal rise in CSFP (bars represent S.E. of the mean)

CMRO$_2$ occured early and was maintained throughout the 4 h. Five possible mechanisms alone or in combination may be responsible for the changes in rCBF: a rise in general intracranial pressures with decreased perfusion pressure and decreased rCBF; a local increase in intracerebral pressure due to the focal mass effect; a spread of edema fluid from the lesion to the tissues manifesting a decrease in rCBF; local reduction of electrical activity, reduction of local metabolism, and reduction of rCBF due to metabolic autoregulation; and finally a neurogenic factor.

In 3 monkeys there was a large rise in SSWP and CSFP, diminished cerebral perfusion pressure, and a general reduction in CBF and metabolism. In 8 monkeys no such increases in intracranial pressures were found and no reduction in CPP occurred. It is quite possible that a local increase in intracerebral pressure in the perilesion area occurred and led to compression of blood vessels and diminished rCBF in this area. Whether it is possible to explain the flow changes in the contralateral area on this basis must await the completion of further experiments in which we are measuring intracerebral pressures. There was no evidence of increased water content in the brain under the perilesion probe at 4 h and no evidence of spread of Evans blue to that area in any of the 8 animals in whom a minimal increase in intracranial pressure occurred. The EEG in the perilesion area showed slowing and decreased amplitude at 1 h, and similar changes were observed in the contralateral probe in some monkeys at 2 h. Whether these electrical changes are the result or the cause of the rCBF changes must remain speculative at present. Finally, we have no evidence for or against a neurogenic mechanism being operative.

Summary

Using an acute cold lesion of the occipital cortex to simulate a cerebral contusion we have demonstrated significant decreases in rCBF in the perilesion area and in the homologous area of the contralateral hemisphere. There were minimal changes in the precentral probe on the side of the lesion and no change in the 3 most distal probes. A small decrease in CMRO₂ occurring within the first 2 h was noted and minimal increases in CSFP and SSWP were recorded. The rCBF changes could not be explained by local increase in water content, and mannitol given at 2 h had no effect on rCBF or CMRO₂. There were EEG changes in the perilesion area and in the contralateral area. The time course of these changes was closely related to the time course of the rCBF changes.

Key Words: Cold injury, rCBF, CMRO₂, EEG, edema.

References

1. BRUCE, D. A., MILLER, J. D., LANGFITT, T. W., GOLDBERG, H. I., STANEK, A. E., VAPALAHTI, M.: CBF and Intracranial Pressure in Comatose Patients. (In press.)
2. FREI, H. J., PÖLL, W., REULEN, H. J., BROCK, M., SCHÜRMANN, K.: Regional Energy Metabolism, Tissue Lactate Content and rCBF in Cold Injury Oedema: In: Ross Russell, Brain and Blood Flow, p. 125–129. London: Pitman 1971.
3. REULEN, M. J., SAMII, M., FENSKE, A., HEY, O., HASE, U.: Energy Metabolism, Fluids and Electrolyte Distribution in Cold Injury Oedema: In: Head Injuries, p. 232–239. Edinburgh and London: Churchill Livingstone 1971.

Energy State of the Brain during and after Compression Ischemia[1]

B. Ljunggren, L. Granholm, H. Schutz[2], and B. K. Siesjö

Introduction

The effects of total ischemia on the energy state of the brain are well documented. These changes consist in a rapid disappearance of available substrates (glucose and glycogen) and of high energy compounds (phosphocreatine and ATP), and in an accumulation of AMP, inorganic P (Pi), and lactate. The magnitude of the increase in the lactate concentration is determined by the preischemic levels of glucose and glycogen which usually suffice to increase the tissue lactate content from about 1.5 to about 15 mMoles/kg of wet tissue. The increase in lactate is maximal within a few minutes of ischemia. Therefore, 3–5 min of total ischemia leads to a state of severe and maximal tissue acidosis and of complete energy depletion [1, 2, 3, 4, 5, 6].

Until recently, it has been assumed that a complete interruption of the cerebral circulation for more than 5–7 min leads to irreversible cell damage in the brain, reflecting the vulnerability of the CNS cells to oxygen lack [7, 8, 9]. Normalization of the energy state of the brain has been reported after total ischemia of 8 min, but in the cerebrum and cerebellum certain metabolites (adenine nucleotides, lactate) are not normalized until after several hours [10].

Recent studies have indicated that vascular changes with permanent closure of individual vessels play a crucial rôle in the pathogenesis of ischemic injuries in the brain [11, 12, 13]. It is thus possible that, provided the tissue can be adequately reperfused in the restitution phase, the brain cells may tolerate longer periods of total ischemia than was previously thought before cell death occurs [14, 15].

It is not yet known whether a deficient reperfusion of individual vessels in the post-ischemic period is due to minute intravascular thrombi or to swelling of the endothelial and the perivascular glial cells. However, certain results indicate that the presence of blood in the intracerebral vessels during the ischemic period aggravates the tendency to capillary obstruction ("no-reflow phenomenon").

1 Supported by grants from the Swedish Medical Research Council (Project No. B72–14X–2179–04 and B72–14X–263–08B), from the Swedish Bank Tercentenary Fund, and by U.S. PHS Grant No. 5 R01 NS 07838–03 from NIH.
2 On leave of absence from the Department of Surgery (Neurosurgery), University of Toronto, Toronto, Canada.

The objective of the present work was to study the maximal ischemic periods compatible with restitution of brain function by using an ischemic model which gives an essentially bloodless cerebral vasculature. In this communication we will describe the metabolic state of the brain during and after ischemic periods of 1–15 min.

Methods

The experiments were performed on 300–400 g male rats which were anesthetized with 70% N_2O and 30% O_2, paralyzed and artificially ventilated so as to give arterial CO_2 tensions of 35–40 mmHg. The body temperature was maintained at 37° C and care was taken to prevent a fall in brain temperature. Cerebral ischemia was induced by increasing the CSF pressure above the arterial blood pressure. The artificial CSF infused into the cisterna magna was prewarmed to body temperature and equilibrated with oxygen and carbon dioxide to physiological tensions. Deleterious vasopressor responses were prevented by the intravenous infusion of trimetaphane camphor-sulfonate (Arfonad) before and during the elevation of the CSFP [16]. The presence of complete cerebral ischemia was controlled by injecting a suspension of carbon black particles and by examining the brains for traces of the suspension. A control group of animals was treated by perfusion of the cisterna magna with artificial CSF at normal pressure.

At the end of the experiment the brain was frozen *in situ* and a frontoparietal portion of cerebral cortex and underlying white matter subsequently analyzed for phosphocreatine (PCr), ATP, ADP, AMP, glucose, lactate, pyruvate, α-ketoglutarate, glutamate and NH_4^+, using specific enzymatic (fluorometric) techniques [2, 17]. In order to evaluate the balance between energy production and energy utilization the energy charge potential ECP

$$\text{ECP} = \frac{[\text{ATP}] + 0.5\,[\text{ADP}]}{[\text{ATP}] + [\text{ADP}] + [\text{AMP}]}$$

was calculated [18].

Results

With the ischemic model used the tissue was essentially depleted of PCr even after 1 min, while some ATP persisted for 5 min (Fig. 1). The derived ECP values indicate that no useful metabolic energy was present after 5–7.5 min (Fig. 1). Most of the glucose content had disappeared after 1 min and the constancy of the tissue lactate content after that time indicates that the tissue was depleted of substrates (glucose and glycogen) after 1–3 min (Fig. 2). Since the total CO_2 content of the tissue remained constant in all ischemic groups it may be concluded that the tissue CO_2 tension must have increased to values exceeding 150 mmHg, and the intracellular pH must have fallen from 7.05 to about 6.2 [6].

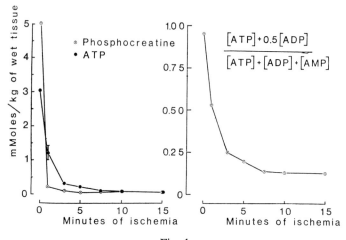

Fig. 1

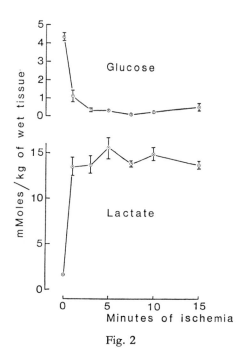

Fig. 2

The table gives the control values for the metabolites analyzed as well as those measured after 90 min of restitution following ischemic periods of 1 and 15 min. The results show that both there was a slight remaining lactic acidosis in the tissue and a very moderate decrease in the energy charge potential in both groups. It is interesting to note that the ECP values showed the same degree of normalization after 15 min of ischemia as after 1 min (see also ADP and AMP values). Thus, since no functional restitution was obtained following ischemic periods of 5 min or longer, the failure of function could not be related to a deficient restitution of the ECP values. However, the longer ischemic periods were accompanied by other metabolic changes which could possibly bear some relation to the deficient function. Thus, the individual ATP values and the sums of the adenine nucleotides decreased progressively as the ischemia continued and, most unexpectedly, a corresponding decrease occurred in the glutamate values.

Table. Metabolic state of rat brain measured after 90 min of restitution following total cerebral ischemia of 1 and 15 min duration. The tissue concentrations of phosphocreatine (PCr), ATP, ADP, AMP, lactate, pyruvate, α-ketoglutarate, glutamate and NH_4^+ are expressed in mMoles/kg of wet tissue (means $\pm$ S.E.M.). Σ Ad = sum of adenine nucleotides. ECP = energy charge potential according to ATKINSON (1968)

Period of ischemia (min)	0 (n = 6)	1 (n = 4)	15 (n = 6)
PCr	5.04 $\pm$ 0.04	4.59 $\pm$ 0.05	4.66 $\pm$ 0.18
ATP	3.06 $\pm$ 0.02	2.99 $\pm$ 0.03	2.49 $\pm$ 0.07
ADP	0.270 $\pm$ 0.002	0.310 $\pm$ 0.008	0.262 $\pm$ 0.020
AMP	0.030 $\pm$ 0.001	0.044 $\pm$ 0.012	0.030 $\pm$ 0.003
Σ Ad	3.36 $\pm$ 0.02	3.34 $\pm$ 0.05	2.78 $\pm$ 0.08
ECP	0.951 $\pm$ 0.001	0.941 $\pm$ 0.004	0.942 $\pm$ 0.001
La	1.60 $\pm$ 0.10	2.22 $\pm$ 0.24	2.57 $\pm$ 0.23
Py	0.105 $\pm$ 0.005	0.089 $\pm$ 0.001	0.115 $\pm$ 0.006
αKG	0.105 $\pm$ 0.005	0.087 $\pm$ 0.009	0.078 $\pm$ 0.005
Glut	12.59 $\pm$ 0.12	12.29 $\pm$ 0.09	9.86 $\pm$ 0.52
NH_4^+	0.25 $\pm$ 0.02	0.30 $\pm$ 0.03	0.21 $\pm$ 0.02

Discussion

The present results have shown that although the present ischemic model induces complete energy depletion in the tissue after about 5 min, an ischemic period of 15 min is followed by an almost complete restitution of the energy state of the tissue, judging from the energy charge potential of the adenine nucleotide system, and disappearance of the lactic acidosis. Thus, since the animals did not regain consciousness after more than 5 min of ischemia there is a poor relationship between the energy state and the functional condition (c. f. Reference [10]). It cannot be stated at present whether or not the loss of function is in some way related to the decrease in ATP, or to other metabolic changes such as the decrease in glutamate. Since glutamate is considered to be an excitatory transmitter, there is a remote possibility that the ischemic period may lead to a derangement of the pathways which lead to synthesis of substances of key importance in nervous transmission. Further experiments are required to gain more information on these points.

Summary

Complete cerebral ischemia was induced in rats for 1–15 min by means of an increase in the intracranial CSF pressure, and the cerebral metabolic state was studied during the ischemia, as well as after 90 min of restitution of the cerebral circulation. After 5 min of ischemia the tissue was depleted of substrates and energy-rich compounds. In spite of this, 15 min of ischemia was followed by an almost complete restitution of lactate and phosphocreatine, as well as of the energy charge potential of the adenine nucleotide pool. Since no functional restitution was obtained after ischemic periods of 5 min or longer it is concluded that there was a poor relationship between the energy state and the functional state.

Key Words: Intracranial pressure, CBF, cerebral energy state, ischemia, restitution after ischemia.

References

1. Thorn, W., Scholl, H., Pfleiderer, G., Muldener, B.: Stoffwechselvorgänge im Gehirn bei normaler und herabgesetzter Körpertemperatur unter ischämischer und anoxischer Belastung. J. Neurochem. **2**, 150–165 (1958).

2. Lowry, O. H., Passonneau, J. V., Hasselberger, F. X., Schultz, D. W.: Effect of ischemia on known substrates and cofactors of the glycolytic pathway in brain. J. biol. Chem. **239**, 18–30 (1964).

3. Schmahl, F. W., Betz, E., Talke, H., Hohorst, H. J.: Energiereiche Phosphate und Metabolite des Energiestoffwechsels in der Großhirnrinde der Katze. Biochem. Z. **342**, 518–531 (1965).

4. Müller, U., Isselhard, W., Hinzen, D. H., Geppert, E.: Regionaler Energiestoffwechsel im Kaninchengehirn während kompletter Ischämie in Normothermie. Pflügers Arch. ges. Physiol. **320**, 168–180 (1970).

5. Maker, H. S., Lehrer, G. M.: Effect of ischemia. In: Lajtha, A. (Ed.): Handbook of Neurochemistry Vol. 4, p. 267–310. New York: Plenum Press 1970.

6. Siesjö, B. K., Plum, F.: Pathophysiology of anoxic brain damage. In: Gaull, G. (Ed.): Biology of Brain Dysfunction. New York: Plenum Press. (In press 1972.)

7. Weinberger, L. M., Gibbon, M. H., Gibbon, J. H.: Temporary arrest of the circulation to the central nervous system. Arch. Neurol. Psychiat. (Chic.) **43**, 961–986 (1940).

8. Hirsch, H., Euler, K. H., Schneider, M.: Über die Erholung und Wiederbelebung des Gehirns nach Ischämie bei Normothermie. Pflügers Arch. ges. Physiol. **265**, 281–313 (1957).

9. Schneider, M.: In: Gastaut, H., Meyer, J. S. (Eds.): Cerebral Anoxia and the Electroencephalogram, Chap. 13. Springfield, Ill.: C. C. Thomas 1961.

10. Müller, U., Isselhard, W., Hinzen, D. H., Geppert, E.: Electrocorticogramm und regionaler Energiestoffwechsel des Kaninchengehirns in der postischämischen Erholung. Pflügers Arch. ges. Physiol. **320**, 181–194 (1970).

11. Ames, III, A., Wright, R. L., Kowada, M., Thurston, J. M., Majno, G.: Cerebral ischemia. II. The no-reflow phenomenon. Amer. J. Path. **52**, 437–454 (1968).

12. Chiang, J., Kowada, M., Ames, III, A., Wright, R. L., Majno, G.: Cerebr al ischemia. III. Vascular changes. Amer. J. Path. **52**, 455–476 (1968).

13. Cantu, R. C., Ames, III, A.: Distribution of vascular lesions caused by cerebral ischemia. Neurology **19**, 128–132 (1969).

14. HOSSMAN, K.-A., SATO, K.: Recovery of neuronal function after prolonged cerebral ischemia. Science **168**, 375–376 (1970).
15. HOSSMAN, K.-A., OLSSON, Y.: Suppression and recovery of neuronal function in transient cerebral ischemia. Brain Res. **22**, 313–325 (1970).
16. KRAMER, W., TUYNMAN, J. A.: Acute intracranial hypertension – an experimental investigation. Brain Res. **6**, 686–705 (1967).
17. MACMILLAN, V., SIESJÖ, B. K.: Brain energy metabolism in hypoxemia. Scand. J. clin. Lab. Invest. (In press 1972).
18. ATKINSON, D. E.: The energy charge of the adenylate pool as a regulatory parameter. Interaction with feedback modifiers. Biochemistry **7**, 4030–4034 (1968).

The Function of Brain Mitochondria after Increased Intracranial Pressure

H. Schutz, P. R. Silverstein, M. Vapalahti, D. A. Bruce, L. Mela, and T. W. Langfitt

Introduction

The brain has a high resting energy consumption but low reserves of high-energy compounds – adenosine triphosphate (ATP) and phosphocreatine. All 3 major foodstuffs are ultimately oxidized by the Krebs cycle via the activated derivative, acetyl Co-A. For each revolution, there are 4 dehydrogenation steps and thus 4 pairs of electrons are extracted from the intermediates of the cycle. Nicotinamide adenine dinucleotide (NAD) and flavoprotein act as electron carriers. They donate their electrons to enzymes (cytochromes) which constitute the respiratory chain. The cytochromes are fixed in geometric assemblies in the mitochondria. Each cytochrome is reduced as it accepts an electron which can, in turn, donate its electron to the next carrier in its oxidized form and so on. Only the last one, cytochrome oxidase, can give up its electron directly to molecular oxygen to form water. At each electron transfer, the decline in free energy is conserved by the phosphorylation of ADP to ATP.

Mitochondrial ATPases (uncoupler-activated ATPase and spontaneous-Mg^{++} activated ATPase) regulate the equilibrium reaction whereby ADP is phosphorylated to ATP. Oxidative phosphorylation is "coupled" when the reaction is principally in the direction of ATP synthesis. "Loose coupling" occurs when ATP hydrolysis is accelerated in the mitochondria due to an increase in spontaneous ATPase activity. Under these conditions, oxygen utilization and electron transfer continue at a greater rate (dissipated as heat) without the coupled formation of adequate amounts of energy.

During ischemia, there is a lack of O_2 and glucose. Consequently, oxidative phosphorylation cannot continue because substrate, in the form of electrons from the Krebs cycle, is not supplied in adequate amounts. Also, the lack of O_2 shifts the various redox systems to their reduced states. The anaerobic formation of ATP in the Embden-Meyerhof pathway stops because of the lack of glucose. Lack of energy results in loss of function and loss of structural integrity.

Material and Methods

61 rabbits were anesthetized with sodium thiopental, tracheostomized, curarized and ventilated with O_2 and N_2O. The systemic arterial pressure (SAP)

was measured from the femoral artery. The cerebrospinal fluid pressure (CSFP) was measured from the cisterna magna. Arterial pO_2, pCO_2, pH and the rectal temperature was measured until a physiological steady state was obtained. Arfonad was infused via the femoral vein to modify the marked pressor response when mock CSF was infused into the cisterna magna. Cerebral ischemia was complete when the CSFP exceeded the SAP. After 5, 10, 20, 30 and 40 min of compression ischemia, the animals were decapitated and the brain was quickly suspended in ice-cold isolation medium. In 10 animals, 20 min of compression ischemia was followed by 60 min of circulatory recovery. In the recovery period the animals were subjected to normotensive normocapnia, hypercapnia (pCO_2 greater than 80 mmHg) and hypocapnia (pCO_2 less than 15 mmHg), respectively.

Brain mitochondria were isolated by a modification of the techniques of CLARK [1] and OZAWA [2]. After light homogenization and incubation, the brain was subjected to differential centrifugation and several washings. The respiratory function of the mitochondrial pellet was assayed in a Clark oxygen electrode in a closed, stirred cuvette in air-saturated testing medium. Uncoupler-sensitive ATPase activity was measured by a recording pH meter.

The respiratory control ratio (RCR) was calculated from the ratio of State 3 and State 4 [3]. Utilization of O_2 in State 4 respiration represented electron transfer in the cytochrome oxidase system in the presence of substrate only. Utilization of O_2 in State 3 respiration represented electron transfer in the presence of substrate plus ADP and thus was an indicator of oxidative phosphorylation.

Results

Figures 1 and 2 show the mean control RCR, State 3, State 4, uncoupler-activated and spontaneous ATPase activities. After 5 and 10 min of compression ischemia, the RCRs and State 3 rates increased slightly, indicating a tendency to "tighter coupling" and a lack of inhibition of oxidative phosphorylation. There was a decline in RCR and State 3 activity after 20 min, but the changes reached statistical significance only after 30 and 40 min. The decrease in RCR was due to inhibition of State 3 respiration and an increase in State 4 respiration. The decline in ADP utilization was not due to inhibition of uncoupler-activated ATPase, but due to a significant increase in spontaneous Mg^{++}-activated ATPase, suggesting loose coupling and heavy inhibition of oxidative phosphorylation (Fig. 1 and 3).

The RCR, State 3 and State 4 activities were normal in those animals where circulatory recovery was allowed after 20 min of compression ischemia, even if the recovery period was complicated by severe systemic hypercarbia or hypocarbia. However, neurological recovery was not possible after only 10 min of compression ischemia.

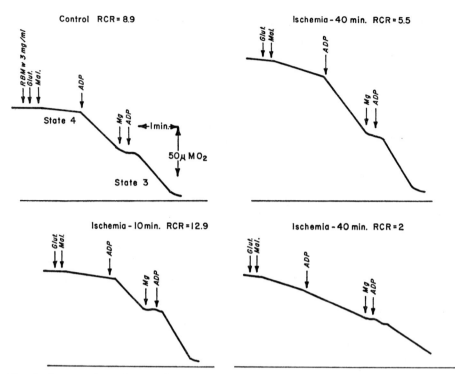

Fig. 1. Oxygen electrode recordings showing O_2 uptake in representative preparations of rabbit brain mitochondria. The RCR was increased after 10 min of ischemia due to increased State 3 respiration. After 40 min of ischemia, some mitochondrial preparations were "loosely coupled" (RCR = 5.5) and others were "uncoupled" (RCR = 2)

Discussion

During the period of total ischemia, mitochondrial metabolism stops completely (see preceding paper), yet mitochondrial function and therefore oxidative metabolism is able to recover after 20 min and possibly 30 min of ischemia, if the mitochondria are resupplied with substrate and oxygen. Secondary deterioration of mitochondrial function does not occur. Neurological recovery is not possible despite full restitution of energy metabolism. Therefore, lack of energy in the recovery period cannot be held responsible for irreversible brain bamage. Instead, the lack of energy during even short periods of ischemia is the cause of irreversible changes in cellular organelles other than the mitochondria, possibly the cell membrane [4].

The fact that mitochondrial metabolism was normal after 30 min of ischemia and remained normal for at least 1 h after restitution of the cerebral circulation is evidence against the "no reflow phenomenon". If the no reflow phenomenon is as extensive as it is described by Ames et al. [5] (50% no reflow after 15 min of ischemia), then oxidative metabolism should be greatly reduced.

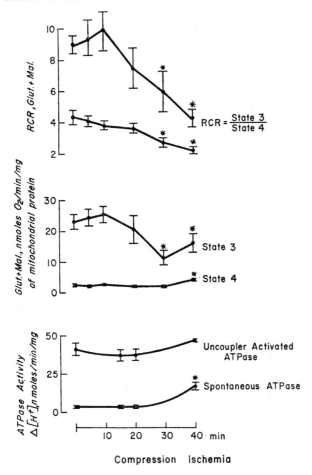

Fig. 2. Effect of compression ischemia on RCR (with and without Mg^{++} and bovine serum albumin), State 3, State 4, uncoupler-activated and spontaneous-Mg^{++}-activated ATPase activities. The decline in RCR after 30 and 40 min of ischemia was due to a decrease in State 3 respiration, an increase in State 4 respiration and an increase in spontaneous ATPase activity suggesting "loose coupling" of oxidative phosphorylation after 40 min of compression ischemia. Values given are mean, $\pm$ SE, * $p < 0.005$

Summary

The effect of compression ischemia on brain mitochondrial activity was examined in 61 rabbits. We found that the RCR increased initially due to an increase in State 3 respiration. The RCR was significantly decreased only after 30 and 40 min of ischemia due to inhibition of State 3, an increase in State 4 and an increase in spontaneous-Mg^{++} activated ATPase, suggesting loose coupling.

Secondary deterioration of mitochondrial function did not occur.

Our findings suggest that alterations in constituents of the cell, other than the mitochondria and therefore oxidative metabolism, are responsible for the lack of neurological recovery.

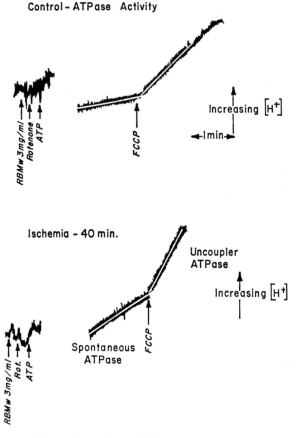

Fig. 3. pH meter recordings of maximum ATPase activities. Uncoupler-sensitive ATPase was activated by the addition of uncoupling agent FCCP. After 40 min of compression ischemia there was a significant increase in spontaneous ATPase, indicating a high degree of "loose coupling" and ATP hydrolysis

Key Words : Mitochondrial function, increased intracranial pressure, ischemia, oxidative metabolism.

References

1. Clark, J. B., Nicklas, W. J.: The metabolism of rat brain mitochondria. J. biol. Chem. **245**, 4724–4731 (1970).
2. Ozawa, K., Seta, K., Takeda, H., et al.: On the isolation of mitochondria with high respiratory control from rat brain. J. Biochem. **59**, 501–510 (1966).
3. Chance, B., Williams, G. R.: Respiratory enzymes in oxidative phosphorylation. Part 3, The Steady State. J. biol. Chem. **217**, 409–427 (1955).
4. Swanson, P. D.: The effects of oxygen deprivation on electrically stimulated cerebral cortex slices. J. Neurochem. **16**, 35–45 (1969).
5. Ames, III, A., Wright, R. L., Kowanda, M., et al.: Cerebral ischemia. II. The no-reflow phenomenon. Amer. J. Path. **52**, 437–453 (1968).

Comments to Session 3

U. Ponten and J. D. Miller

In the discussion of the paper by Nagai et al., Lundberg reemphasized the message of Evans in the opening lecture by pointing out to what a remarkable extent the experimental findings of today coincide with the hypotheses of the last century by citing the 4 stages of increasing intracranial pressure formulated by Duret in 1878 [1].

"The first grade is characterized by the expansion being compensated by absorption of CSF and compression of intracranial veins and utilization of the elasticity of the walls of the craniospinal space. During the second and third degree of hypertension the blood circulation is impaired with cerebro-bulbo-medullary symptoms, including increase in the blood pressure and bradycardia, as a consequence. In the final stage, when the intracranial pressure exceeds the arterial pressure, the blood circulation in the cerebral vessels stops, the cerebral centers are paralysed with fall in blood pressure and respiratory standstill as a consequence."

The hyperventilation seen at the beginning of stage 3 in Nagai's study was discussed by Zwetnow as a possible cause for the simultaneous decrease in CBF. In his own experiments, in which the animals were kept at a constant $PaCO_2$, the vasopressor response came at the same time as the autoregulation started to fail. The increase in arterial pressure thus delayed the fall in perfusion pressure and CBF for a while.

Siesjö questioned the CSF analysis of lactate and acid base parameters if the sampling was done after infusion of saline into the cistern. The samples were obtained, however, only in those experiments in which a balloon was expanded. The fact is that these are two entirely different experimental models. The cisternal saline injection will give a uniform rise in ICP, while the expansion of a balloon will give a mass displacement as well. The effects of these two models upon ICP, CBF and other parameters are not necessarily the same. Conclusions regarding $CMRO_2$ cannot be made from AV oxygen differences representing the total brain, especially when local flow is measured while mass displacements are occurring.

Hamer reported the effects of increased ICP (due to cisternal infusion) on CBF and glucose/oxygen metabolism in dogs. With a moderate reduction in CPP (from 110 to 72 mmHg) CBF and $CMRO_2$ were not significantly changed, but there was a significant increase in the cerebral AV-difference for lactate.

With a marked reduction in CPP (38 mmHg), CBF was decreased significantly, but $CMRO_2$ was not. There was, however, a significant decrease in CMR glucose, and excess lactate production rose from 7–17%.

The last 2 papers of the session demonstrate that complete restitution of the oxidative metabolism in brain tissue as well as in brain mitochondria is possible after compression ischemia for more than 15 min, while functional recovery was impossible after as little as 5 min of ischemia.

WALTZ reported that he had sometimes found some functional recovery after middle cerebral artery occlusion. This model, however, does not necessarily give total ischemia, which is guaranteed in the compression ischemia model.

The question of whether the poor functional recovery was due to the no reflow phenomenon first described by AMES et al. in 1968 [2] was raised by KINDT and MATAKAS.

As pointed out by LANGFITT and SIESJÖ the compression ischemia model has the advantage that the intracranial vascular bed will probably be almost completely emptied by the uniform increase of ICP above the systolic arterial pressure. Direct evidence that no large unperfused areas occur is given by the high energy charge potential values after restitution in the study by LJUNGREN et al. These values are compatible with only a few percent of devitalized tissue.

The same argument can be used to exclude the possibility that the poor functional recovery depends upon a loss of neurons, while the metabolic recovery occurs mostly in the glial cells.

The possibility still exists, however, that irreversible damage has occurred in the brain stem, since these studies so far only refer to the supratentorial parts of the brain.

Furthermore, it is essential to achieve prolonged survival of these animals and to analyze the cause of death before it can be stated that functional recovery of the brain cells is impossible after periods of compression ischemia longer than 5 min.

These findings of a dissociation between functional and metabolic recovery present a new challenge and strongly suggest that the experimental models used to study metabolic events in the brain should also be analyzed with regard to prolonged survival, detailed electrophysiological studies and higher cerebral function.

References

1. DURET, H., 1878, cited by LUNDBERG, N.: Continuous recording and control of ventricular fluid pressure in neurosurgical practice. Acta psychiat. scand. (Suppl. 149), **36**, 65 (1960).
2. AMES, III, A., WRIGHT, R. L., KOWADA, M., THURSTON, J. M., MAJNO, G.: Cerebral ischemia. II. The no-reflow phenomenon. Amer. J. Path. **52**, 437–453 (1968).

Session 4

Focal Brain Damage
(Experimental)

Intracranial Pressure Changes during Experimental Cerebral Infarction[1]

M. D. O'Brien[2] and A. G. Waltz

The role of intracranial pressure gradients in the development of neurologic deficits after cerebral infarction has not been evaluated adequately, partly because of technical problems with measurements of regional intracranial pressure (ICP). The presumed cause of post-infarction ICP gradients is ischemic cerebral edema; as a preliminary to a study of edema and its modification by treatment, ICP was measured in cats after occlusion of one middle cerebral artery (MCA).

Methods

Measurements of ICP. ICP was measured by:

1. A miniature strain gauge of the Wheatstone bridge type (Konigsberg Instrument Co., P-22), cemented into a burr hole over the dura in the parietal region of the skull after calibration with a manometer;

2. Flaccid latex membranes attached to shallow stainless steel cylinders, with internal volumes ranging from 8–25 μl, implanted epidurally and connected to Statham P23Bc strain gauges;

3. Crenelated, open-ended polyethylene catheters implanted epidurally or subdurally and connected to calibrated pressure transducers;

4. A crenelated catheter introduced into one lateral ventricle and connected to a calibrated pressure transducer;

5. A needle placed in the cisterna magna and connected to a calibrated pressure transducer, to compare cisternal pressures with ICP values obtained by other methods.

Production of the Infarct. Unselected adult cats were anesthetized with phencyclidine HCl and Na-pentobarbital injected intraperitoneally. After preliminary measurements of ICP by one or more of the above methods, the left MCA was occluded either immediately or after the animal was allowed to recover for several days of additional measurements. Under anesthesia, a poly-

1 Supported in part by Research Grant NS-3364 from the National Institutes of Health, U.S. Public Health Service.
2 Recipient of an International Postdoctoral Research Fellowship from the National Institutes of Health, U.S. Public Health Service. On leave from the Regional Neurological Centre, Newcastle General Hospital, Newcastle-upon-Tyne, England.

ethylene catheter was passed transfemorally into the aorta for measurements of blood pressure and withdrawal of samples for determinations of arterial pH, PCO_2, PO_2, and hematocrit. The left MCA was exposed through the orbit [1] by collapse of the eye, separation of the lateral muscles, section of the optic nerve, and enlargement of the optic canal. The dura was incised, and the MCA was freed and occluded at its origin with a bipolar coagulator. The enlarged optic canal was sealed so that pressure gradients could develop inside an intact cranium.

Results

Measurements of ICP.

1. Preliminary ICP measurements with the miniature strain gauge appeared reasonable; later measurements were erratic. Therefore, the instrument was placed in a fluid-filled pressure box and calibrated daily for 2 weeks. Even after correction for changes of atmospheric pressure there was an unacceptable and unpredictable base-line drift which varied from 2–5 mmHg per day. Because of the base-line drift and because the strain gauge could not be calibrated *in vivo*, no data obtained with the instrument were used.

2. When implanted epidurally, the balloon devices recorded changes of ICP caused by vascular pulsations, respiration, abdominal compression, and the infusion of physiologic saline solution (PSS) into the cisterna magna; the magnitudes of the ICP changes were similar to those recorded from a needle in the cistern. However, the numerical values for ICP varied with the amounts of PSS used to fill the pressure chambers. Because the devices appeared to detect changes of ICP, the first measurement after implantation was taken as a base, and subsequent ICP measurements were expressed as mmHg above or below this value.

3. Reliable ICP measurements could not be made with the epidural or subdural catheters; despite crenation of the ends, the catheters repeatedly became obstructed. Values for ICP could be obtained after flushing, but the values were questionable because of the introduction of PSS into the small spaces.

4. Cannulation of a lateral ventricle caused considerable brain damage so that changes of ICP could not be related specifically to ischemia.

5. Cisternal pressures could be measured reliably but ICP gradients could not be detected.

Excluding operative failures, 18 cats were used; reliable ICP measurements were obtained after MCA occlusion from only 4. Methodologic difficulties accounted for 11 failures; 3 cats died of cerebral infarction before ICP could be recorded.

Effects of Ischemia. In 3 cats, ICP measurements were made at intervals after MCA occlusion. Increases of ICP were first recorded on the side of occlusion at 8, 15 and 21 h, and were maximal at those times. In one cat with severe neurologic deficits, the maximal recorded epidural ICP on the side of MCA occlusion was 59 mmHg above the base pressure; in this animal, there was also an increase of ICP on the opposite side to 16 mmHg. In another cat with only mild neurologic deficits, the maximal ICP on the side of occlusion was 17 mmHg above the base, and ICP opposite the occlusion appeared to decrease. The third cat, with moderate neurologic deficits, had maximal epidural ICPs recorded at 30 mmHg on the side of occlusion and 4 mmHg on the opposite side. In each animal, epidural ICP decreased as the neurologic deficits lessened; however, ICP remained greater on the side of occlusion for up to 7 days. A fourth cat died 26 h after MCA occlusion, with severe neurologic deficits. Fortuitously, epidural ICP was recorded at the time of death from the side opposite the infarct. Oscillations of pressure related to vascular pulsations increased greatly in amplitude, and ICP increased from 13/5 mmHg above the base to 50/40 mmHg in 3 min; respirations then became irregular and stopped.

Discussion

Methodology of ICP Measurement. None of the methods used for measurement of ICP was satisfactory. The balloon devices were the most reliable, when implanted extradurally; comparisons with measurements of cisternal pressure indicated that changes of epidural ICP reflected changes of intradural ICP. However, the values for pressures recorded epidurally were dependent on chamber volumes; thus, it appeared that the relatively dense, tight dura of the cats distorted the recordings of ICP. Measurements of ICP provided only estimates, not absolute values, for intradural ICP.

Ischemia and ICP. The data from this study show that focal cerebral ischemia can cause intracranial pressure gradients, with the greater pressures on the side of ischemia; similar results have been found with a less satisfactory model [2]. Moreover, in 3 cats the magnitudes of the increases of epidural ICP directly were related to the animals' neurologic deficits. In one cat, a massive increase of ICP (to 59 mmHg) must have interfered with perfusion, and may have contributed to severe neurologic deficits. Measurements of intracerebral oxygen availability and EEG after MCA occlusion have also shown that increases of ICP are associated with evidence of severe ischemia [3].

Increases of epidural ICP after MCA occlusion are probably related to edema around the resulting cerebral infarct. Changes of ICP may provide an index of the development and resolution of ischemic cerebral edema, but because of variability, studies of therapeutic measures would require comparisons and statistical analyses of results from large numbers of animals. At present, it does not appear possible to measure absolute intradural ICP in animals, and any measure of ICP is technically difficult; thus, the usefulness of ICP measurements for studies of experimental cerebral ischemia and infarction is limited.

Summary

One middle cerebral artery was occluded in cats, without craniectomy. In 3 cats variable increases of intracranial pressure (ICP) were recorded epidurally on the side of occlusion, and were directly related to the severity of the neurologic deficits. On the side opposite to occlusion ICP increases slightly or not at all. In one cat a rapid increase of ICP preceded death. ICP gradients presumably were caused by ischemic cerebral edema. Methodologic and technical problems were severe; ICP measurements probably will be of limited value for studies of experimental cerebral ischemia, infarction, and edema.

Key Words: Cerebral edema, cerebral ischema, epidural pressure, intracranial pressure, middle cerebral artery occlusion.

References

1. O'BRIEN, M. D., WALTZ, A. G.: Transorbital approach for experimental occlusion of middle cerebral artery without craniectomy. (In press.)
2. BROCK, M., BECK, J., MARKAKIS, E., DIETZ, H.: Intracranial pressure gradients associated with experimental cerebral embolism. Stroke 3, 123–130 (1972).
3. HALSEY, J. H., Jr., CAPRA, N. F.: The course of experimental cerebral infarction – the development of increased intracranial pressure. Stroke 3, 268–278 (1972).

Intracranial Pressure Changes in Acute Ischaemic Regions of the Primate Hemisphere[1]

N. W. C. Dorsch and L. Symon

Introduction

Since the demonstration by McDowall and his colleagues [1] and by Langfitt et al. [2] of pressure gradients between the supra- and infratentorial compartments, there has been interest in the development of such gradients and the various pathological circumstances.

The experiments to be described set out to investigate the following aspects:

1. Development of pressure gradients between the cisterna magna and other sites.
2. Their importance in intracranial hemorrhage and other mass lesions.
3. Relationship of intracranial pressure (ICP) to steal and counter-steal – are they independent of pressure change or not?
4. What happens to reactivity patterns with raised ICP.

Material and Methods

In this study, 14 baboons were used. They were kept anaesthetised and paralysed, and systemic blood pressure, central venous pressure, endtidal CO_2 and arterial blood gases were monitored. An extradural transducer [3], as demonstrated at this meeting, was implanted over one, or in 2 cases both, hemispheres, and the cisternal pressure was also monitored. Blood from Labbé's vein was passed via an electromagnetic flowmeter to the right atrium and the skull closed with acrylic resin. After control measurements of intracranial pressures, cortical venous flow (CVF) and CO_2 reactivity, the skull was re-opened, the middle cerebral and terminal internal carotid arteries clipped during hypotension induced by bleeding, and the skull then re-closed.

4 animals died before adequate infarction occurred. Of the other 10, one had a persistent leak from the artificial skull, leaving 9 sets of pressure data. In one other animal the flowmeter failed, so flow data are also available from 9, the same group except for one.

---

1 This work was supported by the Medical Research Council.

Results

Intracranial Pressure

Before occlusion, there was no difference between extradural pressure (EDP) with its mean of 7.34 mmHg (S.D. 2.49), and cisternal pressure (CP) at normal arterial pCO_2. During hypercapnia, 3 animals developed differential pressures, EDP being higher; over the whole group the difference was not significant.

After occlusion, EDP rose steadily over several hours to a mean maximum of 38.39 mmHg (S.D. 26.83), becoming significantly greater than control levels ($p < 0.01$). CP also rose, but not as much, to a maximum of 32.78 mmHg (S.D. 26.2), differential pressures developing in 6 out of the 9. The difference between maximum EDP and CP was significant with a p between 0.05 and 0.01.

In the 2 animals where extradural pressure was measured bilaterally, EDP over the infarcted hemisphere rose more than CP, which in turn was greater than EDP on the other side. In one case, the 3 pressures were respectively 25.4, 18, and 8.9 mmHg, and in the other, 88, 71, and 59. It is noteworthy that in one case the EDP on the control side did not rise significantly from normal.

Cortical Venous Flow

In the 9 animals in this group, baseline flow from Labbé's vein was 0.77 ml per min (S.D. 0.25). Vascular occlusion produced an acute fall to a mean of 0.38 ml per min (S.D. 0.17), this difference being significant with a p value of < 0.01. Flow then showed a gradual recovery from this level, and, in fact, came to exceed the control level pre-occlusion in 5 cases. Thus, mean recovery flow was 1.01 ml per min (S.D. 0.20); this differs from immediate post-occlusion values with a p of < 0.01, and is greater than the mean baseline value before occlusion, though not significantly so.

Carbon Dioxide Reactivity

In ICP, reactivity is expressed in mmHg of pressure change per mmHg of pCO_2 change. Prior to clipping, the mean change in intracranial pressure was 1.61 mmHg per mm of pCO_2 (S.D. 2.68). Afterwards, this dropped to 0.79 mm per mm of pCO_2 (S.D. 0.89), having decreased in 4 and risen in 5; this change was not significant.

Reactivity of flow, expressed as percentage change in flow per mmHg change in pCO_2, behaved differently. In control conditions, the mean change with hypercapnia was 8.2% per mmHg pCO_2 change (S.D. 5.69); after occlusion it fell to -0.2% per mm (S.D. 2.50), the difference being significant with a p of < 0.01.

There was no obvious relationship between the level of ICP reached and change in reactivity of pressure, but with CVF the reactivity decreased as ICP rose. Figure 1 shows the relationship of maximum EDP reached with CO_2 with change in flow per mm of pCO_2 change at that time. The correlation coefficient is —0.75, and the correlation is significant with a p of < 0.001. In isolated cases, in fact, increasing the pCO_2 led to a great increase in EDP and a reduction in flow, the reverse also occurring. Figure 2 shows loss of reactivity of CVF to either an increase or a decrease of pCO_2, while in Figure 3 a reversal of reactivity is seen, CVF falling as pCO_2 and, consequently, ICP are increased.

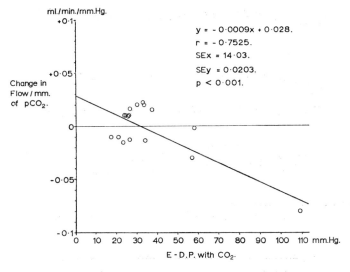

Fig. 1. Graph showing a decrease in reactivity to CO_2 of CVF as ICP increases

Hemisphere Weight

At the end of 6 experiments, the hemispheres were removed and separately weighed. On the control side the mean weight was 65.82 g (S.D. 2.74), while on the infarcted side the mean was 68.2 g (S.D. 2.49); the significance of this difference is between 0.05 and 0.01.

Discussion

A significant difference has been shown between EDP and CP following infarction; although the significance is only between the 1 and 5% confidence levels it is felt that with a greater number of experiments this would come down, and likewise, that there would be an even more significant difference between EDP on infarcted and control sides.

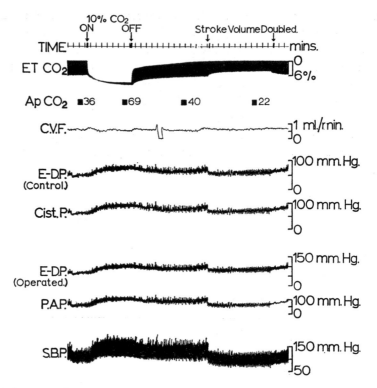

Fig. 2. Effect of increase and decrease of pCO₂ on intracranial pressures and Labbé's vein
flow in an infarcted area of the baboon hemisphere

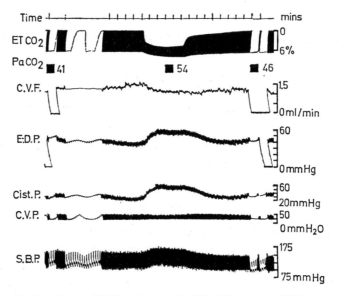

Fig. 3. Reversal of reactivity of CVF to increased pCO₂ following establishment of an infarct

This demonstrates, then, that pressure gradients can exist within the cranial cavity, and also in the supratentorial compartment alone. The reason for this is that the brain is physically more or less solid, and also enclosed by a membrane, the pia, with a certain tensile strength; and that CSF shifts are not enough to neutralise large differences in pressure resulting from local increases, even without obstruction to fluid pathways.

The cause of the increased pressure is undoubtedly spreading oedema in the infarcted hemisphere. This results in increasing brain bulk until there is no longer room in the pia or cranium, and then in increasing local pressure. Evidence for this is seen in the increased weight of the infarcted hemispheres in the 6 cases tested.

It is interesting that the expected drop in CVF on occlusion was followed by a rise to levels higher than control, despite loss of input pressure to the vascular bed and increasing ICP. This suggests maximal dilatation of vessels in and around the infarcted area, and there is further evidence for this in the decreased reactivity of flow to hypercapnia.

A possible explanation for the loss, and in some cases reversal of reactivity of flow, could be considered in the cerebral steal phenomenon. It is felt, however, that in these cases with the re-created skull, it is related more to the increased ICP, with a further increase of this pressure in hypercapnia causing a lesser increase or a decrease in flow, mainly through a reduction of perfusion pressure. Thus, where ICP was reduced or increased by removal or infusion of CSF, with pCO_2 kept constant, similar effects on flow were seen.

Also worthy of mention is an earlier series of experiments where the skull was not re-closed after the infarct was produced. In these, although there was some loss of flow reactivity to hypercapnia, the mean falling from 3.9 to 2.8% per mm of pCO_2 change, it was much less marked, and mean reactivity did not become negative as it did in the present series with the skull closed and pressure allowed to build up.

Summary

After production of an infarct in one hemisphere, differential pressures occurred between it and the opposite hemisphere, and between it and the cisterna. CVF showed a fall followed by recovery, and under conditions of raised ICP there was a reduction, or in some cases a reversal, of reactivity of CVF to pCO_2 changes.

Key Words: Extradural pressure, cortical venous flow, reactivity of flow.

References

1. LANGFITT, T. W., WEINSTEIN, J. D., KASSELL, N. F., SIMEONE, F. A.: Transmission of increased intracranial pressure, I. Within the craniospinal axis. J. Neurosurg. **21**, 989–997 (1964).

2. FITCH, W., McDOWALL, D. G.: Vasodilating anaesthetics and pressures in different compartments of the skull. In: BRIERLEY, J. B., MELDRUM, B. S. (Eds.): Brain Hypoxia, p. 113–117. London: William Heinemann 1971.
3. DORSCH, N. W. C., STEPHENS, R. J., SYMON, L.: An intracranial pressure transducer. Biomed. Engng. 6, 452–457 (1971).

Extradural Pressure and Regional Oxygen Availability in Experimental Cerebral Infarction

J. H. HALSEY and N. F. CAPRA

Introduction

The outcome of a major cerebral arterial occlusion is difficult to predict. We have all seen, both in our patients, and in our experimental animals, death, complete recovery, and all degrees of clinical disability resulting from identical arterial occlusions. This is a progress report of our continuing effort to understand cerebral infarction. We have come to view it as a process which evolves over a considerable period of time and has many determinants. Some of these determinants are known. They include: blood pressure, pCO_2, the nature of the arterial lesion itself, the competence of the collateral circulation and intracranial pressure. We wish to present for your consideration evidence that there may be another determinant. We do not know what it is. We shall be glad to hear your opinions about it.

Material and Methods

Cats were paralyzed and artificially ventilated under pentobarbital anesthesia. Respiratory CO_2 was maintained constant for the duration of the experiment. Arterial pO_2, pCO_2, pH, and hematocrit were measured every 4 h. In regular rotation, experiments were performed at low (15–20 mmHg), normal (28–32 mmHg) and high (40–60 mmHg) pCO_2. Arterial pO_2 was maintained between 120 and 150 mmHg. Rectal temperature was between 36 and 38° C. Mean arterial blood pressure was monitored continuously but allowed to fluctuate spontaneously except that infusion of metaraminol was used in some cases to prevent reduction below 80 mmHg.

Cerebral ischemia was caused by surgical occlusion of the middle cerebral artery by the retroorbital approach. The dura was left open at the site of exposure of the middle cerebral artery but the cranium and dura were otherwise intact. Regional oxygen availability was monitored continuously from chronically implanted bare platinum electrodes [1, 2]. Three had been placed in the cortical convexity, one in the caudate nucleus of the ischemic hemisphere, and one in the convexity of the normal hemisphere. EEG was monitored from the oxygen electrodes. Extradural pressure was measured by an electro-mechanical transducer as the manometric pressure required to separate a pair of electric contacts on the dura overlying the convexity of the ischemic hemisphere [1]. The transducer was placed about 2 h prior to occlusion and sealed in place with acrylic, overlying the ischemic hemisphere.

Results

14 animals developed increased extradural pressures of more than 25 mmHg at some point post occlusion, while in 13 the extradural pressure was continuously less than 15 mmHg. There was no difference between the 2 groups of animals in pCO_2, blood pressure, temperature or hematocrit either at occlusion or at any time subsequently. In the animals which ultimately developed increased extradural pressure, the regional ischemia at the time of occlusion was more severe as indicated by a greater decrease in oxygen availability as well as by EEG changes.

For this discussion we have matched the two groups of animals for severity of initial ischemia [2]. This was achieved by arbitrarily excluding from the group which developed increased extradural pressure the 4 animals with the most severe initial ischemia, and from the group which did not develop increased extradural pressure the 3 with the least severe ischemia. These 2 subgroups did not differ in pCO_2 or blood pressure at occlusion or at any time subsequently. Although initial ischemia was the same, there were very important differences between the 2 groups in their subsequent course.

Figure 1 reveals the successive extradural pressure changes. Slight but significant differences in extradural pressure are evident from the second hour post occlusion onward, and substantial increases become evident after 9 h post occlusion.

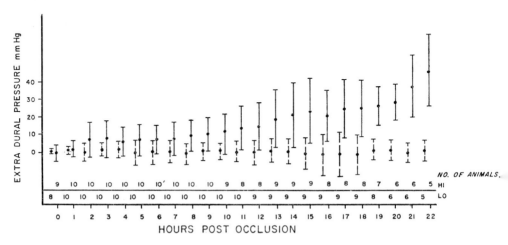

Fig. 1. Mean and standard deviation of extradural pressure changes at successive hours after occlusion. Solid line represents animals developing increased extradural pressure (Hi), interrupted line represents animals which did not (Lo)

In Fig. 2 are summarized the successive oxygen availability changes. There was no difference at occlusion. In the animals which did not go on to develop increased extradural pressure recovery of oxygen availability occurred rapidly.

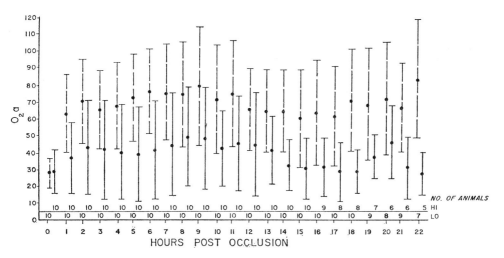

Fig. 2. Mean and standard deviation of oxygen availability changes at successive hours after occlusion

In the animals which did subsequently develop increased extradural pressure, this was slower and less complete, and followed by progressive decline.

Discussion

From the ninth hour onward, progressively declining oxygen availability in the high extradural pressure animals is clearly attributed to the rising extradural pressure. (The oxygen availability rise during the nineteenth and twentieth hours may be an artifact of several animals dying at this time in the high extradural pressure groups).

From the second hour onward, the extradural pressure differences are statistically significant. Though small, they are probably physiologically significant too. Though 5 or 6 mmHg is small in comparison with the systemic arterial pressure, it may be a very substantial fraction of the pressure in the middle cerebral artery distal to the occlusion [3]. The important question, we think, is how to account for the slower recovery of the collateral circulation during the first hour before this pressure difference was evident. During this period there may be significant local tissue pressure or capillary resistance differences which are not reflected in the extradural measurement. Assuming there are, we would like to know why did they occur in one group of animals which is so nearly identical to the other group in which they evidently did not.

Summary

2 groups of cats were subjected to middle cerebral artery ligation. One group developed markedly increased extradural pressure due to infarction. In the other group, infarctions were small or absent and no increase occurred in extradural pressure. The 2 groups were identical in blood pressure, pCO_2, hematocrit, temperature, and severity of the initial ischemic insult. There appears to be an additional determinant of the evolution of local tissue pressure and extension of infarction. Its nature is unknown.

Key Words : Progressive ischemia, pCO_2, blood pressure.

References

1. Halsey, J. H., Capra, N.: The course of experimental cerebral infarction – the development of increased intracranial pressure. Stroke **3**, 268–278 (1972).
2. Halsey, J. H., Capra, N.: Physiologic modification of immediate ischemia due to experimental middle cerebral artery occlusion – its relevance to cerebral infarction. Stroke **2**, 239–246 (1971).
3. Symon, L.: Regional cerebrovascular responses to acute ischemia in normocapnia and hypercapnia. J. Neurol. Neurosurg. Psychiat. **33**, 756–762 (1970).

Studies on the Water Content of Cerebral Tissues and Intracranial Pressure in Vasogenic Brain Oedema

J. W. F. Beks and H. P. M. Kerckhoffs

Introduction

Though there have been many investigations on the problems around cerebral edema and raised intracranial pressure in the last few years and valuable contributions have been made to the solution of these problems [1–9], numerous questions still remained unanswered.

In an excellent study in 1967, Klatzo [4] suggested a classification on practical and theoretical grounds. He divided brain edema into a vasogenic and a cytotoxic form.

The vasogenic form of cerebral edema was supposed to develop as a result of changes in permeability of the cerebrovascular wall, enabling certain chemical substances to penetrate from the circulating blood into the cerebral tissue, thus causing an increase in its water content and therefore brain edema.

Brain edema developing as result of a cold-induced lesion of the cerebral cortex may be used as an experimental model of the vasogenic form because, as was shown by Beks et al. in 1967 [10], this causes increased permeability of the cerebral vessels in the area of the lesion.

This form of cerebral edema is of great clinical importance, because it can occur as a dangerous complication of head injuries, brain tumours, inflammatory conditions etc. . . . .

The therapeutic approach to these complications is still the subject of continual discussion. The question as to whether or not it is desirable to administer hypertonic solutions by the intravenous route to patients suffering from vasogenic brain edema is still a matter of controversial views amongst various authors.

We therefore tried to establish the relationship between the water content of the cerebral cortex and that of the white substance below it in an experimentally-induced form of vasogenic cerebral edema and the influence of some hypertonic solutions, namely solutions of urea and mannitol on the water content of the cerebral tissue and its influence on the intracranial pressure.

We induced cerebral edema by the method described in 1953 by Clasen and his co-workers [11]. The application of cold to a localized area of the cerebral cortex covered by dura mater resulted in a region showing every property of hemorrhagic infarction. In most cases this infarction remained confined to the cerebral cortex, but in some cases it extended to the subcortical white substance.

On microscopical examination the white substance beneath the cerebral cortex, showed the spongioid structure typical of cerebral edema. The brain edema extended over a considerable part of the affected hemisphere and was not confined only to the area beneath the cortex which had been injured by application of cold. The way this form of cerebral oedema propagates, was described by Go and his co-workers in 1969 [12]. Histological examination of the damaged cerebral cortex revealed hardly any oedema. Therefore the increase in volume of the oedematous hemisphere had to be ascribed almost completely to the swelling of the white substance. The oedematous fluid was not evenly distributed throughout the white substance. Some parts, for instance the semi-oval centre, showed no aberrations. According to Go and his co-workers this could possibly be due to the course of nervous fibers in the affected area.

Materials and Methods

For our experiments we used 40 full-grown cats, varying in weight from 1600 to 4400 g. As narcotics we used phenobarbital and a nitrous oxide-oxygen mixture. The animals were intubated and breathed spontaneously. By stereotactic means a needle was inserted into the cella media of the right lateral ventricle and connected with a Statham physiological-pressure transducer.

In the left frontal area a burr-hole 13 mm in diameter was made in exactly the same place in each cat. The dura mater was left intact. A cooling thermode was inserted into the opening made by trepanation in such a way that the basis of the thermode came into contact with the dura mater. After the intraventricular pressure had been recorded for 1 h, the cerebral cortex was cooled locally to a temperature of $-30°$ C. This affected permeability of the cortical vascular walls, inducing brain edema, which in turn entailed an increase in intracranial pressure and therefore in intraventricular pressure.

When the intraventricular pressure had reached a certain level, hyperosmotic solutions of urea or mannitol were administered to a number of test-animals, after which the intraventricular pressure fell. When this had reached its lowest level the animals were sacrificed with the aid of an intra-arterial injection of 10 ml thiobarbital.

As hyperosmotic agents we used 3.3 ml per kg body-weight of a solution containing 30% urea in 10% invert sugar and 10 ml per kg body-weight of a 20% mannitol solution. The dose indicated was administered within 4 min.

After the death of the animals the brains were removed, the dura mater being left intact. Immediately afterwards, the left and right hemisphere were transferred separately into carefully pre-weighed vials.

Samples of grey and white matter were taken from the left and right hemispheres in an air-conditioned, humid room. The samples from the left hemisphere were always taken from the area where the cold injury had been applied. For this purpose the edematous territory was divided into 4 fragments. Samples of grey and white substance were taken from two opposite fragments and again transferred into weighed vials. The samples were dried at 30 °C, for 1 h, 1 h at 50° C, 1 h at 70° C and then for 12 h at 103° C. The samples were then dried until the difference between two consecutive weighings was not more than $1/_{1000}$ of the initial weight of the sample being examined.

The weighing was performed on a semi-microbalance. All water content values are indicated as percent weight volume (w.v.); the water content is expressed in relation to the weight of the wet material.

Results

40 experiments were performed and divided into 4 groups.

Group A

In these test animals no cerebral lesion was induced and no hypertonic solutions were administered. They served as a control group. After premedication and induction of narcosis the animals were sacrificed after 1 h as described above. Then the brain was removed and prepared as above. The results are recorded in Table 1.

Table 1

Cat No.	Weight (grams)	Water Content (%) Cortex		White Matter	
		left	right	left	right
122b	4345	80.50	80.32	72.15	72.40
146	2550	81.00	81.30	73.42	73.50
147	1600	81.43	81.19	73.16	73.51
148	2850	80.88	80.72	72.76	72.18
149	2850	80.20	81.49	73.75	73.29
128	3150	80.30	80.41	72.38	72.49
129	3620	81.24	81.13	73.20	73.18
130	2870	80.78	80.61	72.51	72.46
119	2980	80.55	80.70	72.33	72.28
120	3050	81.10	81.25	73.08	73.18
		80.80	80.91	72.87	72.85

Group B

These 10 animals were sacrificed when the brain oedema, following infliction of an injury by application of cold, had raised the intraventricular pressure to 40 mmHg above the initial value. In this group the animals were not given hypertonic solutions (Table 2).

Table 2

Cat No.	Weight (grams)	Intraventricular pressure (mmHg)		Water Content (%) Cortex		White Matter	
		start	end	left	right	left	right
139	2945	8	48	80.18	81.00	78.22	73.22
140	3250	5	45	80.61	80.74	77.81	73.47
141	2900	10	50	81.33	81.61	78.93	72.13
142	3900	9	49	81.41	80.67	78.02	72.97
144	4400	9	48	80.79	80.28	77.11	73.64
170	2830	7	47	80.31	80.73	78.34	72.98
171	2750	10	50	81.27	81.54	77.92	72.14
174	3200	4	44	81.18	81.67	78.01	72.84
175	3130	5	45	80.44	80.13	78.44	73.05
177	2870	6	46	80.12	80.07	77.19	72.87
				80.76	80.84	78.00	72.93

Group C

In this group the animals received hypertonic urea solution as soon as the intraventricular pressure had risen by 40 mmHg. The intraventricular pressure then fell and the animals were sacrificed when the pressure had reached its lowest level (Table 3).

Table 3

Cat No.	Weight (grams)	Intraventricular pressure (mmHg)			Water Content (%) Cortex		White Matter	
		start	highest	lowest	left	right	left	right
133	3750	5	45	2	81.02	78.31	72.21	71.52
137	4350	10	50	13	81.17	79.23	73.07	71.18
138	3500	9	49	7	80.00	78.89	72.85	72.22
131	3095	10	50	12	80.96	78.68	73.64	72.01
132	4050	12	52	6	81.62	79.78	73.77	72.51
164	3280	9	49	9	80.08	78.14	72.18	71.77
166	3100	9	49	9	80.73	79.18	73.21	72.36
167	2980	7	47	10	81.18	78.88	72.54	71.88
168	3130	6	46	5	80.54	78.19	71.99	71.02
169	2540	9	49	4	81.33	79.02	72.48	71.33
					80.86	78.83	72.79	71.78

Group D

In this group the animals were given hyperosmotic mannitol solution as soon as the intraventricular pressure reached a level 40 mmHg above the initial value. After this, the intraventricular pressure decreased and the animals were killed when it had reached its lowest level (Table 4).

Table 4

Cat No.	Weight (grams)	Intraventricular pressure (mmHg)			Water Content (%) Cortex		White Matter	
		start	highest	lowest	left	right	left	right
155	2530	2	42	5	82.07	78.51	74.05	71.03
159	2850	12	52	46	82.05	80.74	79.98	73.21
162	2550	5	45	30	80.25	80.19	77.71	72.97
163	2500	10	50	17	81.21	79.23	73.78	72.49
150	3080	9	49	18	81.03	79.44	74.31	71.81
151	2970	6	46	13	81.88	80.01	78.31	73.34
152	3120	5	45	9	80.93	78.24	76.24	73.01
153	2940	10	50	18	80.74	78.33	77.51	72.51
154	3080	10	50	16	80.51	79.05	76.22	72.24
157	2640	7	47	14	80.44	79.21	75.18	71.83
					81.11	79.30	76.33	72.53

Discussion

Like NAKAZAWA [13], and in contrast to PAPPIUS [14], we found no evident increase in water content in the injured cortex as compared to the undamaged tissue in our experiments. In each case we measured a water content of 80.76% on the left and 80.84% on the right side. There was, however, a considerable increase in the water content of the white substance beneath the damaged cortex. In this tissue we found an average water content of 78.00%, as compared to 72.93% in the control hemisphere.

In 1967 BEKS [15] and co-workers showed that the application of cold to the cerebral cortex led to leakage of PAS-positive fluid from its vessels and that this penetrated into the white substance.

As early as 1939 STEWART-WALLACE [9] pointed out that in cases of traumatic human cerebral edema there was an increase in the water and electrolyte content of the brain which was proportinally equal to the increase in serum filtrate. This fact is also supposed to support the view that, in traumatic cerebral edema, the edema is derived from the circulating blood. KLATZO based his classification of brain edema into vasogenic and cytotoxic forms [4] partly on these observations.

The above observation that permeability of the cortical vessels is increased by the application of cold is very much in keeping with the results of our later observations. It has become apparent, namely, that after the administration of hyperosmotic agents there is no decrease in water content and, therefore, no dehydration in the damaged part of the cerebral cortex, whereas fluid is derived from the intact cortex. The average fluid content of the intact cerebral cortex amounted to 80.84% (Table 2), whereas after the administration of a hyperosmotic solution of urea or mannitol the water content was 78.83% (Table 3), or 79.30% (Table 4), respectively.

The water content of the damaged cortex amounted to 80.86% (Table 3) or 81.11% (Table 4) after administration of the agents mentioned.

The average water content of the white substance beneath the injured cortex was 78.00% (Table 2), whereas the water content in the control hemisphere was 72.93% in the white substance. After administration of hyperosmotic urea solution the water content was 72.79% (Table 3), which is a fairly normal value. After a comparable dose of mannitol solution the average water content fell to 76.33% (Table 4). This proves that the dehydrating power of a hyperosmotic urea solution is higher than that of a hyperosmotic mannitol solution. The individual range was also more extensive in the group treated with mannitol.

In 1967 Beks and Ter Weeme [15] established that raised intraventricular pressure resulting from a cold injury falls more rapidly and to a lower level after administration of a hyperosmotic urea solution than after administration of an equivalent amount of mannitol. The application of hyperosmotic agents in brain edema results in dehydration of the edematous tissue as long as the walls of the vessels are intact and the chemicals administered cannot pass the vascular wall; this is self-evident if one bears in mind that the effect of these agents is based on the osmotic difference between blood plasma and the surrounding tissue. In the edematous white substance, in contrast to the cold-injured cortex, the vascular wall has not been damaged [4].

This tissue is bound to become dehydrated after administration of a hyperosmotic solution, which is completely in keeping with our findings (Table 3 and Table 4). Pappius and Dayes [16], however, found no evident fall in the water content of the edematous white substance after application of hyperosmotic agents in their experiments.

Our investigations also indicate that the increased intraventricular pressure in experimental brain oedema has to be ascribed largely to the increase in the water content of the injured hemisphere. The intraventricular pressure fell considerably when dehydration of the edematous white substance resulted from the administration of a hypertonic agent, (Table 3 and Table 4). We have been able to establish a moderate degree of direct correlation between the water content of the brain and the increase or decrease in intraventricular pressure. This supports the concept of Reed and Woodburry [17].

According to these authors, the decrease of pressure resulting from the decrease in cerebral volume occuring as a consequence of dehydration after intravenous administration of hyperosmotic agents is partly compensated by an increased production of cerebrospinal fluid and a decrease in the absorbtion of this fluid.

Summary

Vasogenic brain oedema was induced in adult cats by means of application of cold to the cerebral cortex via an intact dura mater. The changes in the water content of the cerebral cortex and in the white substance beneath the cortex were subsequently analyzed. The changes in intraventricular pressure were also measured.

After the application of hyperosmotic solutions the water content of the damaged cerebral cortex, in contrast to that of the intact cortex, appeared not to decrease. However, evident dehydration of the edematous white substance beneath the damaged cortex occurred, which appeared to be more pronounced after the administration of a urea solution than after the use of an equivalent amount of mannitol.

Correlation between the rise in intracranial pressure and the water content of the brain appeared to be only moderate.

Key Words: Brain oedema, intracranial pressure, water content of the brain.

References

1. BAKAY, L., LEE, J. C.: Cerebral Edema. Springfield, Illinois: C. C. Thomas 1965.
2. FRENCH, L. A., GALICICH, J. H.: The use of steroids for control of cerebral edema. In: MOSBERG, W. H. (Ed.): Clinical Neurosurgery, p. 212–223. Baltimore: The Williams & Wilkins Co. 1964.
3. JAVID, M.: Urea – new use of an old agent. Reduction of intracranial and intraocular pressure. The Surg. Clinics of North America, 1–2 (1958).
4. KLATZO, I.: Neuropathological aspects of brain edema. J. Neuropath. exp. Neurol. **26**, 1–14 (1967).
5. PAPPIUS, H. M., GULATI, D. R.: Water and electrolyte content of cerebral tissues in experimentally induced edema. Acta neuropath. **2**, 451 460 (1963).
6. REULEN, H. J., MEDZIHRADSKY, F., ENZENBACH, R., MARGUT, F., BRENDEL, W.: Electrolytes, fluid and energy metabolism in human cerebral edema. Arch. Neurol. **21**, 517–525 (1969).
7. SCHEINKER, J. M.: Zur Histopathologie des Hirnödems und der Hirnschwellung bei Tumoren des Gehirnes. Dtsch. Z. Nervenheilk. **147**, 137–162 (1938).
8. SHENKIN, H. A., GOBULOFF, B., HAFT, H.: The use of mannitol for the reduction of intracranial pressure in intracranial surgery. J. Neurosurg. **19**, 897–900 (1962).
9. STEWART-WALLACE, A. M.: A biochemical study of cerebral tissue, and of the changes in cerebral edema. Brain **62**, 426–438 (1939).
10. BEKS, J. W. F., EBELS, E. J.: Alterations in the intraventricular pressure in cats after cold-induced edema. In: SEITELBERGER, F., KLATZO, I. (Eds.): Brain Edema, p. 564–568. Wien-New York: Springer Verlag 1967.
11. CLASEN, R. A., BROWN, D. V. L., LEAVITT, S., HASS, G. M.: The production by liquid nitrogen of acute closed cerebral lesions. Surg. Gynec. Obstet. **96**, 605–616 (1953).
12. GO, K. G., WOUDENBERG, F., WOLDRING, M., EBELS, E. J., BEKS, J. W. F., SMEETS, E. H. J.: The penetration of ^{14}C-urea and ^{3}H-water into the rat brain with cold-induced cerebral oedema. Acta neurochir. **21**, 97–122 (1969).
13. NAKAZAWA, S.: Biochemical studies of cerebral tissues in experimentally induced edema. Neurol. **19**, 269–276 (1969).

14. Pappius, H. M.: Biochemical studies on experimental brain edema. In: Seitelberger, F., Klatzo, I. (Eds.): Brain Edema, p. 445–460. Wien-New York: Springer Verlag 1967.
15. Beks, J. W. F., ter Weeme, C. A.: The influence of urea and mannitol on increased intraventricular pressure in cold-induced cerebral oedema. Acta neurochir. 16, 97–107 (1967)
16. Pappius, H. M., Dayes, L. A.: Hypertonic urea. Arch. Neurol. 13, 395 (1965).
17. Reed, D. J., Woodburry, D. M.: Effect of hypertonic urea on cerebrospinal fluid pressure and brain volume. J. Physiol. 164, 252–264 (1962).

Delayed Brain Swelling after X-Irradiation of the Visual Cortex in the Macaca Mulatta

W. F. Caveness, M. Kato, A. Tanaka, K. H. Hess, M. O. M. Tso, and L. E. Zimmerman

Introduction

For the past ten years we have studied the effect of 3,500 rads of x-irradiation, in a single exposure, on the cerebral cortex of the young adult Macaca mulatta. The geometry of the exposure and the dosimetry of the absorption area was determined at Brookhaven National Laboratory, in conjunction with Arland L. Carsten. The irradiation site, since 1966, has been the right visual cortex. This permits a precise measurement of functional changes as expressed in the visual evoked response. Attention has been directed to the ultrastructural evidence for cellular changes in carbohydrate and protein metabolism within days of exposure and, by light microscopy, to alteration in the dendritic plexus within four to twelve weeks, and the proliferative and degenerative changes of radionecrosis in the exposed area *four* to *five months* following irradiation [1]. Long-term functional alterations have included unilateral, succeeded by bilateral depression of the evoked response and behavioral blindness. Long-term structural changes have included periodic brain swelling and retrograde transsynaptic degeneration within the visual system. The purpose of the current series is to more precisely delineate, in time and degree, the delayed brain swelling following exposure to ionizing irradiation.

Materials and Methods

12 monkeys, 24 months of age (3 kg in weight) received successful implantations of spinal catheter-reservoir systems in July and August 1971. The catheter, .065 cm O.D., .030 cm I.D., made of medical grade silicone rubber, was inserted in the subarachnoid space at L2–3. The cephalad projection was 18–22 cm and it approached or entered the cisterna magna. The caudal end was connected to a modified side inlet Ommaya Reservoir 1.5 cm in diameter, which was then secured beneath the skin. For the measurement of the CSF. pressure in the spinal subarachnoid space near the cistern, the animal is placed in a prone position with the head fixed, the limbs comfortably restrained, the eyes covered, and the environment quiet. With sterile technique, a 22 gauge needle is passed through the skin into the reservoir. The needle is connected to a closed mano-

metric system that permits pressure measurements above the level of the heart. Readings are carried out over a thirty minute period to obviate effects of agitation (Fig. 1.).

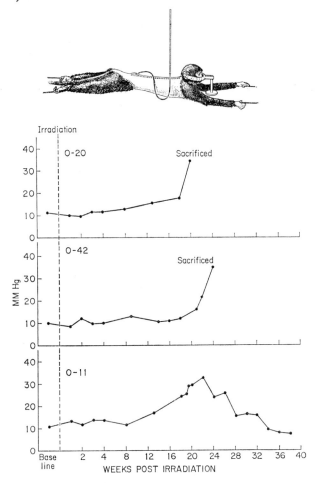

Fig. 1. Catheter-reservoir system for measuring spinal subarachnoid CSF pressure and sequential recordings in monkcys, No. 0–20, No. 0–42, and No. 0–11

6 weeks (4–8) after the implantation of the catheter-reservoir system, the right visual cortex, and the immediate subjacent white matter to a depth of 1 cm, was exposed to 3,500 rads of x-irradiation. The source was a General Electric Maxitron X-Ray machine, operating at 250 KVP and 30 mA. The target to skin distance was 9 in., and the dose rate was 300–350 rad/min. An 0.5 mm copper filter and an aluminum parabolic filter resulted in an x-ray beam having a half value layer equal to 2.15 mm copper.

Sequential observations, prior to and subsequent to irradiation, included each second week the CSF pressure readings, fundoscopic examination, and where indicated, photography with a Zeiss Fundus Camera. Functional changes in the visual system are monitored by evoked EEG responses from photic stimulation of the retina with single and multiple light flashes. The responses are subjected to averaging and frequency analyses, respectively [2].

4 additional monkeys received identical implantation of spinal catheter-reservoir systems, without subsequent exposure to x-irradiation. This control series is receiving similar observations, as to CSF pressure, fundoscopic examination, and visual evoked responses, as the irradiated animals.

Results

The pre-irradiation pressure, with minor variations, was 10 mmHg in 9 of the animals, 13–14 mmHg in 2 and 7 mmHg in 1. In the 20–30 weeks following irradiation, 5 animals have shown little or no increase in pressure, 3 have shown increases from 10–15 mmHg, and four have shown dramatic increases 20–24 weeks following irradiation of 22–38 mmHg.

6 animals, representative of the changes in the first 20–30 weeks following irradiation, have been sacrificed. The remaining six, along with the controls, will be observed for an additional 30 weeks. 1 h prior to sacrifice, Evans Blue, 2 cc per kilo, was injected intravenously. The animals were perfused with paraformaldehyde and their brains and eyes are being subjected to a definitive histological examination.

The first monkey, No. 0–7, with an elevation of only 8 mm at 17 weeks and a return to baseline at 20 weeks, the time of sacrifice, showed early papilledema on the right, no change in visual evoked response, no gross brain lesion and no brain swelling. The only abnormal finding to inspection was a faint blue tinge from the Evans Blue in the white matter of the right occipital lobe.

The second monkey, No. 0–5, with an elevation of 10 mmHg at 20 weeks at the time of sacrifice, showed no papilledema but bilateral disc pallor, dilated pupils, behavioral blindness, and bilateral absence of visual evoked response. The brain was grossly swollen, the right hemisphere greater than the left, together with tentorial herniation. There was evidence of parenchymal destruction in the irradiated right occipital lobe.

The third monkey, No. 0–37, with an unknown pressure because of failure in the catheter-reservoir system prior to sacrifice, at 24 weeks, showed bilateral papilledema and pronounced unilateral (right) depression of the visual evoked response. The right hemisphere was grossly swollen with distortion of midline structures to the left and tentorial herniation on the right. The irradiated area was deeply, but unevenly stained with Evans Blue.

The fourth monkey, No. 0–20, with an increase in pressure of 7 mmHg at 18 weeks and 23 mmHg at 20 weeks, the time of sacrifice, showed bilateral papilledema, obliteration of the evoked response on the right and marked depression on the left, gross brain swelling most prominent in the right hemisphere, and deep staining with Evans Blue in the irradiated area fo the right occipital lobe (Fig. 2).

The fifth monkey, No. 0–42, with an increase in pressure of 6 mmHg at 21 weeks and 25 mmHg at 24 weeks, the time of sacrifice, exhibited behavioral blindness, dilated pupils, a right 6th nerve palsy, bilateral disc pallor and absence of the visual evoked response. Earlier, at 18 weeks, the evoked response was normal bilaterally. At 20 weeks, there was a moderate depression over the right, irradiated cortex. The background EEG in this region showed some delta activity and random high amplitude spikes. On one occasion, a focal seizure, 50 sec in duration, was recorded. At 24 weeks, in addition to the absence of the visual evoked response, there was bilateral delta activity, higher in amplitude and continuous on the right. The brain was grossly swollen with deep Evans Blue staining in the region of irradiation, and right medial temporal lobe herniation through the incisura (Fig. 3).

The sixth monkey, No. 0–41, with an increase in pressure of 11 mmHg at 24 weeks, 26 mmHg at 25 weeks, and 38 mmHg at 28 weeks, had a drop in pressure to zero at 29 weeks, evidently the result of occlusion of CSF circulation above the cistern. The visual evoked response showed a marked depression on the right, accompanied by background delta activity, at 24 weeks. At 28 weeks, just prior to sacrifice, the evoked response was obliterated and the delta activity was bilateral. The animal appeared in distress, refused food and occasionally vomited. Behaviorally blind, the discs were pale, with blurring of the margin on the right, and hemorrhages in the right fundus. The brain was grossly swollen, predominantly on the right, with uncal herniation, and deep staining of the irradiated area in the right occipital lobe, The ventricular system was distorted to the left with obliteration or narrowing on the right and enlargement of the left ventricular spaces.

Of the 6 irradiated animals still being observed, one monkey, No. 0–11, has shown an increase in pressure of 22 mmHg at 22 weeks followed by a decline of 25 mmHg over the next 16 weeks. The increase in pressure was accompanied by alterations in the visual evoked response, and by bilateral papilledema. The recovery from the increase in pressure was accompanied by a resolution of the papilledema and a return in part of the evoked response. (Fig. 4.) The 4 non-irradiated control animals have shown no significant alterations from their baseline findings.

Comment

The delayed relatively abrupt rise in intracranial pressure is thought to be the result of the delayed proliferative and degenerative changes in the brain at the site of exposure to x-irradiation. The local impairment in blood vessels, with the disruption of the blood-brain barrier, permits an outpouring of plasma constituents into the surrounding parenchyma. The extravasation continues,

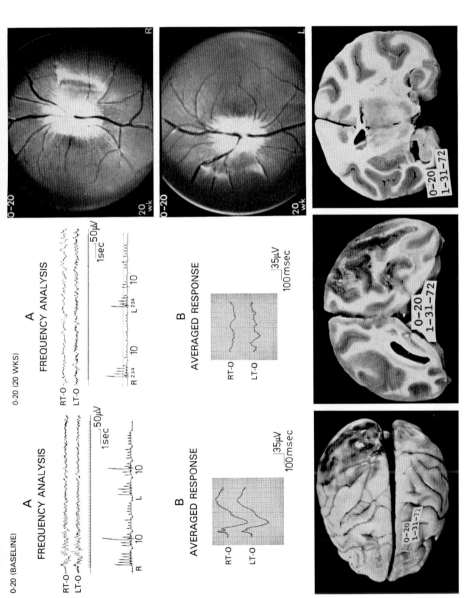

Fig. 2. Obliteration of visual evoked response, papilledema, and gross brain swelling, with Evans Blue stain in the irradiated area, in monkey No. 0–20, 20 weeks after exposure

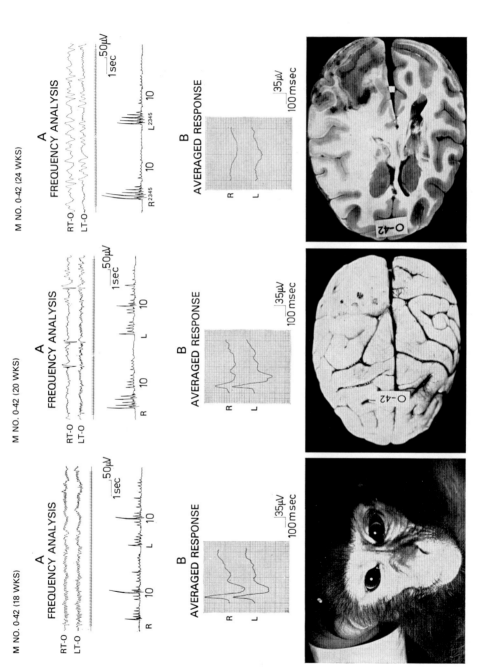

Fig. 3. Reduction in visual evoked response and paroxysmal activity on the right in monkey No. 0–42 at 20 weeks. At 24 weeks, there was no evoked response, but bilateral delta activity in the EEG; dilated pupils and internal rotation of the right eye; and gross brain swelling predo-

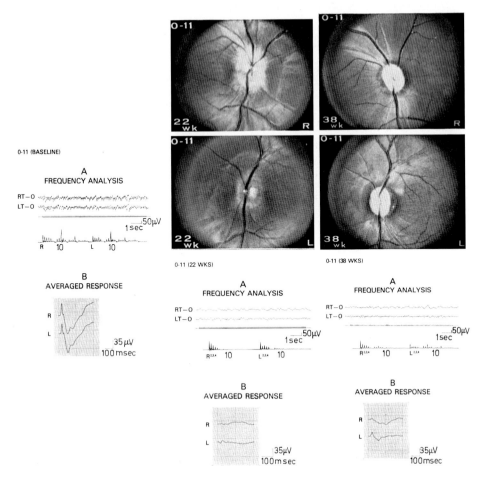

Fig. 4. Monkey No. 0–11, under continuing observation, has shown papilledema and bilateral depression of the visual evoked response at the peak of the elevation (22 mmHg) in CSF pressure, at 22 weeks, followed by appreciable recovery in all parameters by 38 weeks

with the fluid migrating primarily in the extracellular spaces of the white matter, until there is a volumetric increase in the ipsilateral and to some degree the contralateral hemisphere. This mechanism has been described as "Vasogenic Edema" by IGOR KLATZO, [3]. The swelling is compounded by distortion of the ventricular system, with embarrassment of the CSF circulation. The papilledema is secondary to the increase in intracranial pressure. Cranial nerve compression is responsible for the pupillary and oculomotor changes. The unilateral depression in the visual evoked response is related to the destructive lesion, attributable to the x-irradiation, in the right visual cortex. The bilateral obliteration of the evoked response and behavioral blindness is the result of the papilledema and/or the effects of swelling on the visual system within the cranium.

Summary

In six out of twelve Macaca mulatta, 18–22 weeks following 3,500 rads of x-irradiation to the right visual cortex, there is an increase in spinal CSF pressure that may be 2 to 4 times the baseline recording. This is accompanied by bilateral papilledema and obliteration of the visual evoked response. At sacrifice there is gross brain swelling. The mechanism is thought to be a delayed breakdown in the blood-brain barrier with loss of fluid into the brain parenchyma. From the site of exposure, the fluid migrates throughout the ipsilateral and to some extent the contralateral hemisphere. 4 control preparations showed none of the preceding.

Key Words: Delayed brain swelling, X-irradiation, spinal CSF pressure.

References

1. Caveness, W. F., Carsten, A. L., Roizin, L., Schade, J. P.: Pathogenesis of x-irradiation effects in the monkey cerebral cortex. Brain Res. **7**, 1–120 (1968).
2. Hess, K. H., Kato, M.: Comparison of techniques for analyzing visual evoked responses. Electroenceph. clin. Neurophysiol. (In press.)
3. Klatzo, I.: Neuropathological aspects of brain edema. J. Neuropath. exper. Neurol., **26**, 1–14 (1967).

Comments to Session 4

A. K. Ommaya and J. Hekmatpanah

This session consisted of reports on 3 types of experimental models for brain injury. The first 3 papers were concerned with the changes in ICP produced by *experimental infarctions* as recorded by extradural techniques. The fourth paper reported correlations between ICP and tissue water content after *cold lesions* in the cortex, and the final paper dealt with the ICP changes after *x-irradiation* as an index of delayed brain swelling produced by radio-necrosis.

In the first group, the paper entitled "Intracranial Pressure Changes during Experimental Cerebral Infarction" was given by WALTZ. Using the transorbital approach the MCA was occluded in cats and the extent of subsequent infarction correlated with ICP changes measured extradurally. Two groups developed, one in which the infarcts were minimal (good collateral flow), the second with large infarcts. ICP changes were marked in the second group with significant *gradients* of ICP between the infarcted and non-infarcted hemispheres.

The second report, by DORSCH and SYMON, concentrated particularly on the development of ICP gradients between a supratentorial extradural transducer of a new simplified construction and the CSF pressure in the cisterna magna. MCA occlusion in 6 out of 8 animals (baboons) resulted in elevated EDP (24–44 mmHg) within 90–180 min. In *half* of these 6, there was an ICP *gradient* of up to 15 mmHg between the EDP and cisternal CSFP. A good correlation was observed between progressive ICP rise after infarction, hemispheric weight gain (due to edema?) acute reduction of CBF in the MCA ischemic zone paralleling the reduction of perfusion pressure and its improvement after hyperventilation increased the perfusion pressure.

The third report in this group of papers was by HALSEY and CAPRA, on EDP and O_2 availability after MCA occlusion in cats. A good correlation was found between rise in EDP and delay in recovery of O_2 availability markedly reduced after the experimental infarction in the affected brain area. This was particularly true of the period after the ninth hour post-infarction when EDP rose progressively as O_2 availability declined.

Extensive discussion on the validity and value of EDP recording techniques followed these reports and the consensus was that intracranial pressure gradients would develop between zones of expanding lesions (such as an infarcted area) and more normal parts of the brain but that such gradients would dissipate as soon as the lesion stopped growing. However, there were some participants who expressed the opinion that even in such a case ICP gradients should persist. The chairman and other members of the symposium felt this was physically impossible. The need for further data on this point was recognized, particularly with simultaneous recording of subdural or brain tissue pressures before, during and after development of experimental brain lesions.

The fourth paper in the session dealt with a different experimental model, i. e. an area of brain edema produced by freezing a zone of cerebral cortex. Good correlation was found between the extent of edema developed in the white matter and the rise in ICP recorded from the ventricular CSF.

The final paper, by Caveness, reported on the chronic measurement of CSF pressure via a lumbar-cisternal catheter as an index of delayed brain swelling produced by a single dose of x-irradiation (3500 rad, 250 KV). The technique was successful in about 50% of animals and good correlation was found between rise of ICP and the delayed onset of radio-necrosis brain swelling in some of the animals.

Session 5

Brain Compresssion
(Experimental)

The Munro-Kellie Doctrine and the Intracranial Venous Space at the 'Limit' of Raised Intracranial Pressure – an Hydrodynamic Experimental Approach[1]

R. Tym, S. Lichtenstein, and J. Leutheusser

Introduction

Within the frame work of the Munro-Kellie doctrine this paper asks a teleological question: Why does the intracranial pressure (ICP) (defined as measured in any nonvascular space) rise in the presence of a growing space occupying lesion (SOL)?

The author's concept of the Munro-Kellie doctrine is as follows:

The spino-cranial anatomical compartment is rigid and cannot expand: the physiological spaces within it, viz: 1. extradural spinal venous space, 2. intracranial venous space (ICVenS) (being the venous return of the cerebral blood flow (CBF), 3. arterial space, 4. intra- and 5. extracellular fluid spaces, and 6. CSF space, are all changeable but incompressible: an increase or decrease in size of one or more spaces must be compensated for by equal and opposite changes in the sizes of other spaces.

An inexorably growing SOL demands that *compensating mechanisms* be brought into play until, for any instantaneous level of systemic blood pressure (BP) a *'limit'* is asymptotically approached, at which stage the SOL virtually ceases to grow and the ICP virtually ceases to rise – the *'limit'* represents a maximum. The pressure source for the growth of the SOL is directly related to and less than the same BP that sustains the CBF. If the BP rises further after a *'limit'* has been approached then the ICP rises further, the SOL increases in size and a higher *'limit'* is approached. If the BP falls the ICP falls and the SOL may or may not shrink. (It is important to note that the SOL may be *extrinsic* – tumour or blood clot, *intrinsic* – an increase above usual of one or more physiological spaces, e.g. hydrocephalus or cerebral edema, or any combination of these).

Two riders to this doctrine which concern the behaviour of the intracranial venous space (ICVenS) are propounded by the present authors, viz:

1. That the main teleological "purpose" of the rise in ICP is to impart kinetic energy to the blood flowing in the ICVenS. This space can then shrink in

1 Work made possible by National Research Council of Canada Grant No. A-1541 to Professor Hans J. Leutheusser.

size – and play its role as a "front line" compensating mechanism – but at the same time carry its venous blood at a greater velocity and hence have a minimal effect in decreasing CBF.

2. That no matter what the rise in ICP due to a SOL, though CBF may be reduced it cannot be reduced to zero.

By the definition of the Munro-Kellie doctrine given above the *in-vivo* state is never stable but always approaching asymptotically *a limit*. To study the ICVenS at the limit requires an *in vitro* fluid – mechanical simulation.

Materials and Methods

The apparatus is shown schematically in Fig. 1 to which the following description and results refer.

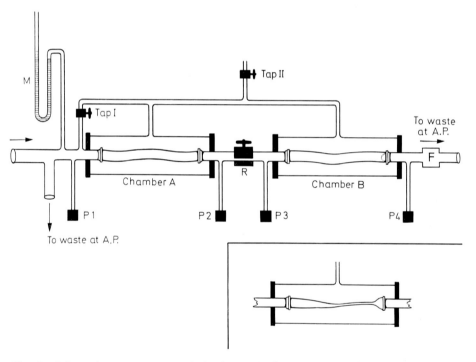

Fig. 1. Schematic representation of simulation fluid mechanics model. F = flowmeter; R = resistance to flow; P 1–4 = pressure transducers; M = Mercury manometer; A.P. = Atmospheric pressure: Inset shows shape of collapsable teflon tube in chamber B at high pressure (SOL) steady state

Water was pumped from a constant volume pump (not shown). The majority of water from the pump escaped to waste, the minority passed through the main pipe from left to right. The main pipe passed through two rigid chambers which, being interconnected remained at equal pressures. As the main pipe passed through each chamber the rigid walls of the main pipe were replaced by flimsy, collapsable teflon tubing. That portion of collapsable tubing in chamber A simulated the arterial space and that in B the ICVenS. The two interconnected chambers simulated the rigid spinocranial anatomical compartment and the pressure within it, the ICP.

A resistance to flow was placed at R.

The opening of tap I with tap II closed enabled water to flow into the chambers – an inflow which simulated an inexorably growing SOL. Its accommodation by a decrease in the calibre of the collapsable tube in chamber B simulated the only compensating mechanism available to this model, i.e. a decrease in the ICVenS. The small calibre and the site of the departure point of the pipe carrying water through tap I ensured that the pressure in it, and hence the pressure in the chambers supplied by it, was always directly related to, but less than the pressure at the site of its departure (i.e. the simulated ICP was related to and less than the BP).

Results

A. Initial Steady State

With tap I closed and tap II open the apparatus was filled with water. Adjustments to the constant volume pump and the resistance to flow at R were made. Tap II was then closed. The following readings were obtained.

1. Flow rate at $F = 56$ (arbitary units on a linear scale)
2. Pressure at $P1 = 130$ $P2 = 130$ $P3 = 78$ $P4 = 78$ (arbitary units on a linear scale). i.e. the pressure drop was across R.
3. Manometer reading $+ 1$ cmHg
4. The appearance of the teflon tubes was as shown in Fig. 1.

B. Pressure Increase

Tap I was opened. Water flowed into chamber B and the shape and calibre of the teflon tube within it changed (see inset Fig. 1 and Fig. 2). The following readings were taken when a steady state was reached.

1. Flow rate at $F = 12$
2. Pressure at $PT_1 = 390$ $PT_2 = 316$ $PT_3 = 316$ $PT_4 = 64$ (i.e. pressure drop across each teflon tube, none across R).
3. Manometer reading $+ 50$ cmHg.

C. Return to Initial Steady State

Tap I was closed and tap II was opened. Fluid (the SOL) escaped and the readings of the initial steady state [(A), above] were re-obtained.

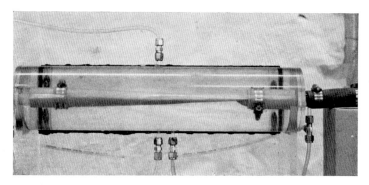

Fig. 2. Photograph through perspex wall of chamber B at high pressure (SOL) steady state

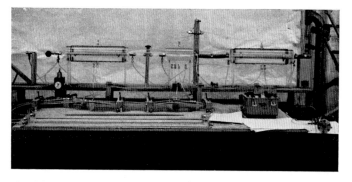

Fig. 3. Photograph of general lay-out of simulation fluid mechanics model

Discussion

If fluid is to flow along a pipe then there must be a down gradient of pressure in the direction of flow. If the pipe is of the consistency of a collapsable vein wall – or, in this present context, the consistency of a collapsable teflon tube – and the pressure of the fluid surrounding the tubing everywhere the same, then the transmural pressure gradient must be equal everywhere. This means that there can be no pressure gradient within the tube. This appears to be a paradox.

No statisfactory explanation for this paradox has appeared so far, and fluid-mechanical data are accumulating: further experiments and changes in design are continuing. For the time being, however, there is some justification for putting constraints on the use of the word "pressure" when it is applied to fluid flowing in collapsable tubes.

Summary

A teleological answer is no more than a phenomenon. The model and the simple experiment described have demonstrated a phenomenon *in vitro* which might occur *in vivo*. The potential energy of high ICP appears to be countered by the kinetic energy of high velocity in the veins at the CSF/ICVenS interface. Despite the absence of any explanation, the authors feel that for the time being it is both useful and justifiable to include their two riders in the hypothesis that is the Munro-Kellie doctrine.

A Critical Rate of Cerebral Compression

S. NAKATANI and A. K. OMMAYA

Introduction

A rapid increase in intracranial mass provokes a Cushing Reflex as an emergency reaction to maintain adequate perfusion of cerebral tissues. Slower expansion of mass induces a less dramatic reaction. Although these observations are very common in neurosurgical practice, it is surprising to find a lack of previous systematic studies on an extremely important variable implicated in these phenomena, i.e., the rate or speed of brain compression by the extra mass in the head.

Because intracranial tissues are incompressible like water; brain compression means brain distortion. We believe that such changes in brain shape, rather than changes in intracranial pressure per se, and the speed of such changes in shape are what determines the gravity of effects on cerebral functions. This report concerns the acute effects of brain distortion by an intracranial mass at controlled rates. We were particularly interested in determining the critical rate at which compensatory functions supporting the brain were most likely to be threatened. A second aim was to assess the significance of the changes in intracranial pressure (ICP) as indices of the severity of such effects.

Methods

Experiments were carried out in 50 Rhesus monkeys under pentobarbital-sodium and flaxedil anesthesia with controlled respiration. A latex rubber balloon was placed epidurally over the cerebral convexity in the central parasaggital area. This balloon was inflated with water continuously by an infusion pump at one of the following rates: 0.5, 0.2, 0.1, 0.05, 0.02, 0.01, and 0.005 ml/min. Inflation was terminated and the balloon was deflated when the continuously monitored EEG became flat and pupils dilated. This was regarded as the end point for decompensation of brain functions protecting cerebral perfusion. Intracranial pressures were recorded from 3 sites: supratentorial subdural space (STP), supratentorial saggital sinus wedge (SSWP) and infratentorial cisterna magna (ITP). For STP minitoring the ventricular end of a V–A shunt tube was gently placed in the subdural space. Systemic arterial pressure (SAP) was recorded from the abdominal aorta via a catheter introduced through the femoral artery. Periodic samples of arterial blood were taken from the same source for estimation of pH, pCO_2 and pO_2. EEG was recorded with needle electrodes placed in the frontal skull and from bilateral ear electrodes. EKG was recorded from standard limbs leads.

Results

Figures 1 and 2 show typical pressure responses to the epidural balloon inflation at faster and slower rates. The critical rate of cerebral compression at

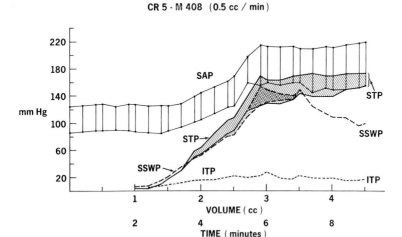

Fig. 1. The effect of rapid inflation of the epidural balloon at a constant rate of 0.5 ml/min under controlled respiration. Great increase in STP is seen concomitant with rise in SAP. End-point was reached in 24 min with 4.8 cc of balloon volume

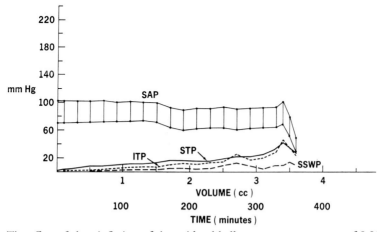

Fig. 2. The effect of slow inflation of the epidural balloon at a constant rate of 0.01 ml/min under controlled respiration. No rapid or significant rise in STP with no rise in SAP. End-point was reached in 360 min with 3.6 cc of balloon volume

and below which the Cushing reflex was not provoked was 0.02 ml/min for expansion of an extradural mass in rhesus monkeys. Balloon inflation at faster rates (0.5, 0.2, 0.1 and 0.05 ml/min) induced an initial vasodepressor response followed by a vasopressor response in which STP and SSWP rose to diastolic SAP levels. ITP rose concomitantly until dissociation from supratentorial pressure resulted in ITP decrease. End points were reached with 4–6.5 ml of balloon volume. Slower rates (0.01 and 0.005 ml/min) of cerebral compression by the balloon did not result in this vasopressor response nor was there a dissociation between STP and ITP. STP, SSWP and ITP rose together to only 20–50 mmHg and then decreased with decreasing SAP. End points were reached with 3.5–4.5 cc of balloon volume. Figure 3 shows typical balloon volume-STP relationships at varying rates of balloon inflations.

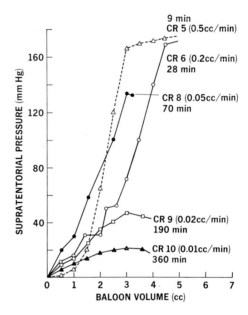

Fig. 3. Volume-Pressure (STP) relationships in epidural balloon inflations at varying rates under controlled respiration. Clear dissociation of ICP ist noted between faster and slower inflation. The critical rate was 0.02 ml/min

Discussion

Rates of balloon expansion not exceeding 0.02 ml/min cause flattening of EEG and dilated pupils without significant rise in ICP. More rapid inflations induced marked Cushing reflex associated with great increases in ICP before a similar end point. Our volume-pressure relationship curves (Fig. 3) show clear dissociation of ICP dependent on rates of inflation. This indicates that the Cushing reflex of increased SAP is a determinating factor for rapid rise in ICP in later phases of extraneous mass expansion. Raised ICP associated with increased SAP is thus seen as a defense mechanism of the brain against rapid expansion of mass; it is not per se a critical factor in brain dysfunction under such conditions. In our opinion the essential factor is not the absolute height of ICP, but the volume of extra mass and the speed of brain distortion, i. e., the rate of growth of such mass[1].

It is therefore misleading to claim that slow inflations of an extradural balloon will result in progressively greater increases of ICP when the added volume exceeds displacable intracranial volume [2, 3]. Blood, CSF and even brain tissue can be reversibly lost from the intracranial volume. What matters is the ability of residual volumes to support cerebral functions and their defense by the dynamic responses evoked at rates of mass growth exceeding 0.02 ml/min[2]. In order to determine the significance of clinical measurements of ICP, therefore, we would suggest the urgent necessity for data on *relative volumes* of the three intracranial compartments during alterations induced intrinsically or extrinsically. Observations in man are practically non-existent[3].

Summary

1. A critical rate of cerebral compression at and below which the Cushing reflex is not provoked is 0.02 ml/min for expansion of an extradural mass in the rhesus monkey. 2. Rapid expansion of mass provoked a Cushing reflex associated with rapid rise in ICP whereas slower expansions did not induce the

---

1 The threshold for detection of volume growth rates and absolute amounts of extra volume tolerated will vary at different sites in the brain and positions of the head [1]. End volumes of the balloon at which EEG became flat and pupils dilated (4–6 cc) were larger in more rapid inflations than at slower inflation. Whether the 10–15 sec delay in EEG activity reflecting cerebral metabolic arrest allowed the greater expansions at higher rates or whether the compensatory rise in ICP allows the experimental animal to live longer is not clear from these experiments.

2 CSF volume can be displaced at any rate without threat to brain functions. Loss of a critical blood volume would of course be irreversible. However, even cerebral dysfunction due to significant decrease in blood and brain tissue volumes is reversible if the rate of blood and brain tissue loss has been very slow as is found in "normal pressure" hydrocephalus [4]. Growth of a mass extrinsic to the brain as studied in this experiment will behave mechanically in the same manner as growth of any of the intrinsic compartments of the intracranial volume, e. g., of the CSF in hydrocephalus, except for the local effects of distortion produced by the mass [5].

3 It is interesting to extrapolate these data obtained in rhesus monkeys to humans. Intracranial volume of the rhesus monkey is about 100 cc, of which 80 cc is brain tissue, 10 cc is blood volume and 10 cc is CSF. End volume of the extradural balloon was 4–6 cc, i. e., about 5 % of intracranial volume. In man intracranial volume is about 1400 cc, of which approximately 1120 cc is brain tissue volume, 140 cc is blood volume and 140 cc is CSF. An equivalent end volume for extrapolated extradural mass in man is 70 cc. If the same data on critical speed were applicable, then 0.3 cc/min of extradural mass expansion is the rate at and below which the Cushing reflex will not be induced in man. It should be emphasized that at slower rates even greater volumes could be tolerated without irreversible failure of brain functions.

Cushing response and the mass grew without great increase in ICP. 3. Critical volume terminating brain function (flat EEG and dilated pupils) was 4–6 cc of extradural mass in a central supratentorial location. 4. We believe that the location and speed of changes in brain tissue volume and shape rather than changes in ICP are more fundamental determinants of the gravity of brain dysfunction in the presence of space occupying lesions.

Key Words: Brain compression, Cushing reflex, intracranial pressure, tolerance, critical rate.

References

1. Hoff, J. T., Reis, D. J.: Localization of regions mediating the Cushing Response in CNS of cat. Arch. Neurol. **23**, 228–240 (1970).
2. Langfitt, T. W., Kassel, N. F., Weinstein, J. D.: Cerebral vasomotor paralysis produced by intracranial hypertension. Neurol. **15**, 622–641 (1965).
3. Langfitt, T. W., Weinstein, J. D., Kassel, N. F.: Vascular factors in head injury. In: Caveness, W. F., Walker, A. E. (Eds.): Head Injury, pp. 172–194 (1968).
4. Salmon, J. H., Armitage, J. L.: Surgical treatment of hydrocephalus ex-vacuo. Ventriculo-atrial shunt for degenerative brain disease. Neurol. **18**, 1223–1226 (1969).
5. Ommaya, A. K., Metz, H., Post, K.: Observations on the mechanics of hydrocephalus. In: Harbert, J., Thomas, C. (Eds.): Isotope Cisternography and Hydrocephalus. (1972).

Irreversible Damage and Cerebral Death in Increased Intracranial Pressure

J. Hekmatpanah

Introduction

The high morbidity and mortality that exist following marked increased intracranial pressure have long been a matter of great concern and a subject for numerous investigations. Mortality is particularly high when both pupils become dilated, in spite of prompt decompression with reduction of pressure to a normal range.

In an attempt to study further the causes or factors which influence this mortality and morbidity, cerebral compression was done in animals by gradual inflation of an extradural balloon. 40 cats and 10 monkeys were studied. Intracranial pressure, vital signs and electroencephalogram (EEG) were monitored. Cerebral blood flow was observed through a cranial window under magnifications of 25–100 times and measured in 5 monkeys with Xenon injected into the internal carotid artery. Some of the earlier results have been previously published [1, 2].

Material and Methods

The experiments were done under general anesthesia with Dibutal or Nembutal (20–25 mg/kg). All animals had a tracheostomy or tracheal intubation. The intracranial pressure was measured from the epidural region next to the burr hole for the cranial window and on the opposite side from the inflating epidural balloon. Further details of the technique can be found in previous papers [1, 2].

Results

The alteration of vital signs occurred in a rather sequential manner as the intracranial pressure was raised. The ipsilateral EEG altered first, followed by slowness of respiration, and then pulse. Later, the ipsilateral pupil began to dilate. The blood pressure rose in the terminal stage almost concurrent with, or even after, both pupils were dilated.

When the balloon was inflated approximately every 5 min with increments of 0.2 ml of saline for cats and 0.5 ml for monkeys, usually a total of 3 and 5 ml, respectively, was sufficient to cause bilateral dilation of pupils, apnea, and death within $1^1/_2$ to 3 h.

In 25 cats, cerebral perfusion with dyes gradually decreased as the intracranial pressure rose, with practically no capillary perfusion when both pupils were dilated (Fig. 1).

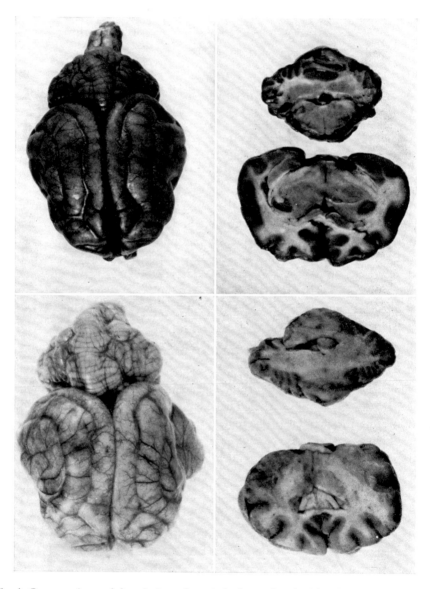

Fig. 1. Cross section and dorsal view of a cat's brain, perfused with india ink when cerebral compression began to give bilaterally dilated pupils (upper photographs), compared with a normal brain perfused under similar conditions. Note the lack of capillary perfusion in the upper photographs

Observation through the microscope revealed that the cerebral cortical blood flow decreased as the intracranial pressure increased, and the flow stopped almost completely when both pupils were dilated. This process occurred gradually, from smaller to the larger vessels, and in veins prior to arteries. Essentially, and contrary to common belief, the veins rather than the arteries dilated. As blood flow slowed, the red cells sludged and formed microemboli. These microemboli from inside, and compressing adjacent tissue from outside, gradually occluded the vessels. The flow was reduced or stopped in some vessels long before the others.

In earlier experiments, the respiration was not supported when apnea occurred, to study the animals at different stages or rising pressure [2]. The respiration, however, was supported in 10 monkeys in order to study the effect of resuscitation with urea [3] and decompression. With these measures the animals did not die immediately, as they usually did when both pupils were dilated, EEG was flat, and apnea remained for several minutes. But they all died within 24–36 h. Following administration of urea, the blood flow returned in a certain proportion of vessels if the drug was given before complete cessation of the flow. Deflation of the balloons further improved the blood flow. The detailed description of these resuscitation measures is avoided here because of limitations of space and will be the subject of later communications [3]. But, in regards to return of the blood flow following resuscitation, 3 observations are of great interest to this paper: a) while blood flow returned in many vessels, reflow did not occur in all, and some remained obstructed; b) the reflow of the blood was associated with forward movement of sludged red cells and microemboli which had casted the vessels. Many of these vessels were occluded for periods between 30–60 min (Fig. 2). c) Cerebral blood flow gradually slowed and stopped again in some vessels, especially when there was associated hypotension, in spite of low intracranial pressure.

The cerebral blood flow studies with Xenon could well be correlated with the cortical blood flow seen under the microscope. The washout curve was practically flat when the vessels were occluded.

The light microscopic studies of tissue in 10 monkeys reveals laminar cortical necrosis, shrunken nerve cells and increased perivascular space throughout the cerebrum, with a lesser degree in the cerebellum. The alterations were more severe when the animal was kept longer on the respirator. Electron microscopic studies revealed large astrocytic processes in the pericapillary region; torn cytoplasmic membrane with scattered cellular organelles; and swollen, disorganized, mitochondria with distorted cristae (Fig. 3).

Discussion

The high mortality of marked cerebral compression with bilaterally dilated pupils in man is also observed in experimental animals when cerebral compression is produced by an expanding epidural balloon. At the late stage, death occurs in man irrespective of the pathological nature of the lesions causing cerebral compression. This is thought to be due to tentorial herniation [4, 5], secondary brain stem hemorrhage [5], and/or marked cerebral swelling [6].

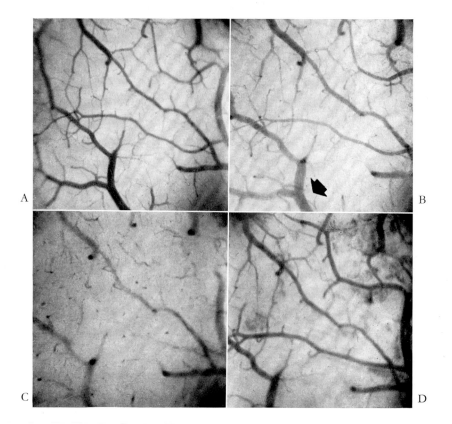

Fig. 2. Small cerebral blood vessels, magnified 60 times. Please note: normal vessels before cerebral compression in the monkey (A), early increase in intracranial pressure when EEG and respiration altered (B), complete obstruction of capillaries and larger vessels when the second pupil began to dilate (C), and the return of flow in some vessels about one hour after the administration of urea. Note dilatation of the vein (arrow)

However, the frequently found uncus or cerebellar tonsil herniation on contrast studies and at operation in conscious patients, the often found lack of secondary brain stem hemorrhage and even marked cellular swelling in animals (and sometimes in man) might indicate that these alterations could be (at times) the associated rather than the causal factor for disability and death. Observation of cortical vessels under magnification shows beyond any reasonable doubt that cerebral blood flow decreases and finally stops in advancing cerebral compression. One would carry skepticism too far in thinking that this phenomenon would differ in man.

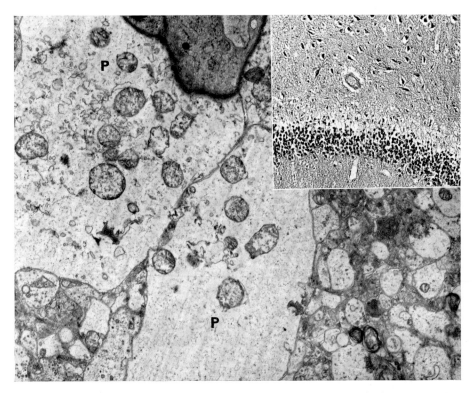

Fig. 3. Electron micrograph of the cerebral cortex in the monkey 48 h after resuscitation (urea and deflation of the balloon). The respiration was artificially supported. Note swollen pericapillary astrocytic processes (P). Note torn mitochondrial membrane and distorted cristae. The inlet shows light microscopic study of hippocampus gyrus. Note shrunken, anoxic nerve cells with widened pericapillary space

The question might arise that the observations through a burr hole would only show a small surface of cortex, not representing the entire cerebrum. However: a) in earlier experiments, several burr holes on different locations showed the same vascular alterations; b) in cerebral perfusion, different dyes showed essentially similar vascular fillings throughout the brain, except for somewhat more uptake in the content of the posterior fossa; c) the flow studies with Xenon correlated well with the direct observation; and finally, d) the burr hole for the observation of vessels was made on the opposite side of the compressing balloon. Therefore, it is concluded that the observed alterations were samples of what went on in the entire cerebrum, except for the very early stages of rising pressure.

The gradual slowing of blood flow; the progressive one by one occlusion of vessels; the absence of reflow in some vessels; and the return of flow in others (after periods of ischemia far beyond the ischemic tolerance of the nerve cells) might clarify the diffuse cerebral damage and its effect on morbidity and mortality at different stages of increased intracranial pressure. On the basis of these experiments, the author believes that bilaterally dilated pupils in the presence of, and as a result of, generalized increased intracranial pressure is analogous to infarction of the entire cerebrum.

Summary

Increased intracranial pressure and cerebral compression is studied in cats and monkeys. Cerebral death, high mortality, and morbidity are thought to be due to: a) vascular occlusions and total brain infarct during rising intracranial pressure, and b) no reflow in some vessels or a prolonged ischemic period in the others after resuscitation.

Key Words : Cerebral death, cerebral compression, capillary obstruction, no reflow.

References

1. Hekmatpanah, J.: Sequence of alterations in vital signs during acute experimental increased intracranial pressure. J. Neurosurg. **32**, 16–20 (1970).
2. Hekmatpanah, J.: Cerebral circulation and perfusion in experimental increased intracranial pressure. J. Neurosurg. **32**, 21–29 (1970).
3. Hekmatpanah, J.: The effect of urea on cerebral blood flow in the monkey following cerebral compression (in preparation).
4. Jefferson, G.: The tentorial pressure cone. Arch. Neurol. Psychiat. (Chic.) **40**, 857 (1938).
5. Scheinker, I. M.: Transtentorial herniation of the brain stem. Arch. Neurol. Psychiat. (Chic.) **53**, 289 (1945).
6. Scheinker, I. M.: Cerebral swelling and edema associated with cerebral tumor. Arch. Neurol. Psychiat. (Chic.) **45**, 117 (1941).

Kinetics of Arterial and Venous Hemorrhage in the Skull Cavity[1]

J. Löfgren and N. N. Zwetnow

Introduction

In a previous communication from our laboratory [1] we reported on an experimental study on the course of arterial hemorrhage in various compartments of the intracranial cavity. It was demonstrated that bleeding from an intracranial artery is usually an extraordinarily shortlived event compared with arterial bleeding in other regions of the body. Moreover such bleeding seems fundamentally to be an eminently survivable condition even when bleeding occurs from major arteries such as the middle cerebral artery.

The aim of the present study was to define the mechanical characteristics of intracranial arterial and venous bleeding in canine experiments. The basic mechanics involved were evaluated in experiments on a physical analogue.

Material and Methods

Experimental data were obtained in 52 dogs weighing 8–20 kg, anesthetized with sodium pentobarbital (25 mg per kg). The animals were intubated, some of them breathing spontaneously, and some ventilated with a respirator pump. In some experiments the animals were heparinized. The hemorrhage was produced by transsection, under direct vision, of the middle cerebral artery or one of its branches, the longitudinal sinus and/or the straight sinus. A brass cylinder was screwed into a burr hole, the dura was opened and the transsection made. The cylinder was then plugged with a rubber stopper with a central cannula through which the bleeding could proceed freely. By switching a 3-way stopcock the cannula was connected to a pressure transducer and the intracranial cavity thus closed. In some experiments bleeding was routed through an extracorporeal shunt from the external carotid artery into the cisterna magna or into the supratentorial subdural space where an electronic drop recorder measured rate and volume of bleeding. Pressures were recorded in the femoral artery, the inferior vena cava, the superior longitudinal sinus, the lateral ventricle, the cisterna magna and in the developing hematoma with Statham P23 transducers and they were displayed on a Grass Model 7 Polygraph. The reference level was the

1 This study has been supported by grants B 72-17X-3500-01 and B-73-17X-3500-02, which herewith is gratefully acknowledged.

mid-spine in the lateral position. Increased outflow of cerebrospinal fluid (CSF) during bleeding was demonstrated by the recording of an increased clearance of radioactive iodinated serum albumin injected into the cisterna magna.

The *physical model* consisted of a series of Latex rubber tubes in a fluid-filled plexiglass container, perfused with fluid from an external pressure reservoir. The tube system was divided into high pressure and low pressure sections by flow resistance. Leakage simulating arterial and venous bleeding was initiated and the various pressures and rate of bleeding measured.

Results

Model Experiments. When a vessel in this system was allowed to "bleed" into the extravascular space of the container the various pressures and rate of bleeding followed courses schematically described in Figure 1. The pressure in the bleeding vessel fell rapidly due to the sudden loss of flow resistance and was in proportion to this loss. The intravascular and extravascular pressures then rose simultaneously towards the external driving pressure of the system representing the systemic arterial pressure. This rise was steep at first and then levelled out exponentially, approaching the driving pressure as an asymptote. The rate of bleeding was an inverse function of the extravascular pressure. These changes were essentially the same but with different time characteristics in bleeding from both the high-pressure and the low-pressure parts of the system. These events are readily explained in simple physical terms. The bleeding pressure is appropriately defined as the difference between the driving pressure-head and the extravascular pressure of the container. The rate of bleeding is proportional to this exponentially-decreasing gradient and inversely propor-

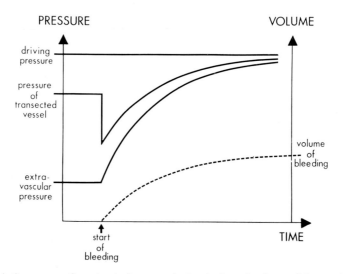

Fig. 1. Summary of mechanical events during leakage in the model experiments

tional to the series of resistances from the pressure reservoir to the extravascular space of the container. One may note that the bleeding pressure is equivalent to the perfusion pressure in this hydraulic system.

Canine Experiments. Transsection of small arterial and venous vessels resulted in insignificant bleeding and change in the intracranial pressure, presumably due to high resistance to bleeding and rapid blood coagulation. In bleeding from the middle cerebral artery ICP increased steeply to 50–100 mmHg within 15–30 sec (Fig. 2). Thereafter ICP attained a plateau, and remained at this level for about two minutes before it started to decrease exponentially and was reduced to half in about 10 min. In 2 out of 16 experiments this fall in pressure did not occur but instead the pressure continued to rise, soon reaching the level of the arterial pressure. In these cases a marked arterial pressure response occurred and respiratory arrest ensued. All other dogs survived for the experimental period of approximately 5 h. Heparinization, however, resulted in 100% mortality, usually within 10–20 min, ICP continuously increasing exponentially towards the arterial pressure.

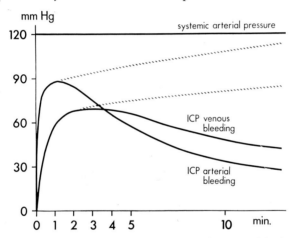

Fig. 2. Schematic outline of ICP changes in arterial and venous bleeding. Dotted lines show the courses in heparinized dogs

In venous hemorrhage from large venous sinuses ICP changed in various ways. It increased fairly rapidly within $^1/_2$–1 min to 30–90 mmHg. In some experiments there was practically no change at all in the pressure. A plateau was reached and maintained for 4–8 min before the pressure fell again but more slowly than in arterial bleeding. After 2 h mean ICP in venous hemorrhage was 34 mmHg (range 15–60) whereas the corresponding value in arterial hemorrhage was 18 mmHg (range 12–25). The high ICP after the bleeding episode in venous hemorrhage also showed marked instability with repeated spontaneous pressure waves sometimes attaining levels of about 100 mmHg. In heparinized venous bleeding ICP rose steadily, ultimately approaching the arterial pressure and resulting in the death of the animals in about 4 h.

Discussion

Hemorrhage from major vessels in other parts of the body results in continuing loss of blood and the eventual cessation of bleeding is usually dependent upon a fall in blood pressure permitting the development of a firm clot. Severe bleeding from a leak in the cerebral vascular bed, in contrast, is rapidly controlled by the buildup of a counterpressure which transforms the initially furious bleeding in less than 30 sec to a slow ooze more reminiscent of capillary than large vessel hemorrhage from a mechanical point of view. A clot will evidently form under these conditions, effectively arresting the hemorrhage within a few minutes. There were some suggestions of more rapid clotting in arterial than in venous bleeding.

The basic hydrodynamics seem essentially the same in both arterial and venous hemorrhage. If blood coagulation is prevented ICP will increase ultimately to the level of the arterial pressure irrespective of the type of vessel bleeding. It might have been expected that significant venous leakage would be impossible in the skull cavity because of rapid elimination of the small transmural pressure gradient in this case. The mechanical reason seems to be that the rising ICP compresses the distal part of the intracranial venous system causing a concomitant increase in the lateral pressure in the vascular bed proximal to the obstruction. The gradient of pressure between the bleeding vessel and the extravascular (CSF) pressure is thus maintained but is successively reduced as the pressures rise higher and higher, approaching the arterial pressure asymptotically, a course usually interrupted by the development of a clot. In cases of both arterial and venous hemorrhage the effective "bleeding pressure" is therefore the pressure differential between the systemic arteries and CSF. The rate of bleeding is determined by the ratio of this pressure differential and the resistance to the movement of blood through the various sections of the vascular bed leading up to and including the leak. This resistance is generally higher in venous bleeding due to the interposed capillary bed.

It was not possible to evaluate the influence of vasoconstriction in these experiments. Its effect should be a delay of bleeding due to the increased resistance. A comparison of heparinized and non-heparinized bleeding shows that the arrest of bleeding is, however, related to the intracranial counterpressure and the formation of a clot. On the other hand, a vasodilatory response to the increased ICP might contribute to the pressure changes, possibly in venous hemorrhage in particular, due to interference with the drainage conditions in this case.

The sequential course of events is modified continuously by a diminishing CSF volume due to the mechanism of "CSF overflow" [2]. ICP is therefore lower than it otherwise would have been throughout the course. To some extent this outflow may have the effect of delaying hemostasis and permitting a larger accumulation of blood intracranially.

The ICP level attained during bleeding is probably determined primarily by the resistance to bleeding and the efficiency of the CSF outflow mechanism. The subsequent exponential fall of pressure was more rapid in arterial bleeding and the pressure fell to lower levels than in venous bleeding. This might to some extent be explained by varying effects on the CSF outflow system.

Summary

The unique "closed space" dynamics of hemorrhage in the skull cavity were studied experimentally in dogs and in a physical model. In severe uncontrolled hemorrhage of both arterial and venous origin ICP increased exponentially, approaching the arterial pressure as an asymptote. Usually, however, the counterpressure acts as a tamponade, permitting formation of an effective clot within minutes. Simultaneous outflow of cerebrospinal fluid modifies the pressure course and results in an exponential fall in pressure after clot formation.

Key Words: Intracranial venous hemorrhage, intracranial arterial hemorrhage, bleeding pressure, volume of bleeding, physical model, intracranial pressure.

References

1. Löfgren, J., Zwetnow, N. N.: Experimental studies on the dynamic course of intracranial arterial bleeding. Acta neurol. scand. 48, 252 (1972).
2. Löfgren, J., Zwetnow, N. N. (in manuscript).

Regional Cerebral Blood Flow in Increased Intracranial Pressure Produced by Increased Cerebrospinal Fluid Volume, Intracranial Mass and Cerebral Edema[1]

H. P. LEWIS and R. L. McLAURIN

Introduction

At least 3 different mechanisms may elevate intracranial pressure (ICP): an increased cerebrospinal fluid (CSF) volume, the addition of an intracranial mass or an increase in cerebral mass. Clinically elevated ICP is hazardous only when it produces herniation or reduces cerebral blood flow (CBF) but the pressures at which these events occur have not been defined. In an effort to define ICP/CBF relationships, experiments have been performed to study CBF with increased ICP produced by increased CSF volume, an expanding mass, and by producing cerebral edema.

Material and Methods

Nineteen rhesus monkeys weighing 4–8 kg were similarly prepared after being tranquilized with phencyclidine (3 mg/kg). ICP was monitored by means of a subminiature electronic pressure transducer implanted within the right frontal lobe [1].

Regional cerebral blood flow (rCBF) was measured by the ^{133}Xe washout technique. A single one-inch sodium iodide crystal detector was placed over the intact scalp of the left fronto-parietal region. The detector was provided with a parallel collimator which allowed it to "see" 30.6 cm^3 with 50% or better efficiency. A bolus of ^{133}Xe was injected through a 22 Ga polyethylene catheter placed in the left internal carotid artery. The 16 min washout curve was subjected to compartmental analysis [2] and adjusted to PaCO$_2$ 40 [3].

Ventilation was controlled by a Bennett MA-1 respirator. Continuous end tidal CO$_2$ monitoring allowed maintenance of PaCO$_2$ 40 by addition of CO$_2$ to inspired air. Systemic arterial pressure, lumbar subarachnoid pressure, blood gases and hemoglobin concentration were determined throughout each experiment.

In 6 macaques baseline CBF determinations were performed prior to infusing sterile saline into the lumbar subarachnoid space. Repeated CBF

1 This work was supported by Grants NS 07253-04 and HD-05221 from the National Institutes of Health.

measurements were performed at 15 mmHg increments of ICP and continued until pupillary dilatation occurred.

In 6 macaques a 10 mm subdural balloon was inflated at 4 ml/h after baseline CBF measurements had been made. Repeated CBF determinations were continued until bilateral pupillary dilatation occurred.

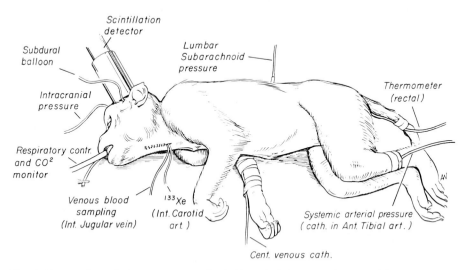

Fig. 1. Preparation of rhesus macaques for balloon inflation experiments. All other animals were prepared in a similar fashion except that the subdural balloon was not introduced

In 5 macaques cerebral edema was produced by intravenous sterile water infusion. After baseline rCBF determinations the infusion proceeded (1 ml/min) until pupillary dilatation occurred. rCBF determinations were performed every 30 min.

The 2 control macaques prepared as above were subjected to rCBF determinations hourly for the average experiment duration of 5 h.

Results

Subarachnoid Infusion. ICP rose as soon as the saline infusion began. No change in compartmental rCBF occurred until ICP had reached 74 mmHg. Precipitous reduction in rCBF accompanied further ICP elevation. Reduction in perfusion pressure (mean SAP minus mean ICP) below 35 mmHg was also accompanied by CBF reduction. Fully dilated pupils were noted when ICP reached 100–110 mmHg.

Invariably perfusion pressure (PP) had been reduced below 35 mmHg when dilated pupils appeared. CBF had been reduced 50% at that time.

Balloon Inflation. Progressive reduction in compartmental rCBF accompanied ICP elevation. No relation between rCBF and PP could be demonstrated.

Unilateral pupillary dilatation occurred in all animals at an ICP of 45–50 mmHg and when CBF was 60% of baseline. Bilateral pupillary dilatation occurred at an ICP of 80 mmHg. CBF was 50% of baseline at this occurrence.

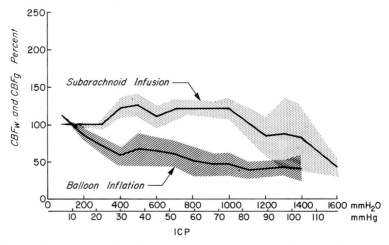

Fig. 2. Statistical representation (mean ± one standard error) demonstrating maintenance of CBF during subarachnoid infusion and the progressive reduction in CBF accompanying balloon inflation

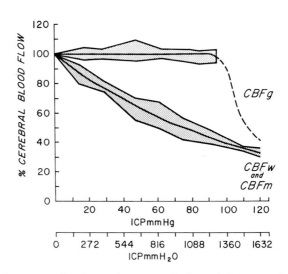

Fig. 3. Statistical representation (mean ± one standard error) demonstrating maintenance of fast compartment CBF and progressive reduction in slow compartment CBF accompanying cerebral edema

Cerebral Edema. Disparate results in rCBF compartments were noted as ICP rose. Maintenance of fast (gray) compartment rCBF at baseline levels in spite of rising ICP was apparent. Progressive reduction in slow compartment rCBF accompanied increasing ICP. Bilateral pupillary dilatation occurred at an ICP of 60–90 mmHg when slow compartment (white) rCBF was 50% of baseline.

Control Group. rCBF during the 5 h observation period averaged 76 ml/ 100 g/min fast compartment, 21 ml/100 g/min slow compartment and a mean rCBF of 40 ml/100 g/min. These measurements agreed with the average baseline values for the experimental groups.

Discussion

Increased ICP due to any of the 3 causes tested produces a reduction in rCBF. That ICP/CBF relationships vary with the cause of increased ICP suggests the involvement of at least another factor. When elevated intracranial pressure results from increased CSF volume an adaptive mechanism maintains CBF at normal levels. This mechanism fatigues when ICP $= 74$ mmHg or when PP is reduced to 35 mmHg.

Cerebral edema produced by intravenous water is basically a white matter disease [4]. The reduction in the slow compartment of CBF seen in edema suggests interference with the adaptive mechanism in the white matter vasculature. A similar failure of the adaptive mechanism is seen in the balloon experiment. It is suggested that distortion of vasculature is the common factor which may explain both phenomena.

Bilateral pupil dilatation occurred when CBF had been reduced 50% in all experiments, while the pressures at which this event occurred varied with the cause of the increased ICP suggesting that CBF rather than ICP was an important factor in pupillary dilatation.

Summary

1. Elevated ICP due to increased CSF volume reduces CBF only when ICP exceeds 74 mmHg or PP falls below 35 mmHg.

2. Mass lesions cause progressive reduction in CBF as ICP rises.

3. Increased ICP secondary to the cerebral edema of intravenous water produces reduction in slow compartment CBF and reduces fast compartment CBF only at very high ICP.

4. The hypothesis is advanced that distortion of vasculature grossly by a mass, or microscopically by edema, causes failure of the adaptive mechanism which maintains CBF as ICP rises.

Key Words : Cerebral blood flow, cerebral edema, intracranial pressure.

References

1. Coe, J., Nelson, W., Rudenberg, F. H., Garzo, R.: Technique for Continuous Intracranial Pressure Recording. J. Neurosurg. **27**, 370–375 (1967).
2. Høedt-Rasmussen, K.: Regional Cerebral Blood Flow, pp. 79. Copenhagen: Munksgaard 1967.
3. Reivich, M.: Arterial pCO_2 and Cerebral Hemodynamics. Amer. J. Physiol. **206**, 25–35 (1964).
4. Herschkowitz, N., MacGilliray, B. B., Cummings, J. N.: Biochemical and Electrophysiological Studies in Experimental Cerebral Edema. Brain **88**, 557–584 (1965).

Perfusion Pressure in Intracranial Hypertension

J. O. Rowan, I. H. Johnston, A. M. Harper, and W. B. Jennett

Introduction

Cerebral blood flow (CBF) is determined mainly by the pressure difference and the sum of the resistances across the cerebral vascular system. This pressure difference or the cerebral perfusion pressure (CPP) as it is commonly called can be varied by a change in inflow pressure (carotid artery blood pressure – CABP) or in outflow pressure (cortical venous pressure, which will also be referred to as cerebral subarachnoid venous pressure – CSAVP). The convention of defining CPP as the difference between mean CABP and mean intracranial pressure (ICP) assumes that ICP is the same as the vascular outflow pressure. It has been shown that raised ICP may substantially reduce CBF [1, 2, 3, 4]. However, vascular resistance changes may sginificantly affect CBF without any change in CPP. These resistance changes may be caused in a complex way by neural, chemical and metabolic factors as well as by transmural pressures. The relationship between CBF and CPP, as presently defined, is not uniform and in the case of intracranial hypertension the authors have shown that this relationship depends on the way in which ICP is raised [5, 6] e.g.

1. With infusion of fluid into the cisterna magna of baboons, in general CBF remained constant until CPP fell to levels in the range 30–85 mmHg and there then followed a period of arterial hypertension and hyperaemia before CBF dropped progressively to zero.

2. The addition of fluid to a latex balloon placed supratentorially resulted in CBF remaining constant until CPP dropped to approximately 40 mmHg when CBF again fell progressively to zero.

3. With the addition of fluid to an infratentorial balloon CBF fell linearly with CPP.

Two questions arise from these results:

1. What is the relationship between ICP and venous outflow pressure during intracranial hypertension?

2. What vascular outflow pressure differences can occur during raised ICP?

This study was initiated in an attempt to answer these questions.

Method

Adult baboons weighing approximately 10 kg were used. Anaesthesia was induced with phencyclidine hydrochloride (10 mg) and sodium thiopentone (60 mg) and maintained with a combination of phencyclidine hydrochloride, suxamethonium and a nitrous oxide/oxygen mixture. Ventilation was controlled throughout using a Starling pump.

Pressures were continuously monitored by means of strain gauge transducers (Bell and Howell, type 4–327–L221) and indwelling catheters in carotid artery, lateral ventricle, cortical vein, posterior end of the superior sagittal sinus and jugular vein and the resultant waveforms were written out on heat sensitive chart recorders (Devices M2 and M4) CBF was measured at intervals using the ^{133}Xe clearance method as previously described from this laboratory [7] and the mean carotid artery flow was measured using using an electromagnetic flowmeter.

As in the previous series of experiments, ICP was raised by three different methods.

1. By cisterna magna infusion of mock CSF[1] from a reservoir maintained at body temperature by a water bath. The reservoir was pressurised using a sphygmomanometer bulb connected to an aneroid manometer.

2. By addition of small quantities of fluid at 30 min intervals to a latex balloon placed supratentorially. Each addition of fluid was adjusted to raise the ventricular fluid pressure (VFP) by 10–20 mmHg.

3. By addition of fluid in a similar manner to a balloon placed infratentorially.

Results

Figure 1 shows a composite plot of 86 paired observations of cortical venous pressure and VFP taken from 11 animals. The regression equation and the boundary lines signifying two standard errors of estimate are drawn and a highly significant correlation coefficient is also indicated. The regression line displayed is closely parallel to the line of identity, $y = x$, and the positive intercept on the cortical venous pressure axis indicates a small shift of 2.5 mmHg away from the VFP axis.

Table 1 indicates the regression equations, correlation coefficients and their significance, together with the standard errors of estimate for the paired observations of cortical venous pressure and VFP when ICP was raised in each of three ways. The regression line for each series of experiments exhibits the same characteristics of a gradient close to unity coupled with a small shift away from the VFP axis relative to the line of identity. A highly significant correlation coefficient was obtained in all cases.

---

1 Formula (in mequiv./l) for mock CSF: Na 145.0, K 3.5, Cl 121.5, H_2PO_4 2.0, HCO_3 25.0.

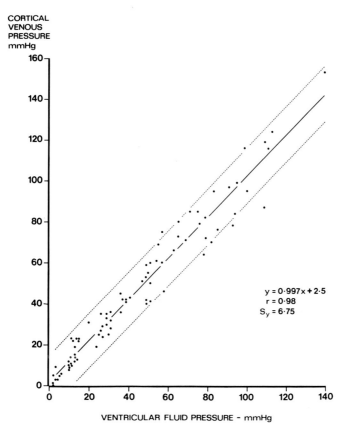

Fig. 1. Composite plot of relationship between cortical venous pressure and ventricular fluid pressure

Table 1. Summary of relationships between cortical venous pressure and ventricular fluid pressure obtained by raising intracranial pressure by three different methods

Method of Raising I.C.P.	Regression Equation	Correlation Coefficient	t	p	Standard error of estimate of y	Number of paired observations
Cisterna Magna Infusion	y = 1.03 x + 2.8	0.98	32	≪0.001	7.95	39
Supratentorial Balloon	y = 0.91 x + 2.7	0.97	22	≪0.001	6.58	33
Infratentorial Balloon	y = 0.89 x + 6.9	0.96	10	≪0.001	2.88	14
All three methods	y = 0.997x + 2.5	0.98	41	≪0.001	6.75	86

Figure 2 shows a graph of CABP, CSAVP, VFP, sagittal sinus pressure (SSP), jugular venous pressure (JVP) and CBF plotted against the times of measurement in one experiment. VFP was raised by infusion of fluid into the cisterna magna. The CABP curve exhibits a vasopressor response at a VFP level of 40 mmHg. The CSAVP and VFP curves follow each other very closely, the maximum difference being 12 mmHg. SSP begins to rise at a VFP level in the region of 54 mmHg and continues to rise with successive increases in ICP until there is no significant difference between VFP, CSAVP and SSP. JVP did not rise above 11 mmHg and CBF remained between 41 and 61 ml/100 g/min throughout the whole experiment.

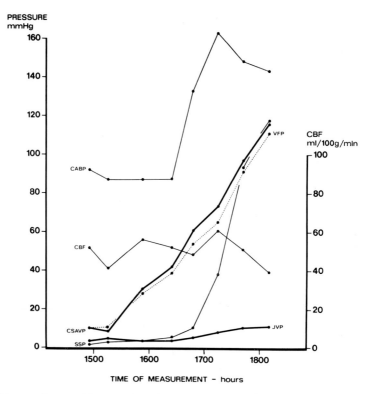

Fig. 2. Changes in carotid artery blood pressure (CABP), cerebral subarachnoid venous pressure (CSAVP), ventricular fluid pressure (VFP), sagittal sinus pressure (SSP), jugular venous pressure (JVP) and cerebral blood flow (CBF) with incremental increases in intracranial pressure. Data from one experiment

With all cisterna magna infusion experiments CABP, CSAVP, VFP and JVP behaved in a similar fashion. However, two other types of SSP response were noted, viz.,

1. SSP remained at JVP levels throughout the time course of the experiment, i.e. in the region of 2–10 mmHg. In these experiments CBF remained

within control limits until the perfusion pressure was such that autoregulation ceased to exist.

2. SSP rose to some intermediate pressure between JVP and CSAVP levels. When this occurred, a hyperaemic phase was observed as well as an increased CABP response.

SSP was observed to rise significantly above JVP levels only with cisterna magna infusion.

Discussion

The highly significant correlation coefficients found with cortical venous pressure and VFP measurements in all three series of investigations suggest that the convention of accepting perfusion pressure as mean arterial pressure minus mean intracranial pressure is realistic. The fact that the regression equations have small positive intercepts on the cortical venous pressure axis is expected, since in order to allow venous drainage the pressure in the veins has to be slightly greater than the pressure surrounding them.

When considering the vascular outflow pressure differences during intracranial hypertension, the situation becomes more complex. While JVP is not influenced by increasing ICP, observations of SSP during cisterna magna infusion indicate that three different physical situations are possible.

1. When there is little difference between SSP and JVP, little resistance to flow exists between the two points of measurement.

2. When SSP rises approximately to cortical venous pressure and VFP levels with control CBF values, then a very high resistance to flow has developed between the points of measurement of SSP and JVP suggesting that complete collapse of the sinus below the point of measurement is imminent and that a no flow situation will develop.

3. When SSP rises to an intermediate value somewhere between cortical venous pressure and JVP during a hyperaemic phase, a resistance has developed between the points of measurement of SSP and JVP such that a pressure drop dependent on the level of CBF is produced.

Conclusion

These experiments have confirmed that it is realistic to consider VFP as the value of the venous outflow pressure and that the definition of CPP as mean arterial pressure minus mean intracranial pressure is valid over a wide range of intracranial pressure and does not depend on the way in which the pressure is raised.

During cisterna magna infusion sagittal sinus pressure may behave in a complex fashion, while JVP in general does not vary significantly.

Summary

Carotid artery, cortical venous, sagittal sinus, jugular venous and ventricular fluid pressures, together with cerebral blood flow, were measured in anaesthetised baboons during incremental increases of intracranial pressure produced by infusion of fluid into the cisterna magna, and by pressurising balloons placed supratentorially and infratentorially. A highly significant correlation was found between cortical venous pressure measurements and VFP measurements between 0 and 140 mmHg. The regression equations for these two variables displayed gradients close to unity with small positive intercepts on the cortical venous pressure axis. Jugular venous pressure remained at control levels in all experiments. While sagittal sinus pressure behaved in a complex fashion during cisterna magna infusion, it remained close to JVP levels in other experiments.

Key Words : Cerebral perfusion pressure, ventricular fluid pressure, cortical venous pressure, sagittal sinus pressure, jugular venous pressure.

References

1. Kety, S. S., Shenkin, H. A., Schmidt, C. F.: The effects of increased intracranial pressure on cerebral circulatory functions in man. J. Clin. Invest. **27**, 493–499 (1948).
2. Greenfield, J. C., Jr., Tindall, G. T.: Effect of acute increase in intracranial pressure on blood flow in the internal carotid artery of man. J. clin. Invest. **44**, 1343–1351 (1965).
3. Langfitt, T. W., Kassell, N. F., Weinstein, J. D.: Cerebral blood flow with intracranial hypertension. Neurology (Minneap.) **15**, 761–773 (1965).
4. Zwetnow, N. N.: Effects of increased cerebrospinal fluid pressure on the blood flow and on the energy metabolism of the brain. An experimental study. Acta physiol. scand. (Suppl. **339**), 1–31 (1970).
5. Johnston, I. H., Rowan, J. O., Harper, A. M., Jennett, W. B.: Raised intracranial pressure and cerebral blood flow. I. Cisterna magna infusion in primates. J. Neurol. Neurosurg. Psychiat. **35**, 285–296 (1972).
6. Johnston, I. H., Rowan, J. O., Harper, W. M., Jennett, W. B.: Raised intracranial pressure and cerebral blood flow. II. Supratentorial and infratentorial mass lesions in primates. J. Neurol. Neurosurg. Psychiat. (In press.)
7. Rowan, J. O., Harper, A. M., Miller, J. D., Tedeschi, G. M., Jennett, W. B.: Relationship between volume flow and velocity in the cerebral circulation. J. Neurol. Neurosurg. Psychiat. **33**, 733–738 (1970).

The Effects of Intra-Carotid Artery Administration of Mannitol on Cerebral Blood Flow and Intracranial Pressure in Experimental Brain Edema

M. N. Shalit

Brain edema following head injury is considered to be a major factor in the generation of the subsequent increase in intracranial pressure (ICP). Moderate brain edema can still be controlled in many cases by various techniques such as hyperventilation, administration of hyperosmotic drugs and steroids, and internal or external decompression of the brain, but severe brain edema is untreatable in most cases.

The present report describes an attempt to reduce brain edema effectively by attaining a high concentration of Mannitol in the blood perfusing the brain. This was achieved by administration of the drug into the carotid artery in experimental animals after head injury.

Materials and Methods

The experiments were carried out on adult cats under pentobarbital anesthesia. The animals were paralyzed with gallamine thriethiodide (Flaxedil) and artificially respirated. Arterial PO_2, PCO_2, and pH were checked intermittently using an appropriate electrode system (Radiometer type pHA 927b). End-tidal CO_2 was continually monitored by the use of a Beckman infra-red CO_2 analyzer. Arterial PCO_2 was maintained within the range of 25–35 mmHg by adjustment of the respirator. Arterial blood pressure was measured in one of the femoral arteries by a pressure transducer. One of the femoral veins was cannulated for the administration of drugs. Intracranial pressure was recorded continuously by the use of a small intra-dural balloon connected to a pressure transducer. Regional cerebral blood flow (rCBF) was repeatedly measured simultaneously on the parietal regions of both cerebral hemispheres by the wash-out curve ^{85}Kr technique [1]. The radioactive substance was injected into the brachiocephalic artery. An EEG was recorded by means of 6 brass epidural electrodes screwed into the bone at the frontal, parietal and occipital regions of each hemisphere.

In the control group (6 animals), 10% Mannitol was administered continuously in relatively high concentrations (20–25 mg/kg/min) into one of the carotid arteries via the cannulated lingual artery by means of a Harvard pump.

The drug was infused over 4–6 h while ICP, rCBF, EEG, and reflex activity were recorded.

In the experimental group (23 animals) head injury was produced by a hammer blow on the occiput. In most cases this trauma had to be repeated several times before ICP began to increase. Administration of Mannitol was begun when ICP exceeded 35 mmHg. In 10 animals, the drug was administered intravenously for 1–2 h at the rate of 4–8 mg/kg/min. This was followed by intra-arterial administration at the rate of 2–8 mg/kg/min for 2–3 h. In 10 animals the drug was administered intra-arterially first and then intravenously. In the other 3 animals, the route of administration was changed several times after short periods of infusion (15–30 min).

Animals found to have an intracranial hemorrhage at autopsy were excluded from this study. Values of the investigated parameters recorded when arterial blood pressure showed marked fluctuation were rejected.

Results

A. Control Group

The continuous intra-arterial administration of high doses of Mannitol for several hours did not significantly affect rCBF, reflex and EEG activity in this group of animals. The rCBF and EEG of the injected hemisphere did not differ from those obtained from the other hemisphere during the administration of the drug.

When the administration of Mannitol was stopped suddenly, no rebound phenomenon of increasing ICP was detected. At the end of the experiment, the administration of gallamine triethiodide was stopped. The animals gradually regained spontaneous respiration and then recovered consciousness.

B. Experimental Group

When ICP was increased after head injury a significant reduction in rCBF was observed in most cases. In 8 of the animals neither the intravenous nor the

---

Fig. 1. A comparison between the effects of intravenous and intracarotid artery administration of Mannitol. The animal had a head trauma one hour before this recording with a persistent increase in ICP in the range of 30–40 mmHg. The intravenous administration of Mannitol 10 % (8 mg/kg/min) for 16 min reduced ICP to about 5 mmHg. rCBF was not significantly affected. ICP subsequently returned to the previous level. Administration of the drug into the right carotid artery at the same rate resulted in a rapid reduction of ICP to about 20 mmHg. rCBF was doubled in the right hemisphere. The relatively low ICP was maintained when the rate of Mannitol administration was reduced to 50 %. When the intravenous route was repeated, ICP gradually increased. 10 min after this recording was taken, ICP reached values above 50 mmHg with rCBF arrest. B.P. = Blood Pressure; ICP = Intracranial pressure; CO_2 (%) = End-tidal CO_2 concentration; rCBF = Regional cerebral blood flow, expressed in ml/g/min

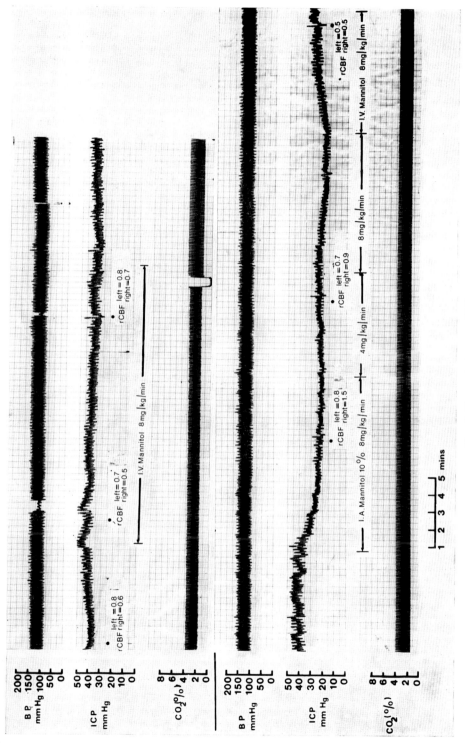

Fig. 1 (Legend see page 172)

intra-arterial administration of Mannitol exerted any detectable effect on ICP or rCBF. In these animals, ICP was usually high (above 50 mmHg). In 4 animals, the administration of the drug was followed by a decrease in ICP in various degrees with no concomitant change in rCBF. In the other 11 animals, the decrease in ICP was accompanied by an increase in rCBF which was usually more marked in the injected hemisphere. The effects of intra-arterial administration of the drug on ICP and rCBF were much more significant than the effects of intravenous administration, even when larger doses were administered intravenously. Furthermore, the drug reached its full effect after a much shorter time when administered by the intra-arterial route than when given intravenously, and smaller doses of Mannitol were required. Once an effective decrease in ICP was achieved by intra-arterial injection, it was possible to maintain ICP at relatively low levels by smaller doses of Mannitol (Fig. 1).

However, when intra-arterial administration of Mannitol was suddenly interrupted, a sharp increase in ICP and a marked decrease in rCBF was usually observed. This process began within a few minutes of withdrawal of the drug. ICP was then raised in a few minutes to extremely high levels, with complete cessation of rCBF. This rebound phenomenon could be controlled to a certain degree only by repeating the intra-arterial administration and then only if it was started while ICP was still moderate. Intravenous administration had no effect at all.

Comment

When Mannitol is administered intravenously to patients suffering from brain edema, the dose level is subject to various limitations such as the fact that at high concentrations, Mannitol overloads the systemic circulation due to the resultant acute shift of fluid from the tissues into the circulation [2].

In an attempt to achieve a constant high concentration of Mannitol in the blood perfusing the brain, rapidly and without a significant increase in the concentration of the drug in the systemic circulation, the intra-carotid artery route was used. This method was found to be significantly more effective than intravenous administration. Furthermore, the intra-arterial technique was found to be non-toxic to the brain, as reflected by EEG and reflex activity, rCBF and the animals' capacity for recovery.

The dissociation of concentration of Mannitol in the brain and in the systemic circulation may be fatal if the intra-arterial administration is interrupted suddenly for any reason. This dangerous rebound phenomenon may still theoretically be controlled by gradually increasing the Mannitol concentration in the systemic circulation by an intravenous infusion while gradually withdrawing the intra-arterial administration.

Another factor to be considered is the possibility of vascular complications associated with any intra-arterial infusions.

These important limiting factors must be considered and controlled before the intra-arterial route is used for Mannitol in patients suffering from severe brain edema.

Summary

The effects of the intravenous and intra-carotid artery administration of Mannitol on regional cerebral blood flow and intracranial pressure were investigated in experimental animals suffering from post-traumatic brain edema.

It was found that the intra-arterial route was by far the more effective for reducing intracranial pressure and improving cerebral blood flow. Furthermore, smaller amounts of Mannitol were required and the optimum effect was achieved in a shorter time.

It is suggested that this method of administration might, under certain circumstances, be considered in the treatment of patients suffering from severe brain edema.

Key Words: Mannitol, intra-arterial, intracranial pressure.

References

1. Betz, E., Ingvar, D. H., Lassen, N. A., Schmahl, F. W.: Regional blood flow in the cerebral cortex, measured simultaneously by heat and inert gas clearance. Acta physiol. scand. **67**, 1–9 (1966).
2. Aviram, A., Pfau, A., Czaczkes, J. W., Ulman, T. D.: Hyperosmolality with hyponatremia, caused by inappropriate administration of mannitol. Amer. J. Med. **42**, 648–650 (1967).

The Effect of Mannitol on Intracranial Pressure and Cerebral Blood Flow

Clinical and Experimental Observations

I. H. Johnston, A. Paterson, A. M. Harper, and W. B. Jennett

Introduction

Mannitol has been shown to be effective in reducing raised intracranial pressure when used in a single large dose [1]. Its use in the control of raised intracranial pressure over longer periods of time, particularly in patients with diffuse brain damage is, however, less well founded and here other effects, for example on cerebral blood flow, may be of importance. This paper briefly reports the results of a clinical study of the effect of small serial doses of Mannitol on intracranial pressure and of an experimental study of the effect of Mannitol on cerebral blood flow.

Method

a) *Clinical*: 20 patients were studied following direct surgery for intracranial aneurysm. Each patient received 6 doses of Mannitol (30 g in 150 ml over 10 min) at 6-hourly intervals starting 18 h from the end of operation. Further 20 patients, matched for mean intracranial pressure levels over the first 18 h after operation were used as a control. Intracranial pressure was continuously monitored for 72 h after operation using an intraventricular catheter inserted during operation.

b) *Experimental*: The effect of Mannitol on cerebral blood flow was studied in 2 groups of anaesthetised baboons using both the ^{133}Xe clearance method and an electromagnetic flow meter placed on the right common carotid artery after ligation of the right external carotid artery. In the first group an intravenous infusion of 1.5 g/kg Mannitol was given over a 10 min period. Cerebral blood flow was measured 5, 20, 40 and 70 min from the start of Mannitol infusion. In the second group intracranial pressure was raised by expansion of a supratentorial subdural balloon and a similar series of blood flow estimations carried out after Mannitol infusion.

Results

a) *Clinical*: 4 series of comparisons were made. Firstly, a comparison was made between mean intracranial pressure levels over the one hour period before and after the first, third and sixth Mannitol infusions. Mannitol reduced intracranial pressure during the first hour after infusion and the effect was maintained with succeeding doses (Table 1). If, however, the patients are divided into those with a mean pre-infusion intracranial pressure level of less than 20 mmHg (9 patients) and greater than 20 mmHg (11 patients), only the first dose of Mannitol reduced the mean intracranial pressure in the group with lower initial intracranial pressure levels, while succeeding doses of Mannitol continued to produce a 20–25% reduction in intracranial pressure in those with higher initial levels.

Table 1. Mean intracranial pressure (ICP) levels over 1 h and 6 h periods before and after 1st, 3rd and 6th of 6 serial infusions of Mannitol. Results from 20 patients after surgery for intracranial aneurysm

Dose No. Mean ICP mmHg	Mannitol 1 before	after	Mannitol 3 before	after	Mannitol 6 before	after
Over 1 h	22.8	17.8	19.0	16.0	20.3	17.0
Over 6 h	23.4	21.0	18.6	17.1	19.0	20.6

Secondly, comparison was made between mean intracranial pressure levels over the 6 h period before and after the first, third and sixth Mannitol infusions. Only the first dose of Mannitol produced a statistically significant reduction in the mean intracranial pressure level for the whole group, and the degree of reduction was small (Table 2). Effective reduction in intracranial pressure occurred only with the first dose in those patients with initial intracranial pressure levels less than 20 mmHg and with the third dose only in those with initial levels greater than 20 mmHg. In both cases the magnitude of the reduction was small and with the sixth dose the mean intracranial pressure level after infusion exceeded that before infusion.

Table 2. Mean intracranial pressure (ICP) levels over successive 18 h periods post-operatively in 20 patients given Mannitol 6-hourly from 18–54 h, and in 20 patients not given Mannitol

Mean ICP mmHg	h post Op. 0–18	19–36	37–54	55–72
With Mannitol	19.3	18.9	20.7	19.0
Without Mannitol	16.2	17.6	17.0	16.3

Thirdly, comparison was made between the mean intracranial pressure levels for succeeding 18 h periods between the group of patients receiving Mannitol and those not receiving Mannitol. There was no statistically significant difference between the mean levels for the two for any of the 18 h periods under consideration (Table 2). The mean level for the group not receiving Mannitol was, in fact, consistently slightly less than that for the group given Mannitol.

In addition, the mean level for each group remained relatively constant throughout the 72 h period.

Fourthly, there was no apparent difference in outcome, in terms of morbidity and mortality, between those patients given Mannitol and those not given Mannitol.

b) *Experimental*: 1. Normal Intracranial Pressure – Mannitol produced a significant increase in cerebral blood flow, from 11.3–78.5% during the first Xenon clearance measurement (Table 3). Blood flow remained slightly above control levels during subsequent measurements but this was not statistically significant. One animal did show a persistently high flow during the hour after infusion, which could not be accounted for by a change in any of the other parameters measured, including intracranial pressure, jugular venous pressure and sagittal sinus pressure $PaCO_2$, PaO_2, PCV. Apart from a transient fall in cerebrovascular resistance during the period of increased flow, values for cerebral perfusion pressure, cerebrovascular resistance and $CMRO_2$ did not show any significant change.

2. Raised Intracranial Pressure – 3 of the 4 animals showed no change in cerebral blood flow with Mannitol infusion, while the fourth animal showed a substantial increase persisting for about 1 h (Table 3). Mean cerebral blood flow levels for all 4 animals did, however, not show any significant increase with Mannitol infusion. Other measured parameters, including cerebral perfusion pressure, remained relatively constant.

Table 3. Effect of Mannitol (1.5 g/kg) on cerebral blood flow (CBF ml/100 g/min) and cerebral perfusion pressure (CPP mmHg) under conditions of normal and raised intracranial pressure (ICP)

	Control		Mannitol + 5 min		Mannitol + 20 min		Mannitol + 40 min		Mannitol + 70 min	
	CBF	CPP	CBF	CPP	CBF	CPP	CBF	CPP	CBF	CPP
Normal ICP	62.5	82.8	86.8	86.8	73.2	87.8	75.7	88.7	74.0	79.4
Raised ICP	36.0	57.0	42.0	58.5	–	68.3	45.0	65.0	37.3	61.3

Comment

The results of the clinical study show that serial Mannitol infusion, in the doses used, had no sustained effect on intracranial pressure levels, although it did continue to cause a transient reduction in pressure immediately after infusion. There was no evidence of a rebound effect on intracranial pressure. What is the significance of these findings? Firstly, it is apparent that serial Mannitol infusions in the present dosage cannot be relied upon to control raised intracranial pressure, particularly as its effectiveness is likely to be greatest in relatively undamaged brain (the majority of patients in the present study) and least in patients with severe diffuse brain damage where the need for control of raised intracranial pressure may be greatest. In deciding on the place of Mannitol in the control of raised intracranial pressure, it would seem worthwhile to assess the effects of larger doses in a similar type of study, although increasing the dosage might well introduce problems of rebound [2] and substantial disturbances of water and electrolyte balance.

Turning to the effect of Mannitol on cerebral blood flow, previous studies have yielded conflicting results [3, 4]. The present study provides clear evidence of a transient but significant increase in cerebral blood flow during and immediately after the period of infusion, associated with a substantial reduction in cerebrovascular resistance, but not dependent on any significant change in cerebral perfusion pressure. The mechanism by which this increase in flow is effected is not clear. Possible contributory factors include changes in cerebral metabolism, leading to changes in the diameter of the cerebral resistance vessels, or changes in the physical properties of the blood, such as plasma viscosity. Under conditions of increased intracranial pressure, however, the increase in cerebral blood flow was seen in only one of the 4 animals studied. A possible explanation for this is that cerebral vasodilatation had already occurred as a result of the increase in intracranial pressure, as in 2 of the 3 animals not showing an increase in cerebral blood flow there had been a substantial reduction in cerebral perfusion pressure prior to the administration of Mannitol. If this is so, it would indirectly suggest that active vasodilatation is the means whereby Mannitol effects an increase in flow.

Summary

The effect of serial 30 g doses of Mannitol on intracranial pressure was studied in 20 patients following surgery for intracranial aneurysm. Mannitol continued to produce a transient reduction of intracranial pressure immediately after infusion, but became progressively less effective with time. Mean intracranial pressure levels in patients given Mannitol did not differ significantly from a further 20 patients who where not given Mannitol. In an experimental study in baboons, Mannitol produced a transient increase in blood flow during and immediately after infusion under conditions of normal intracranial pressure. This effect occurred in only 1 out of 4 animals under conditions of raised intracranial pressure.

Key Words : Mannitol, intracranial pressure, cerebral blood flow.

References

1. WISE, B. L., CHATER, N.: The value of hypertonic Mannitol solution in decreasing brain mass and lowering cerebrospinal fluid pressure. J. Neurosurg. **19**, 1038–1043 (1962).

2. JAVID, M., GILBOE, D., CESARIO, T.: The rebound phenomenon and hypertonic solutions. J. Neurosurg. **21**, 1059–1066 (1964).
3. HARPER, A. M., BELL, R. A.: The failure of intravenous urea to alter the blood flow through the cerebral cortex. J. Neurol. Neurosurg. Psychiat. **26**, 69–70 (1963).
4. GOLUBOFF, B., SHENKIN, H. A., HAFT, H.: The effects of Mannitol and urea on cerebral hemodynamics and cerebrospinal fluid pressure. Neurology (Minneap.) **14**, 891–898 (1964).

Comments to Session 5

G. T. Tindall and H. Nagai

There was considerable interest and discussion concerning the status of vital signs and cerebral hemodynamics during gradual increases in ICP. Hekmatpanah has made continuous observations of the cerebral and pial circulation during increases in ICP and demonstrated these in a film. He emphasized alterations in the micro-circulation as a significant correlate associated with physiological changes. He showed an increase in the diameter of cerebral veins and related this change to an increase in ICP. Administration of urea prior to marked pupillary dilatation resulted in return of blood flow to cortical vessels.

Ommaya and Nakatani showed differing physiological responses depending on the rate of inflation of an extra-cerebral balloon. When they infused at a rapid rate (0.5 ml/min) they obtained a pronounced vasopressor response (Cushing response), whereas with slower rates of infusion (0.02 ml/min) the vasopressor response did not occur. They emphasized the importance of relative volume changes in the intracranial compartment in the interpretation of ICP measurements.

Some interesting studies on experimental intracranial hemorrhage and ICP were reported by Löfgren and Zwetnow. They presented the interesting and somewhat paradoxical finding that intracranial bleeding of venous origin produced a greater rise in ICP than bleeding of arterial nature.

An interesting and intriguing fluid-mechanics-model to illustrate certain features of ICP and the Monro-Kellie doctrine was presented in detail by Lichtenstein and Tym and stimulated a good discussion.

Reduction in CBF (^{133}Xe) with increasing ICP appeared to be dependent upon the method of elevating ICP according to Lewis and McLaurin. The adaptive mechanism which maintains CBF during increasing ICP appears to fail when: ICP elevation is due to a mass lesion; perfusion pressure (SAP-ICP) is reduced below 35 mmHg with ICP elevation accompanying CSF volume expansion; and in the slow compartment of CBF when cerebral edema is produced by intravenous water. The hypothesis was advanced that gross or microscopic vascular distortion is responsible for the failure of this adaptive mechanism. In the ensuing discussion, Zwetnow pointed out the importance of evaluating white matter flow in this situation. Rowan, Johnston, Harper and Jennett found a highly significant correlation between cortical venous pressure and ventricular fluid pressure measurements over a wide range of ventricular fluid pressures (0–140 mmHg) regardless of the method used for raising ventricular fluid pressure. While jugular venous pressure remained low during elevated ICP, sagittal sinus pressure behaved in a complex fashion.

Two interesting papers on mannitol and its effect on ICP were presented. SHALIT showed that intracarotid injections of mannitol caused acute reductions in ICP. However, there was a rebound effect following administration by this route. In the discussion following this paper, the possible toxic effects of the drug administered by this route were mentioned. JOHNSTON, PATERSON, HARPER and JENNETT stated that they had not observed significant decreases in ICP with mannitol, but this may be related to the low dosage and administration schedule used by these authors. In the discussion BECKER emphasized the importance of monitoring serum osmolality in patients who receive frequent dosages of mannitol. He recommended administration of mannitol in dosages of 1 g per kg body weight administered every 3 h or a continuous infusion at 0.3 g/kg/h. He also recommended frequent monitoring of serum osmolality in order to maintain this value below 320 milliosmols/l.

Session 6

Miscellaneous
(Experimental)

Measurement of "Interstitial Fluid" Pressure in the Brain in Dogs

P. Brodersen, K. Højgaard, and N. A. Lassen

Introduction

The interstitial fluid pressure is the hydrostatic pressure of the fluid between the solid tissue elements such as cells, fibers and vessels. Guyton measured negative pressures in chronically implanted perforated capsules, which he considered to be the true interstitial pressure in the subcutis [1]. Others showed that a cotton wick inserted in a needle or catheter recorded a negative pressure in the subcutis within a few minutes just as the Guyton capsule did [2, 3].

Interstitial pressure measurements in the brain appear to be of particular interest in relation to the propagation of edema. The present study was undertaken as an attempt to measure the interstitial fluid pressure in the brain.

Material and Methods

9 mongrel dogs of 20–25 kg body-weight were premedicated with 50–75 mg acepromacine (Plegicil) orally, anesthetized with pentobarbital, 20–25 mg/kg intravenously, intubated and artificially ventilated with 50% N_2O and 50% oxygen using an Engström respirator. Supplementary doses of 5–10 mg/kg of pentobarbital were given at intervals of 2–3 h. The mean arterial blood pressure (MABP), monitored via a catheter in the femoral artery, was 90–110 mmHg in the resting state. The arterial PCO_2 was checked hourly and ranged from 30–45 mmHg, usually 35–40 mmHg. Thin-walled hypodermic needles (outer diameter [o. d.] 1.4 mm) were introduced 2–3 cm into the brain tissue with stylets through bilateral parietal burr holes. The stylet was then removed, a catheter introduced, and the needle withdrawn. The burr hole was closed around the catheter with dental cement. Two types of catheters were used: A polyethylene catheter (Intracath, o. d. 1.0 mm) split into 4 lobes for 5–7 mm at the distal end using a razor blade, or a teflon tube 15 cm long (o. d. 1.1 mm) mounted with $1^1/_2$ cm cotton thread at the distal end, about 2 mm of the cotton thread being outside the tip of the tube. The wick probe was boiled 30 min in 0.9% saline to remove air bubbles. The probes were each connected with an Elema-Schönander (EMT 35) transducer, an Elema-Schönander (EMT 31) pressure manometer, and a Servogor 2 channel recorder by means of a three-

way stopcock. To prevent clotting, the split catheters were flushed with 0.9%
saline containing heparin, 4 IU/ml, before insertion. Both probes yielded identical results in human subcutaneous tissue: —2 to —5 mmHg. Our reference
level was the tip of the probe. A needle was introduced into the suboccipital
subarachnoid space to record the pressure and route the infusions. After resting state recordings, the responses were noted when cisternal fluid pressure was
increased to 50 mmHg by infusion of cisternal saline. Then the responses to
water intoxication (2 l water i. v., i. e. 10% of body-weight) were recorded with
the cisternal needle kept open to the atmosphere. Finally the responses to increased cisternal fluid pressure were repeated. The animals were sacrificed at
the end of the experiments, and the exact position of the catheters checked at
autopsy after fixation.

Results

17 probes were placed in 9 dogs. In 6 probes in 5 dogs we found negative
pressures without pulsations in the range —3 to —12 mmHg, mean —6.5,
SD 3.2. These 6 probes were all situated in the brain tissue without communication with the subarachnoid space. None of these probes contained tissue
plugs or grossly hemorrhagic fluid. The cisternal fluid pressures recorded at
the same time ranged from 6–13 mmHg with a mean of 10. After introduction
of the probes it was often noted that the pressure increased to 5–10 mmHg and
afterwards decreased slowly to a negative pressure plateau within 5–15 min.

In 4 probes we found pulsating pressures which were identical to or differed by only a few mmHg from the cisternal fluid pressure. The autopsy in all
these cases revealed that the catheters communicated with the subarachnoid
space. In 7 cases the catheter was either blocked by a tissue plug or surrounded
by marked hemorrhage, and these measurements were therefore excluded.

The increase in cisternal fluid pressure to 50 mmHg did not change the
negative pressures. During water intoxication the negative pressures approached zero after i. v. administration of about 1 l of water and became positive (+5 mmHg) after 2 l. A new increase in cisternal fluid pressure to 50
mmHg was followed by an increase of 4–5 mmHg in the previously negative
pressure probes. Autopsy showed signs of brain edema. In a few studies we
found that split catheters communicating with the ventricles yielded accurate
recordings even of extreme rises in pressure, indicating that perhaps obstruction is less likely to occur in these catheters than in conventional side-hole
catheters.

Comment

Cotton wick probes were inserted into the brain tissue, and pressure curves
almost identical to intraventricular pressure recordings were obtained [4]. We
only found recordings of this kind when the probe had penetrated into the sub-

arachnoid space or if we injected a minute amount of fluid so that a small fluid pool at the tip of the catheter could act as a small balloon. According to Guy-ton et al. [5] tissue pressure involves both the interstitial fluid pressure and the pressure of solid components, which means this pressure cannot be measured with a wick or a split catheter. The tissue pressure must be measured with a small balloon or possibly in a small intracerebral vein. It is possible that the tissue pressure recordings by Brock et al. [4] might be explained by a fluid pool at the tip of the wick acting as small balloon or by communication between surface liquor and the tip of the probe.

The negative pressures we measured might be interstitial fluid pressures. Negative interstitial fluid pressures have been described in subcutaneous tissue [1, 2, 3], but colloid osmotic forces due to membrane formation and/or macro-molecules in the intercellular substance have been suggested as a possible ex-planation for these values [6, 7]. We have provided evidence for negative inter-stitial fluid pressure in the brain, but our measurements are open to the same criticism. In the lung, however, the existence of negative interstitial fluid pres-sures has been widely accepted. It would be interesting to measure interstitial fluid pressure in a localized brain edema, such as a freeze lesion.

Summary

Using split catheters or wick probes fixed in the brain tissue of dog, we found negative pressures in the range —3 to —12 mmHg, while the cisternal fluid pressure at the same time ranged from 6–13 mmHg. The negative pres-sures only responded minimally to elevations of the cisternal fluid pressure after water intoxication. The study provides evidence for negative interstitial fluid pressure in the brain.

Key Words: Intracranial pressure, tissue pressure, interstitial fluid pressure, brain edema, dogs.

References

1. Guyton, A. C.: A concept of negative interstitial pressure based on pressures in implanted perforated capsules. Circulat. Res. **12**, 399–414 (1963).
2. Scholander, P. F., Hargens, A. R., Miller, S. L.: Negative pressures in the interstitial fluid of animals. Science **161**, 321–328 (1968).
3. Ladegaard-Pedersen, H. J.: Measurement of the interstitial pressure in subcutaneous tissue in dogs. Circulat. Res. **26**, 765–770 (1970).
4. Brock, M., Winkelmüller, W., Pöll, W., Markakis, E., Dietz, H.: Measurement of brain-tissue pressure. Lancet **I**, 595–596 (1972).
5. Guyton, A. C., Granger, H. J., Taylor, A. E.: Interstitial fluid pressure. Physiol. Rev. **51**, 527–563 (1971).
6. Stromberg, D. G., Wiederhielm, C. A.: Effects of oncotic gradients and enzymes on negative pressure in implanted capsules. Amer. J. Physiol. **219**, 928–932 (1970).
7. Kirsch, K., Rafflenbeul, W., Roedel, H.: Untersuchungen zur Ursache des negativen interstitiellen Gewebsdruckes (Guytonkapsel). Pflügers Arch. ges. Physiol. **328**, 193–204 (1971).

Brain Tissue Pressure

W. Pöll, M. Brock, E. Markakis, W. Winkelmüller, and H. Dietz

The changes in regional cerebral blood flow observed in diseased areas of the brain when arterial PCO_2 and/or arterial blood pressure are altered have been attributed to variations in local tissue perfusion pressure (TPP) [1] and to pressure gradients within the brain [2, 3, 4]. Conclusions drawn from "cerebral" perfusion pressure (CPP) calculations appear to possess only a restricted value for the analysis of local circulatory phenomena since CPP is an overall value. Local brain tissue perfusion pressure, however, can only be determined if the blood pressure within the small intraparenchymatous brain vessels and the "interstitial" pressure of the brain tissue are known. While recent papers [5, 6] contain quantitative data on blood pressure in small vessels of the brain, no satisfactory method has hitherto permitted the measurement of brain tissue pressure. Implantable capsules [7] and balloons filled with saline [8] are inappropriate for this purpose since they involve excessive damage to the brain tissue.

The development of the "wick-method" [9] and its successful application to a series of plant and animal tissues [10, 11, 12] led us to try the measurement of pressures within the brain parenchyma by this method [13]. We recorded the normal pressure values and confirmed the above mentioned pressure gradients within the brain tissue under experimental pathological conditions. The present paper is restricted to the presentation of the technique and to reporting normal brain tissue pressures in the cat.

Material and Methods

The data reported were obtained from 15 spontaneously breathing healthy cats of both sexes (average weight: 3200 g) studied under intraperitoneal Nembutal® anesthesia (40 mg/kg body-weight). Following cannulation of one femoral artery and vein, and tracheostomy, each animal's head was fixed in a stereotactor (David Kopf Instruments, California).

Three burr holes (diameter: 3 mm) were made with a conventional dental drill to permit puncturing one of the frontal horns of the lateral ventricles and both internal capsules. Ventricular fluid pressure was continuously recorded from the frontal horn by means of a metal needle (outer diameter: 1 mm) introduced stereotactically. The position of the needle tip corresponded to the coordinates +13, +3, +17 of the atlas of Reinoso-Suarez [14].

Tissue pressure in both internal capsules was measured by means of wick-catheters introduced stereotactically with the aid of metal needles (outer diameter 1,6 mm). The position of the wicks corresponded to the coordinates +11, +9, +13 of the atlas of REINOSO-SUAREZ.

Preparation of the Wick-Catheter

The wicks used are made of "long fiber" cotton wool (Sea Island)[1] with an average fiber length of 6 cm and a width of about 10 micra. Before use the wick is combed to remove shorter and weaker fibers (Fig. 1 A). A thin yarn is then tied around the midpoint of the combed bundle of fibers (Fig. 1 B). This yarn is pulled through a thin polyethylene catheter from its bottom to its tip until the (folded) bundle protrudes 6 mm beyond the tip (Fig. 1 C). The knot and the fold in the bundle are cut off, leaving a wick 4 mm in length (Fig. 1 D).

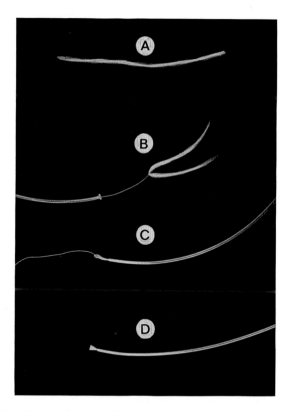

Fig. 1. A: Bundle of combed cotton fibers as used in preparation of the wick-catheter. B, C and D: 3 steps in the preparation of the wick-catheter

1 The authors thank Mr. E. LORD, of the Cotton, Silk and Man-made Fibres Research Association for kindly supplying the cotton fibers used.

The wick-catheter is then rinsed and filled with saline solution containing heparin, and connected to a conventional pressure transducer. The thickness required for the fiber bundle is established empirically according to the size of the catheters used. Wick-catheters prepared as above can be sterilized and stored. We found it unnecessary to boil the wicks, as suggested by others [11], to remove small amounts of air trapped between individual fibers of the wick.

The wick prevents the obliteration of the catheter tip by surrounding tissue, while permitting satisfactory and reliable measurement of tissue pressure (Fig. 2). The theoretical principle of this method has been extensively validated by SNASHALL and coworkers [11].

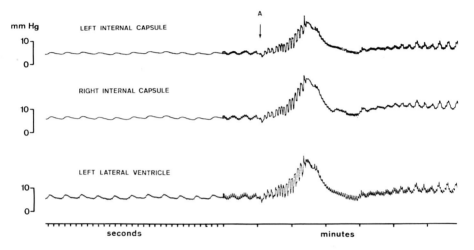

Fig. 2. Pressure recordings from both internal capsules and from the lateral ventricle of a spontaneously-breathing cat (pento-barbitone anesthesia, 35 mg/kg body-weight). AB: tracheal occlusion. [Reproduced from Lancet **II**, 595 (1972) with kind permission]

In the present series zero point calibration was performed through the catheter (or needle) tip at the level of the frontal horns. Following the introduction of the ventricular needle and of both wick-catheters the burr holes were sealed with dental cement and the animals were left undisturbed for at least 30 min. Femoral arterial blood pressure, ventricular and brain tissue pressures were then, measured 3 times at intervals of 5 min and averaged. Pulse, respiratory rate, rectal temperature and pupillary size were also recorded.

Results

The results obtained are presented in Table 1. Ventricular pressure (measured in 14 animals) averaged 6.14 ± 2.45 (SD) mmHg. In the left internal capsule tissue pressure was 5.42 ± 2.59 (SD) mmHg and in the right internal capsule 5.62 ± 2.62 (SD). The above differences are not significant. In no

Table 1. Mean pressures (mmHg)

animal	femoral artery	internal capsule left	internal capsule right	lateral ventricle
1	140	3.00	6.00	6.00
2	120	5.30	5.10	4.70
3	120	9.00	8.00	8.30
4	105	7.00	7.50	6.20
5	145	4.50	5.50	4.00
6	145	6.50	7.50	8.00
7	125	8.00	8.00	7.50
8	115	8.00	8.00	8.00
9	95	2.00	2.50	–
10	100	10.00	10.00	12.00
11	100	5.00	4.50	4.00
12	100	2.50	0.50	3.00
13	125	1.50	2.50	3.50
14	95	3.50	5.50	6.00
15	107	4.50	3.25	4.75
Mean:		5.42	5.62	6.14
SD:		± 2,59	± 2.62	± 2.45

animal were negative pressures observed under physiological conditions. Only in certain pathological states, as when a previously inflated intracranial balloon was being deflated, or following an animal's death, did we record subatmospheric intracranial pressures. Experience indicates that the recording of permanent pressures below 0 mmHg in the brain under normal conditions is artifactual and may be caused by inappropriate calibration, leakage of the recording system or partial withdrawal of the catheter after its introduction. In this latter instance fluid is drawn out of the system by the cleft left in the tissue.

Comments

SNASHALL et al. [11] have shown that the pressure values recorded by means of the "wick-method" are purely hydrostatic and independent of osmotic forces. While this technique permits the reliable detection of relatively slow pressure variations, transmission of very rapid pulsatile pressure changes is dampened to a variable degree depending on the amount of fibers in the wick. "Loose" wicks allow a better transmission of pulsatile phenomena. This technique is suitable for recording the changes in tissue pressure associated with respiration.

Although the introduction of a needle or catheter causes damage to the surrounding tissue, usually the needle track is "neat" and histological studies have shown that edema around the wick develops later than the time at which our measurements were made. On 3 occasions bleeding occurred around the tip of the catheter. This was promptly detected by a slow and steady increase in pressure on the affected side. If bleeding occurs the experiment is abandoned. CO_2-reactivity and autoregulation (Fig. 3) are preserved in the animal preparation described here. Nevertheless, it should be borne in mind that the pressures recorded by this procedure can only be considered approximations of the true interstitial pressure of the brain since the introduction of the wick-catheter disrupts the normal texture of the examined tissue and also damages cellular structures. We consider it more appropriate to speak of brain tissue pressures.

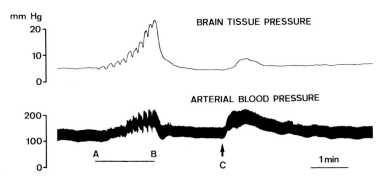

Fig. 3. Before beginning an experiment CO_2-responsiveness (AB: tracheal occlusion) and autoregulation (C: i.v. injection of noradrenaline) of cerebral vessels are tested. Careful stereotactic introduction of the wick-catheters does not appear to alter the physiological properties of the blood vessels within the studied structures. [Reproduced from Lancet **II**, 595 (1972) with kind permission]

The finding of positive pressures within the brain tissue, as opposed to other tissues, under physiological conditions is not surprising since the CNS is encased within a rigid container and surrounded by a liquid milieu whose normal pressure is 10–15 mmHg above zero. It is difficult to conceive that the cells of the CNS, lying, so to speak, between the blood stream and the CSF, both of which have pressures well above atmospheric, could withstand permanent subatmospheric pressures of several mmHg. Nor does it seem possible that the osmotic and oncotic pressures within the nervous parenchyma could uphold such pressure differences. Theoretically, negative tissue pressures are not to be expected in the CNS [16]. The observation that pressure within the brain tissue is on average somewhat lower than CSFP is compatible with the fact that interstitial pressure in other tissues (e.g. in the subcutaneous tissue) is also lower than that of the surrounding milieu (in this case the atmosphere); in the subcutaneous tissue the boundary between the normal and the edematous state is the atmospheric (zero) pressure [7]. We believe that the formation of brain edema is analogously associated with an increase in brain tissue pressure to levels above those of the surrounding CSF. Such a local increase in brain tissue pressure could also be responsible for the well-known propagation of edema fluid, by bulk flow, to the surrounding, non-edematous areas, where tissue pressure is not as high.

The wick-method constitutes a valuable tool for the study of pressure phenomena within the CNS both experimentally and clinically, and our group has also used it with satisfactory results for direct postoperative monitoring of intracranial pressures in man (Fig. 4). For this latter purpose the wick-catheter is left in the tumoral bed for 2–3 days after surgery and is afterwards simply pulled out.

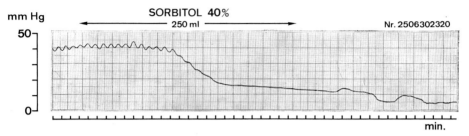

Fig. 4. Effect of intravenous hypertonic (40 %) sorbitol on the pressure within the cavity of an extirpated glioma 24 h following surgery, as measured with a wick-catheter left in situ during surgery

Acknowledgements

The authors are indebted to Miss M. DIETZ, C. KRUSE and I. STAUDIGL for technical assistance and to Mrs. I. HARKINS for typing the manuscript.

References

1. BROCK, M., HADJIDIMOS, A. A., DERUAZ, J. P., FISCHER, F., DIETZ, H., KOHLMEYER, K., PÖLL, W., SCHÜRMANN, K.: The effects of hyperventilation on regional cerebral blood flow. On the role of changes in intracranial pressure and tissue-perfusion pressure for shifts in rCBF distribution. In: TOOLE, J. F., MOOSSY, J., JANEWAY, R. (Eds.): Cerebral Vascular Diseases, p. 114–123. New York: Grune & Stratton 1971.
2. BROCK, M.: Cerebral blood flow and intracranial pressure changes associated with brain hypoxia. In: BRIERLEY, J. B., MELDRUM, B. S. (Eds.): Brain Hypoxia, p. 14–18. Philadelphia: J. B. Lippincott Co. 1971.
3. BROCK, M., MARKAKIS, E., BECK, J., DIETZ, H.: Intracranial pressure gradients associated with cerebrovascular occlusion. Lancet, II, 824 (1971).
4. BROCK, M., BECK, J., MARKAKIS, E., DIETZ, H.: Intracranial pressure gradients associated with experimental cerebral embolism. Stroke, 3, 123–130 (1972).
5. KANZOW, E., DIECKHOFF, D.: On the location of the vascular resistance in the cerebral circulation. In: BROCK, M., FIESCHI, C., INGVAR, D., LASSEN, N., SCHÜRMANN, K. (Eds.): Cerebral Blood Flow, p. 96–97. Berlin-Heidelberg-New York: Springer 1969.
6. SHAPIRO, H. M., STROMBERG, D. D., LEE, D. R., WIEDERHIELM, C. A.: Dynamic pressures in the pial arterial microcirculation. Amer. J. Physiol. 221, 279–283 (1971).

7. Guyton, A. C.: A concept of negative interstitial pressure based on pressures in implanted perforated capsules. Circulat. Res. **12**, 399–414 (1963).
8. Weinstein, J. D., Langfitt, T. W., Bruno, L., Zaren, H. A., Jackson, J. L. F.: Experimental study of patterns of brain distortion and ischemia produced by an intracranial mass. J. Neurosurg. **28**, 513–521 (1968).
9. Scholander, P. F., Hargens, A. R., Miller, S. L.: Negative pressure in the interstitial fluid of animals. Science **161**, 321–328 (1968).
10. Strømme, S. B., Maggert, J. E., Scholander, P. F.: Interstitial fluid pressure in terrestrial and semiterrestrial animals. J. appl. Physiol. **27**, 123–126 (1969).
11. Snashal, P. D., Lucas, J., Guz, A., Floyer, M. A.: Measurement of interstitial 'fluid' pressure by means of a cotton wick in man and animals: an analysis of the origin of the pressure. Clin. Sci. **41**, 35–53 (1971).
12. Ladegaard-Pedersen, H. J.: Measurement of the interstitial pressure in subcutaneous tissue in dogs. Circulat. Res. **26**, 765–770 (1970).
13. Brock, M., Winkelmüller, W., Pöll, W., Markakis, E., Dietz, H.: Measurement of brain-tissue pressure. Lancet, **II**, 595–596 (1972).
14. Reinoso-Suarez, F.: Topographischer Hirnatlas der Katze. Darmstadt 1961.
15. Guyton, A. C.: Personal communication to M. B. in 1970.
16. Brock, M., Markakis, E., Pöll, W., Dietz, H.: In preparation.

Subarachnoid-Pressure-Dependent Drug Effects on CSF Transport and Brain Volume

E. Betz, W. Roos, B. Vamosi, and R. Weidler

Cats or rabbits anaesthetized with Nembutal or Urethan were fixed in a stereotactor, the head in an upright position. A small burr hole was drilled into the skull so that thin tubes of varying lengths could be fixed vertically into the burr hole near to the crossing of the sagittal and coronary sutures. The system was made watertight. The dura in the burr hole was opened. Mock CSF was filled into the vertical tube and the rate of its disappearance was plotted against the hydrostatic pressure. Pressure was increased from 0.5–8 cm H_2O. In this pressure-range the degree of resorbed CSF fluid is linearly dependent on the CSF pressure and even small increases in CSF pressure cause an increase in CSF-resorption [1]. From experiments by Heisey et al. [2] and Bering and Sato [3] it can be concluded that the production of CSF is not significantly changed during such small increases in CSF pressure. Therefore, it seems to us that the disappearance of mock CSF is caused by resorption. The brain volume was recorded with a device consisting of a very light displacement transducer within the tube fixed on the skull. It is possible to take the change in vertical displacement of one point in the brain as a relative measure of its volume variation. According to the law of similar bodies, the volume variations of such bodies are equal to the cubes of their lengths. Thus the vertical displacement of the surface is a relative measure of the brain volume. The displacement transducer was watertight to prevent an escape of fluid. It was possible to occlude it and to record the pressure in the subdural space continuously with a Statham-transducer. Combined measurements of cortical blood flow and brain volume showed pulse-synchronous and respiratory variations in the brain volume when the burr hole was open. Increases of 1–5 cm water in the CSF pressure did not cause significant variations in the mean brain volume. However, in the closed skull the amplitudes of subarachnoid pressure oscillations ranged over several mmHg [1].

The relation of CSF resorption and brain volume can be changed by drugs. We used 2 different substances: one substance, O-(β-Hydroxyethyl)-Rutoside[1] is used in antiedema therapy. Its molecular weight is 742. Intravenous injections of up to 250 mg/kg in 15 cats and 25 rabbits caused no variation in cortical blood flow. The endexpiratory CO_2-concentration and arterial blood pressure

---

1 3′ 4, 7-tri-O-(β-Hydroxyethyl)-Rutoside, manufactured by Zyma-Blaes AG, Munich.

did not change significantly. The action of this substance was compared with the effects of intravenous injections of hyperosmotic Sorbitol.

Figure 1 shows the relation between the dose of the injected substance and the rate of resorption of CSF. Following up to 180 mg/kg of Rutoside the resorption remains constant, increasing with higher concentrations. The

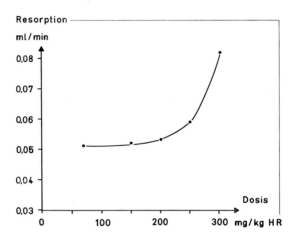

Fig. 1. Relation between dosis and disappearance of CSF after injection of 3′ 4, 7-tri-O-(β-Hydroxyethyl)-Rutoside. Each measuring point represents a mean value of 6 animals. The measuring period lasted 120 min after injection

highest dose we used was 250 mg/kg. Brain volume, CSF resorption, arterial blood pressure and endexpiratory CO_2-concentration were recorded simultaneously. The values were obtained by taking the mean of periods of 10 min. The brain volume decreased with increasing resorption or disappearance of CSF in open-skull experiments. We conducted 15 experiments of this type and observed almost the same pattern of reactions in all of them. CSF disappeared at a faster rate after injections of Rutoside and Sorbitol. The effect of one substance on brain volume was increased by the addition of the other substance. The correlation between brain volume and fluid-resorption in 6 experiments is shown in Fig. 2. There is no linear relation between the disappearance of CSF per unit of time and brain volume. With low doses of Rutoside or Sorbitol the resorption increases in inverse proportion to brain volume. However, with high doses of these substances, the resorption of fluid tends to approach a maximal value, whereas the brain volume continues to decrease. We refrained from following up these reactions with extreme concentrations to avoid disturbing the blood pressure regulation. Therefore, we cannot say at what concentration of Rutoside or Sorbitol the brain volume reaches its minimum. To find the underlying mechanisms of these effects we measured the resorption and osmotic pressure of the blood simultaneously. Figure 3 gives the values obtained in 7 rabbits when an injection of Rutoside was followed by an injection of Sorbitol 1–2 h later. When a dosage of 250 mg/kg Rutoside and 2 g/kg Sorbitol was used the rate of resorption was linearily dependent on the osmotic pressure of the blood. The osmotic effects may be one of the reasons why there was no linear correlation between the brain volume and the rate of disappearance of CSF. If the osmotic pressure exceeds a certain value, an effect upon the CSF production may be combined with resorption. It is, however, impossible to conclude from our experiments whether this is the case in the nonlinear slope of the relation.

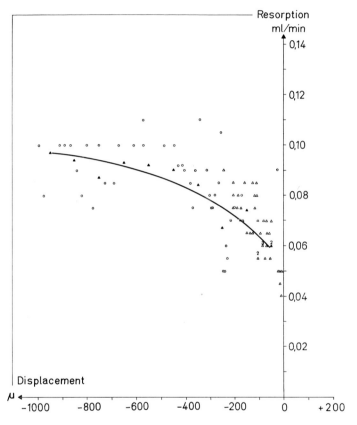

Fig. 2. Correlation between brain volume changes (displacement) and resorption of mock CSF during the action of Rutoside (△) and Sorbitol (○): mean values of 6 animals. Notice a non-linearity between disappearance of CSF and decrease of brain volume. Mean values are characterized by ▲

These experiments lasted no longer than 12 h. During this time the brain volume remained low in the experiment with Rutoside despite a renormalization of the fluid resorption after several hours. In the experiments with Sorbitol the fluid resorption remained high for longer than 8 h.

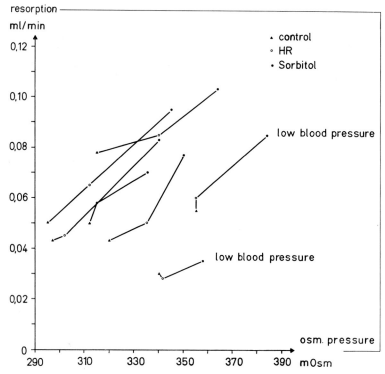

Fig. 3. Correlation between osmotic pressure of the arterial blood and the rate of resorption of Mock CSF. The osmotic pressure was increased by intravenous infusion of Rutoside or Sorbitol in 7 rabbits. In 2 animals the mean arterial blood pressure was between 50–80 mmHg

Conclusion

The experiments demonstrate that subarachnoid CSF-pressure in cats or rabbits with the head fixed in the upright position is not the same at the crossing of the sagittal and coronary sutures as in regions where a hydrostatic pressure is also affecting CSF-pressure. In normal cats or rabbits the mean CSF pressure at the convexity of the brain was about zero when the head was held in the upright position. This can also easily be seen when the dura is opened and no fluid escapes.

An increase in the mean CSF pressure is rapidly compensated by increases in CSF resorption, at least in the CSF-pressure range which we recorded. This points to the conclusion that a pathological increase in intracranial pressure requires an additional mechanism. With regard to the local resorption at the convexity of the brain, it is difficult to understand how CSF can be resorbed under static conditions exept by osmotic forces. Since, however, we demonstrated that in the closed skull high amplitudes of subarachnoid pressure appeared, which were synchronous to the cardiac and respiratory cycle, the findings of WELCH and FRIEDMAN [4] and PROKOP [5] are not in contradiction to our experiments. They found that the transport of CSF into the sinuses is mainly caused by hydrostatic pressure gradients.

Our findings do not allow conclusions as to the role of an active transport of fluid. HAMMERSEN [6] assumes that Rutoside affects the active transport mechanisms (pinocytosis) across the capillary wall. In recently published measurements of brain volume and subarachnoid pressure in combination with continuous recording of local blood flow, mean arterial blood pressure and cortical blood flow, we observed neither a strict correlation between blood flow and brain volume nor a correlation between CSF-pressure and blood flow [1]. It became evident, however, that disturbances of this pattern always influenced the subarachnoid pressure. We cannot expect a direct and linear relation between brain volume, osmotic pressure of the blood and CSF resorption, for we are dealing with at least three compartments in which fluid is exchanged: the CSF-blood system, the blood-brain system and the extracellular-intracellular system.

Summary

In normal, anaesthetized cats and rabbits a burr hole was drilled into the skull at the convexity of the brain. Tubes of different lengths were fixed the burr holes and the effect of increasing hydrostatic pressure was recorded. Between 0 and 8 mmHg hydrostatic pressure the rate of resorption of CSF from the arachnoid space was linearly related to this pressure. β-Hydroxyethyl-Rutoside and Sorbitol caused increases of resorption of the mock CSF in the tube. Continuous recording of CSF resorption and brain volume showed no strict correlation after administration of these substances. Since the rate of resorption varies according to the pressure, it is concluded that an increase in CSF alone cannot cause long-lasting pathological CSF-hypertension.

Key Words: Brain volume, hydrostatic pressure, Sorbitol, Rutoside, resorption.

References

1. BETZ, E., ROOS, W., VAMOSI, B., WEIDLER, R.: Die Medizinische Welt, **23** (N.F.), 579–583 (1972).
2. HEISEY, S. R., HELD, D., PAPPENHEIMER, J. R.: Amer. J. Physiol **203**, 775–781 (1962).
3. BERING, E. A., SATO, O.: J. Neurosurg. **20**, 1050–1063 (1963).
4. WELCH, K., FRIEDMAN, V.: Brain **83**, 454–469 (1960).
5. PROKOP, L. D.: Fed. Proc. **21**, 152 (1962).
6. HAMMERSEN, F.: Proc. Erg. Tagg. Dtsch. Ges. Angiol. 1970 (in Press.).

Cardiorespiratory Interaction during Increased Intracranial Pressure[1]

A. F. HECK

Sinus arrhythmia – the periodic acceleration-deceleration of instantaneous heart rate associated with respiration – is a biphasic phenomenon which may be modified by neural activity above and below the level of the brain stem and by peripheral factors as well. It has been shown that neural mechanisms subserving sinus arrhythmia require anatomic integrity of the brain stem to a point just rostral to the pontomedullary junction [1]. Focal lesions of the neuraxis, especially the brain stem, and general factors known to affect cardiovascular and respiratory function, such as increased intracranial pressure (ICP) or hypoxia, might, therefore, alter normal patterns of sinus arrhythmia and interaction of heart rate with respiration.

FITCH and McDOWALL [2] have recently introduced the concept of sinus arrhythmia index (SAI) in the evaluation of these cyclical changes in heart rate.

$$\text{SAI} = \frac{\text{Maximum heart rate} - \text{minimum heart rate}}{\text{mean heart rate}} \times 100\%.$$

This is a useful concept, since it indicates the relationship of fluctuation in instantaneous heart rate during respiration to the level of mean heart rate about which the fluctuation takes place. FITCH and McDOWALL have found increase in SAI to be an early, consistent sign in expanding intracranial lesions.

Monitoring of heart rate and respiration and observation of alterations in normal patterns of interaction between these parameters, occurring in sequence during the clinical course of patients with brain damage, may better define premonitory signs of evolving change in neurological status and, hopefully, identify points in the clinical course at which therapeutic intervention is indicated.

To test the rationale of this approach to the monitoring of patients, a series of experiments was carried out in cats in which the interaction of heart rate and respiration particularly was evaluated during transient increases in intracranial pressure. Similar evaluation of cardiorespiratory interaction has been carried out in normal conscious humans and in dogs anesthetized with pentobarbital sodium.

1 This work was supported by Public Health Service Grants NS-06779 (NINDS), GM 15700, (Division of General Medical Sciences) and FR 5379-10.

Material and Methods

Transient increases in epidural pressure of 3–60 mmHg were produced in cats anesthetized with pentobarbital sodium by injection via catheter of saline at body temperature into the epidural space. At the conclusion of experiments, brains were examined for pathology. ECG, aortic and central venous pressures, the transthoracic impedance pneumogram and contralateral epidural pressure were monitored continuously. The R-R interval of the ECG – reciprocal of the instantaneous heart rate – and the voltage output of the pneumograph at which each R-R interval was measured were recorded for each heart beat by means of a special monitoring system previously described [3]. R-R interval and respiratory data were listed from magnetic tape, then plotted against diurnal time, reproducing the respiratory signal and sequential R-R interval measurements as time functions. By these means, the maxima and minima of R-R interval measurements (and on instantaneous heart rate [2]) and their relationship to the phase of the respiratory cycle can be evaluated. The exact value of mean heart rate and of sinus arrhythmia index (SAI) from the beginning of one inspiration to the beginning of the next can also be calculated.

Results

Studies show that in normal humans and in anesthetized cats and dogs, the minimal R-R interval that is, the fastest instantaneous heart rate – occurs at or just after the end of inspiration. SAI varied 3–37% from breath-to-breath in conscious humans and from 8–45% in anesthetized dogs. This variation is not related to the duration of the respiratory cycle. In anesthetized cats, the fluctuation is smaller, from 1 to 3%.

Transient increase in ICP of cats in this experimental model produces tachycardia, sometimes preceded briefly by slight bradycardia, but, in later trials, large fluctuations in instantaneous heart rate coincident with respiration occur with little change in mean heart rate [4]. These changes are transient.

Induction of increased epidural pressure and simple tachycardia in cats is not accompanied by changes in SAI, and the relationship of minimum R-R interval to phase of respiration does not change. But in later trials, following induction of increased pressure, initial tachycardia and slowing of respiration is followed for several minutes by increase in SAI by as much as three- to tenfold. This increase is transient. During this time, minimal R-R intervals (i.e., maxima of instantaneous heart rate), which regularly occur during inspiration or early expiration, were found to shift into the inter-respiratory phase after completion of expiration and before the beginning of the next inspiration (Figs. 1–3), i.e., the cyclical changes in instantaneous heart rate were dissociated from

2 Instantaneous heart rate is calculated by dividing the R-R interval measurement into 60,000 milliseconds to obtain the equivalent frequency of heart rate in conventional beats per minute.

the phase of respiration in which they usually occur. Thus far, this dissociation is noted only in conjunction with increase in SAI, but conversely, increase in SAI may occur without dissociation of cardiochronotropic-respiratory phase relationships. The dissociation phenomenon is also transient; cardiorespiratory

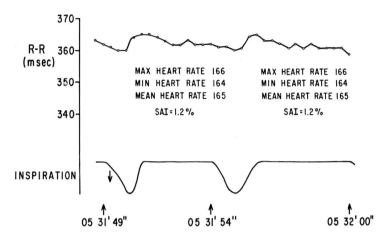

Fig. 1. Plot of individual, sequential R-R interval measurement (top) and impedance pneumogram (bottom) during two respirations from 5 h 31 min 49 sec to 5 h 32 min 00 sec in an anesthetized cat prior to induction of increased ICP. Note that shortest R-R intervals (i.e. maxima of instantaneous heart rate) occur at the end of inspiration

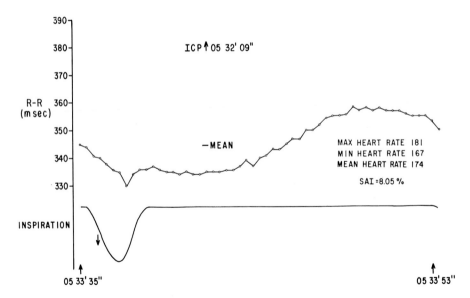

Fig. 2. Plot of sequential R-R intervals and pneumogram during one respiration beginning 1 min 26 sec after induction of transient increase in ICP at 5 h 32 min 09 sec. Duration of this respiratory cycle: 18 sec. Note that the shortest R-R interval occurs just after the end of inspiration

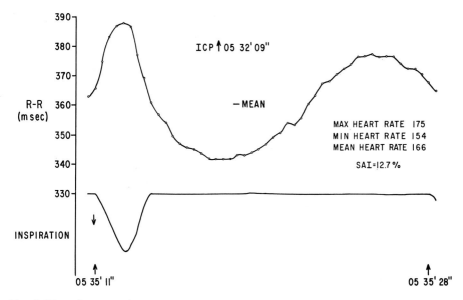

Fig. 3. Plot of sequential R-R intervals and pneumogram during one respiration beginning 3 min 2 sec after transient ICP increase induced at 5 h 32 min 09 sec. Duration of this respiratory cycle: 17 sec. The shortest R-R interval now occurs in the interrespiratory period of the respiratory cycle. SAI, mean heart rate and heart rate-respiratory phase relationships returned to values shown in Fig. 1 by 5 h 39 min 00 sec

relationships return to normal within 5–10 min, despite the fact that pathoanatomic studies, as previously reported [4], often show extensive petechial and confluent hemorrhages and/or edema in the cerebrum and brain stem down to the pontomedullary junction.

Discussion

The results of these studies in cats confirm the observations of FITCH and McDOWALL in dogs [2] that SAI may be increased significantly with induction of intracranial hypertension. It seems significant, however, that the changes in SAI may be transient, even in the presence of extensive neuropathology, and that increase in SAI may occur with little or no change in mean heart rate from levels pertaining prior to induction of intracranial pressure increase.

The observation in these experiments that maximal instantaneous heart rate may be dissociated during increased ICP from the phase of respiration in which it usually occurs has not been previously reported, but is of a genre similar to observations recently noted by MARKAKIS [5] in which the periodic reduction in ICP pulse amplitude occurring during inspiration was found to shift into the expiratory phase of respiration in the presence of intracranial hypertension.

Observation that cyclical changes normally occurring in cardiovascular and intracranial parameters in association with respiration have changed in their amplitudes, or have undergone a dissociation in relationship to the phase of respiration in which they usually occur, may be an important premonitory sign of brain decompensation during changes in intracranial pressure.

Summary

Studies in anesthetized cats during transient increases in ICP confirm the observations of Fitch and McDowall [2] that sinus arrhythmia index (SAI) may increase significantly during intracranial hypertension. Changes in SAI may occur with little or no change in mean heart rate and may be transient even in the presence of parenchymal hemorrhages. Furthermore, cyclical changes in instantaneous heart rate may be dissociated from their usual relationship to phase of respiration. Changes in amplitude and phase relationships to respiration of cyclical changes in cardiovascular and intracranial parameters usually associated with respiration may be useful signs in monitoring during intracranial hypertension.

Key Words: Instantaneous heart rate, sinus arrhythmia index, respiration, brain hemorrhage.

References

1. McCrady, J. D., Vallbona, C., Hoff, H. E.: Neural origin of the respiratory-heart rate-response. Amer. J. Physiol. **211**, 323–328 (1966).
2. Fitch, W., McDowall, D. G.: Vasodilating anaesthetics and pressures in different compartments of the skull. In: Brierley, J. B., Meldrum, B. S. (Eds.): Brain Hypoxia, p. 113–117. Philadelphia: J. B. Lippincott 1971.
3. Heck, A. F., Minter, R., Caggiano, V.: A system for continuous recording of cardiovascular time interval data and respiration. Med. Res. Engr. (in press).
4. Heck, A. F.: Cardiovascular and respiratory changes during transient increase in intracranial pressure. In: C. Fieschi (Ed.), Cerebral Blood Flow and Intracranial Pressure. p. 486–492. Basel: S. Karger 1972.
5. Markakis, E., Brock, M., Beck, J., Dietz, H.: The recording of brain pulsations during intracranial pressure measurements. Acta neurol. scand. **48**, 254 (1972).

The Effect of Hypoxia on the Cushing Response[1]

J. T. HOFF and R. A. MITCHELL

Introduction

Previous investigators have suggested that the systemic arterial pressure (SAP) elevation evoked by elevated intracranial pressure (ICP) – the Cushing response – is due to hypoxia [1], ischemia [2, 3], pressure upon or distortion of the brainstem [4], or a combination of these stimuli. Because of the apparent inseparability of the possible stimuli, efforts to identify the essential stimulus, and thereby the nature of its origin, have been frustrated. Cushing originally proposed ischemia of the medulla as the fundamental stimulus [2]. That the response could be triggered by localized pressure on the dorsal surface of the medulla has also been recognized [5]. Hypoxia was implicated when the typical Cushing response was augmented during asphyxia [1]. While recent works have placed more emphasis upon the pressure/distortion concept, hypoxia has not been eliminated as an essential component of the response. In order to determine the effect of hypoxia upon the Cushing response, the following study was done.

Method

14 adult cats were anesthetized with pentobarbital (30 mg/kg). A cannula was inserted into the femoral artery and attached to a P 23 a Statham transducer for measurement of SAP. A tracheal cannula was placed and connected to a Harvard respirator. Mechanical ventilation, adjusted to maintain end tidal CO_2 (ET CO_2) at 4–5% and monitored by an infrared CO_2 gas analyzer, was begun after the animal was paralyzed with gallamine triethiodide (10 mg/kg). The animal was placed supine in a stereotaxic frame. Body temperature was monitored by a rectal temperature probe and regulated (36–38° C) by a heating lamp.

One phrenic nerve was divided over the scaleneus aticus muscle and the proximal stump placed on a bipolar platinum electrode to record efferent discharge. One sympathetic cervical trunk was divided proximal to the superior ganglion and a few teased fibers of the proximal stump were placed on a mono-polar platinum electrode to record preganglionic efferent discharge. The nerve

1 This investigation was partially supported by Trauma Center Program Project Grant No. GM-18470, NIHNDS Training Grant No. 5593, and Teacher-Investigator Award NS 11051 NSRB.

preparations were bathed in mineral oil (37° C) and their signals were displayed on an oscilloscope.

ICP was measured by an epidural balloon sealed in a parietal burr hole by dental cement and attached to a P 23 a Statham transducer. A second burr hole in the opposite parietal bone was made to accommodate a multiperforated PE50 polyethylene subdural catheter sealed there with dental cement. ICP was elevated by hand injections of 37° C saline into the subdural space and displayed on the oscilloscope. SAP, ICP, ET CO_2 and sympathetic discharge were continuously recorded by a Grass polygraph. Arterial blood gases and inhaled oxygen (F_IO_2) were measured intermittently.

ICP was elevated abruptly (< 1.0 sec) for a brief period (< 2.0 sec) or gradually (> 30 sec) for a long period (15–30 sec). Control blood pressure responses to elevated ICP were obtained during normoxia (F_IO_2 20%, PaO_2 105). Inhaled oxygen was then either reduced to hypoxia (F_IO_2 11%, PaO_2 24) or increased to hyperoxia (F_IO_2 100%, PaO_2 450) and blood pressure responses to elevated ICP observed. The latency, magnitude, duration and threshold of evoked vasomotor responses during normoxia, hypoxia, and hyperoxia were compared.

Results

During normoxia a gradual elevation of ICP evoked an SAP elevation of greater magnitude ($P < 0.01$) and longer latency than did an abrupt elevation of ICP (Fig. 1). Further, the duration of the blood pressure response was usually longer and the threshold lower when ICP was elevated gradually.

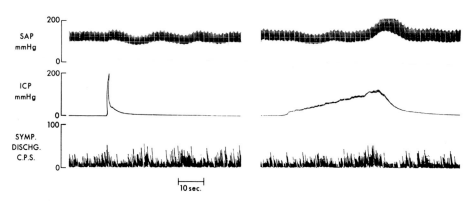

Fig. 1. Cushing response to abrupt (left) and gradual (right) elevation of ICP. A SAP elevation of greater magnitude and longer duration occurred from gradual elevation of ICP. Note the sympathetic discharge resulting from elevation of ICP and coincident with SAP variations

During hypoxia the latency, threshold, and magnitude of SAP elevation following either abrupt or gradual ICP elevation did not differ significantly from responses evoked during normoxia. The duration of blood pressure elevation

Table 1. SAP response to abrupt or gradual ICP elevation during normoxia or hypoxia

Systemic arterial pressure response	Abrupt ICP elevation				Gradual ICP elevation			
	normoxia		hypoxia		normoxia		hypoxia	
	N	BP Response	N	BP Response	N	BP Response	N	BP Response
Magnitude (% of mean SAP)	25	24 ± 18	8	31 ± 21	21	39 ± 18	15	35 ± 27
Latency[a] (seconds)	28	7.6 ± 6.9	10	6.0 ± 3.6	12	15 ± 10	4	12 ± 6.3
Duration[a] (seconds)	15	41 ± 51	11	91 ± 78	11	57 ± 44	3	67 ± 37
Threshold (mmHg ICP	22	136 ± 41	13	128 ± 59	10	126 ± 37	15	128 ± 51

[a] Latency and duration of the SAP response were determined when mean SAP elevation exceeded 10 % of mean SAP baseline.

during hypoxia, however, usually exceeded the duration of the response during normoxia (Table 1).

During hyperoxia SAP elevation produced by increased ICP failed to differ significantly from responses observed during normoxia.

Abrupt elevation of ICP above threshold during normoxia evoked a graded burst of sympathetic discharge (Fig. 2). Usually the discharge occurred within 100 msec, lasted for more than 45 sec, and was associated with SAP elevation that followed the initial sympathetic burst. The latency of the sympathetic response to elevated ICP was similar during normoxia and hypoxia; the background discharge and duration of sympathetic response to elevated ICP were greater during hypoxia.

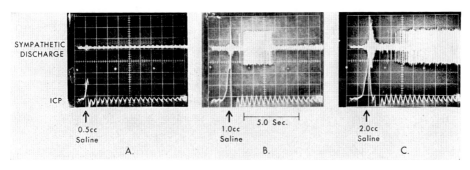

Fig. 2. Sympathetic discharge resulting from abrupt elevation of ICP. Note the brief latency and graded magnitude of the sympathetic response to ICP

Phrenic nerve efferent discharge was rhythmic and independent from the respirator. The rhythm, more rapid during hypoxia, was interrupted consistently when ICP exceeded SAP, but resumed when ICP was reduced.

Discussion

We sought to separate hypoxia as one possible stimulus for the Cushing response from other commonly recognized stimuli, namely pressure, distortion, and ischemia. A significant change in the characteristics of the response during hypoxia was anticipated, provided hypoxia was an essential stimulus. In our study hypoxia had little apparent effect upon the classical response evoked by either an abrupt or gradual elevation of intracranial pressure. Thus, hypoxia was probably not fundamental to the Cushing response.

The relative vulnerability of medullary vasomotor neurons to hypoxia is not known. It remains possible that the degree of hypoxia used in this experiment was insufficient to affect the response produced by vasomotor neurons. Consequently, more severe hypoxia may play a role in the Cushing response, but the vasomotor instability that accompanies severe hypoxia ($PaO_2 < 24$) will likely preclude studies of the response during more profound hypoxia.

We have confirmed mediation of the Cushing response by the sympathetic nervous system [6]. Elevation of ICP evokes a sympathetic discharge of short latency, graded magnitude and long duration, which in turn effects a blood pressure rise.

Pressure upon and distortion of the medullary vasomotor center remains the most likely primary stimulus. Ischemia, the result of progressive elevation of ICP, probably affects the response secondarily by increasing the susceptibility of vasomotor neurons to pressure. Thus, the more profound Cushing response achieved by a gradual rise of ICP, in contrast to an abrupt rise, is probably a response to both ischemia and pressure/distortion of the vasomotor center.

Summary

The Cushing response was evoked by intracranial subdural injections of saline in cats. No significant differences in latency, threshold, magnitude, and duration of the response were observed during normoxia (PaO_2 105), hypoxia (PaO_2 24), and hyperoxia (PaO_2 450). The sympathetic response to elevated ICP was of brief latency and graded magnitude, and was manifested by an elevation of SAP. This study suggests that hypoxia is not an essential component of the Cushing response.

Key Words: Cushing response, hypoxia, sympathetic discharge, intracranial pressure.

References

1. Yesinick, L., Gellhorn, E.: Studies on increased intracranial pressure and its effects during anoxia and hypoglycemia. Amer. J. Physiol. **128**, 185–194 (1939).
2. Cushing, H.: Some experimental and clinical observations concerning states of increased intracranial tension. Amer. J. med. Sci. **124**, 375–400 (1902).

3. Guyton, A. C., Satterfield, J. H.: Vasomotor waves possibly resulting from CNS ischemic reflex oscillation. Amer. J. Physiol. **170**, 601–605 (1952).
4. Thompson, R. K., Malina, S.: Dynamic axial brain stem distortion as a mechanism explaining the cardiorespiratory changes in increased intracranial pressure. J. Neurosurg. **16**, 664–675 (1959).
5. Hoff, J. T., Reis, D. J.: Localization of regions mediating the Cushing response in CNS of cat. Arch. Neurol. **23**, 228–240 (1970).
6. Grimson, K. S., Wilson, H., Phemister, D. B.: The early and remote effects of total and paravertebral sympathectomy on blood pressure. Ann. Surgery **106**, 801–825 (1937).

Arterial pCO_2 Effect at Various Levels of Intracranial Pressure[1]

G. W. Kindt and H. H. Gosch

Introduction

Although hyperventilation has long been known to reduce intracranial pressure, the limits of application are still not defined. As early as 1894, Mosso [1] reported that hyperventilation reduced the tension of the brain in 2 patients with skull defects. Hyperventilation has long been used for brain relaxation during surgery. Recent reports have stated beneficial effects from a lowered arterial partial pressure of carbon dioxide (pCO_2) in patients with head injuries [2, 3]. Some have cautioned the use of hyperventilation because of the possible danger of reduced cerebral blood flow [4, 5]. Also, patients in certain stages of decompensation are known not to respond to reduction in arterial pCO_2 [6]. This study was undertaken to further define the effect of varying arterial pCO_2 at various base levels of intracranial pressure.

Materials and Methods

8 adult Macaca mulatta monkeys were anesthetized with intramuscular phencyclidine hydrochloride. The animals were tracheostomized and ventilated with a modified anesthesia machine capable of delivering any desired mixture of nitrogen, oxygen and carbon dioxide. On some occasions cerebral blood flow was monitored with a Peltier flow device. Intracranial pressure recordings were made with a subdural strain gauge transducer, as well as a subdural fluid manometer. Femoral artery blood pressured were continuously recorded and a mass spectrometer was used to record the arterial pO_2 and pCO_2.

Baseline recordings were made of the effect of varying the arterial pCO_2 by increments from 20–80 mmHg. The intracranial pressure was then elevated by increments of approximately 20 mmHg, and the arterial pCO_2 adjustments were repeated for each increment of raised intracranial pressure. Observations of the clinical status of the animal were made as the intracranial pressure was adjusted. A graphic comparison of intracranial pressure with arterial pCO_2 was made under the conditions described.

---

1 Supported by a gift of Mrs. Arvella Bentley to the neurosurgical research fund.

Results

Intracranial pressure was noted to vary directly with the arterial pCO$_2$ until decompensation occurred. At lower levels of intracranial pressure the changes were small with variations in arterial pCO$_2$. When the baseline pressure was higher, the intracranial pressure changes were more marked with changes in pCO$_2$ (Fig. 1). The greatest changes in pressure occurred in the midrange of pCO$_2$ values, with less response both at lower and at higher levels of pCO$_2$ (Fig. 2).

No significant deleterious effects seemed to occur to the animals until the intracranial pressure reached 70–90 mmHg. At that point the animals' pupils usually dilated and were fixed to light stimulus. After the pupils dilated there was no longer a significant intracranial pressure response to changes in arterial pCO$_2$ (Fig. 2). Even if the baseline intracranial pressure was reduced the pCO$_2$ response did not return. However, further elevations of intracranial pressure could still trigger systemic hypertension (Cushing response).

Discussion

The increase in intracranial pressure with elevated arterial pCO$_2$ is due to the increased intracranial blood volume from the vasodilatation produced by the CO$_2$. At lower baselines of intracranial pressure there is still room for compensation by venous collapse and CSF movement. However, at the higher baselines of intracranial pressure there are no longer compensation mechanisms available and the intracranial pressure rises markedly with changes in pCO$_2$. Certain patients in a comparable category with elevated pressure might benefit greatly from hyperventilation.

The maximum effect from changes in pCO$_2$ occurs at the midrange (30 to 50 mmHg) with less change at the higher and lower levels. This reduced response to pCO$_2$, less than 30 mmHg, has been reported clinically [6]. An explanation can be given by simply relating intracranial pressure to cerebral blood flow. In fact, the curve relating CBF and pCO$_2$ is very similar to those in Fig. 2 [7]. The maximum CBF change also occurs in the midrange of pCO$_2$.

Decompensation occurs at the higher levels of intracranial pressure, and there is cessation of the intracranial pressure response to pCO$_2$ changes. This lack of intracranial pressure response to pCO$_2$ has been described in patients [6]. This occurs when the CBF response to CO$_2$ has ceased and clinically is a morbid condition. In our animals at this stage there was not yet brain stem failure because the Cushing reflex could still be elicited with further elevation of intracranial pressure.

These laboratory studies cannot be easily related to a patient with increased intracranial pressure due to a head injury. This experimental model was an acute preparation of a healthy brain until the point of decompensation.

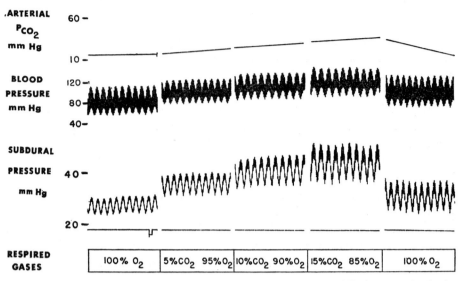

Fig. 1. Arterial pCO₂ and subdural pressure sample tracing in the mildly hypertensive brain. A significant rise of pressure is noted as the pCO₂ level increases with changes in the inspired gas mixture

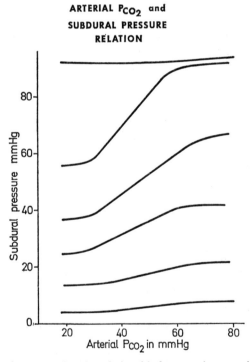

Fig. 2. Profile curves demonstrating the relationship between intracranial pressure and alteration in arterial pCO_2. After decompensation there is no longer a response to pCO_2 as shown by the top line

Patients with head injuries have part of their brain which is healthy and part which is decompensated because of the injury. The reduction in intracranial pressure with hyperventilation occurs because of the CO$_2$ response in the healthy brain. This pressure reduction may be beneficial to some patients because it can prevent the spreading decompensation and necrosis from the damaged brain. Patients with severely damaged and decompensated brain probably would not benefit from hyperventilation.

Summary

The effect of changes in arterial pCO$_2$ on intracranial pressure at various baselines of intracranial hypertension was investigated. Intracranial pressure varied directly with arterial pCO$_2$ until the higher levels of intracranial pressure were reached and decompensation occurred. Changes in pCO$_2$ had a relatively greater effect at higher baselines of intracranial pressure than at lower baselines. The greatest changes in intracranial pressure occurred during the midrange of pCO$_2$ values with less change occurring at the lower and at the higher levels of pCO$_2$.

Key Words : Arterial pCO$_2$, intracranial pressure.

References

1. Mosso, A.: Die Temperatur des Gehirns. Leipzig: Verlag von Veit & Comp. 1894.
2. Gordon, E.: The effect of controlled ventilation on the clinical course of patients with severe traumatic brain injury. In: Russell, R. W. R. (Ed.): Brain and Blood Flow, p. 365 to 369. London: Pitman Medical and Scientific Publ. Co., Ltd. 1970.
3. Rossanda, M.: Prolonged hyperventilation in treatment of unconscious patients with severe brain injuries. Scand. J. clin. Lab. Invest. (Suppl. 102) 22, XIII:E (1968).
4. Cohen, P. J., Alexander, S. C., Wollman, H.: Effects of hypocarbia and of hypoxia with normocarbia on cerebral blood flow and metabolism in man. Scand. J. clin. Lab. Invest (Suppl. 102), 22, XIII:E (1968).
5. Gotoh, F., Meyer, J. S., Takagi, Y.: Cerebral effects of hyperventilation in man. Arch. Neurol. 12, 410–423 (1965).
6. Paul, R. L., Polanco, O., Turney, S. Z., McAslan, T. C., Cowley, R. A.: Intracranial pressure responses to alterations in arterial carbon dioxide pressure in patients with head injuries. J. Neurosurg. 36, 714–720 (1972).
7. Reivich, M.: Arterial pCO$_2$ and cerebral hemodynamics. Amer. J. Physiol. 206, 25–35 (1964).

Comments to Session 6

H. Troupp and M. Brock

The two first papers reported rather contradictory results, presumably because of technical differences. It does seem odd that Brodersen and associates applied a cisternal pressure of 50 mmHg, with little reaction in so-called interstitial pressure; but compare with the paper by Lorenz and Grote (p. 265–269). As clinicians we see two possible applications of recording pressures within brain tissue: to gauge whether a lesion is expanding, i.e. to compare pressure within the lesion with ventricular pressure; and, as Brock suggested, to measure pressure postoperatively in the tumor bed after removal of a tumor.

The paper by Betz and associates touched on a novel method of attacking swelling of the brain by increasing the rate of absorption of CSF; it remains to be seen whether this is applicable clinically. It should be remembered that in conditions where edema of the brain is important, i.e. injuries, infarctions and hemorrhages of the brain, the ventricles and the subarachnoid space are very narrow.

Heck, and Hoff and Mitchell dealt with different types of systemic response to a rise in ICP. Heck used the ratio of respiration to pulse rate and its variations (given as a sinus arrhythmia index – SAI); Hoff and Mitchell used the burst of activity in the cervical sympathetic chain. The latter authors were mainly concerned with finding whether hypoxia was important for the Cushing response and did not find it to be so. Personally, we think attempts at estimating ICP from other parameters are interesting, but all methods must be extensively tested in clinical practice *in patients who have some sort of direct and reliable ICP recording running*. The so-called Cushing response is a laboratory product; by the time it becomes recognizable in human beings it is usually too late to do anything. In the discussion, McGraw said that he had seen an increase in the sinus arrhythmia index (SAI) in patients with slowly rising ICP, but a decrease during plateau waves.

Kindt and Gosch investigated the ICP response to a rise in $PaCO_2$, starting from different baselines of ICP. They found that a rise in $PaCO_2$ caused a pronounced increase within the ICP range between 20 and 40 mmHg. Again, this suggests the importance of maintaining a reasonably narrow range of $PaCO_2$, e.g. 25–35 mmHg.

This session very clearly showed that experimental research is very necessary but the difference between healthy laboratory animals and desperately ill human beings should be borne in mind.

Session 7

Acute Brain Injury
(Clinical)

Minute by Minute Intracranial Pressure Monitoring as a Guide to Management of Pathological Intracranial Pressure[1]

R. M. P. Donaghy and M. Numoto

Intracranial pressure (ICP), mostly epidural, in 65 clinical cases including 56 head injuries, 3 encephalitides, 3 ruptured aneurysms, 2 vascular malformations with rupture and 1 hydrocephalus, has been monitored during 1965 to 1971 by means of the pressure switch (PSW) developed by us. The period of monitoring was up to 14 days.

Method

Currently we are using three types of PSW to measure ICP. The latest one, pressure indicating bag (PIB), is still in the development stage and has not been used in clinical cases. All these three devices depend on the principle of balancing.

The technical aspects of the first one, the electrical PSW [1, 2] and the second, the fiber-optic PSW[2] are described elsewhere.

The third and the most recent one is PIB. This is a flat balloon, 10 mm in diameter and 1 mm thick made of Silastic (Dow Corning) sheet with a metal frame. A semi-rigid vinyl tubing with an inner diameter of 0.5 mm is attached to the balloon. The PIB is filled with a colored liquid to the half way mark of the tubing. The volume of the empty portion of the tubing is slightly larger than the volume of the balloon (ca. 0.08 cc) so that even when the balloon is completely compressed the liquid does not come out from the open end of the tubing. The level of the liquid in the tubing is marked "0" (zero calibration) when the pressure applied on the bag and the pressure applied at the open end of the tubing is equal. The entire system is shown in Fig. 1.

To measure ICP the system is pressurized by the syringe until the liquid level in the tubing reaches the "0". The ICP is now balanced to the pressure indicated on the manometer. The automatic system has a small photo-electric level detector attached at the "0" point and this triggers a servo-pump and automatically records the pressure, as in the system for the electric PSW [2].

1 Supported by the John A. Hartford Foundation.
2 Ladd Research Industries, Inc., U.S.A.

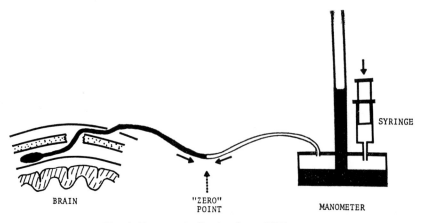

Fig. 1. Pressure indicating bag. (PIB) system

Clinical Results

Head Injury

56 patients monitored by the PSW constituted only approximately 3.5% of our total head injury cases during this period. They were the most severely injured. Criteria for selection were:

1. Comatose or stuporous at entry.
2. Decerebrate or decorticate at entry.
3. Burr hole had been made or was to be made.

As shown in Fig. 2 the highest pressure recorded in the head injury group was 131 mmHg in a patient who died. But a pressure of 123 mmHg was recorded in a patient who recovered.

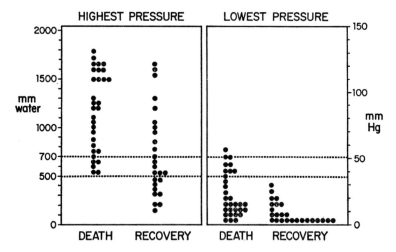

Fig. 2. Highest and lowest pressures in 56 head injuries

The height of pressure alone was not the most important factor, yet high pressure does alter the prognosis in an unfavorable way. 26 of the 31 deaths (84%) had pressures above 50 mmHg at some time. Only 11 of the 25 recoveries (44%) had pressures in this range.

A prompt response to hyperventilation and mannitol which persisted for several (6–8) hours was a good prognostic sign. A fall, however, which lasted about an hour or less was a poor prognostic sign, and these patients had a tendency to have less and less effect from each succeeding dose.

35 mmHg we regard as a critical level which agrees with LUNDBERG's [3] clinical observations. Our animal studies [4] by observing through a cranial window, show that this pressure range produces occlusion of the cortical veins.

All 9 patients whose pressure never fell below this level died. All 25 recoveries fell below this level.

There are a number of negative exceptions to the general rule. That is, patients whose pressures were not high but who did not recover. These were more likely to have severe lacerations and contusions, and less general swelling than those who died with high pressure.

Two Compartment Study

One of the advantages of the PSW is ease of multiple implantations. This makes it possible to monitor the ICP from several compartments simultanously. We have monitored ICP of the middle and the posterior fossae in a few cases. One of them, which is believed to be the most important record, is shown in Fig. 3. A 13 year old boy who had a severe fracture with subdural hematoma had exploration of both middle and posterior fossae. He had a PSW placed in each. Post-operatively pressures ran in the 20 mmHg range for a period of time, but at one point pressure rose in the middle fossa but to a lesser extent in the posterior fossa (A in Fig. 3). It responded to hyperventilation, rose slightly as he shivered, as he was undergoing hypothermia, and fell with *Thorazine* (B in Fig. 3). When hyperventilation was stopped it rose again (C in Fig. 3), but this time it did not rise in the posterior fossa to any significant degree. We wondered if this meant a block at the tentorium or merely retention of carbon dioxide with a greater rise over the large cerebrum than over the small cerebellum. We reasoned that if the latter were the case hyperventilation should reduce the pressure in both areas. If this were a block, hyperventilation should cause pressure to fall in the middle fossa, but it should rise in the posterior fossa as communication was restored. This actually happened (D in Fig. 3), and we believe this graph is the demonstration of a block and its release. We were unaware, during this time, of blood pressure, pulse or pupillary changes or any change in the patient's ICP. We have noted in general a lag of from 5–30 min between the recording of a high ICP and its reflection in blood pressure, pulse or pupillary response.

Encephalitides

3 out of 4 encephalitides were monitored. They were the only cases in which we made a burr hole for the sole purpose of ICP monitoring. One died with ICP as high as 176 mmHg which never responded to therapy. The other two

cases whose highest ICP was 118 mmHg and 17.6 mmHg respectively responded at once to hyperventilation. They recovered fully in a few weeks with Decadron and Mannitol. One who was not monitored died with clinical signs of herniation. Post mortem showed pressure cones both of the temporal lobes and the cerebellar tonsils.

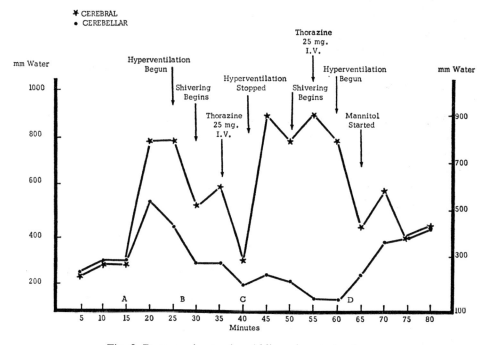

Fig. 3. Pressure changes in middle and posterior fossae

Conclusion

1. The intracranial pressures of 65 neurosurgical cases were monitored by means of pressure switches developed by us.

2. Such monitoring is valuable first of all as to prognosis.

3. It is also valuable in signaling the need for therapy, since rise in pressure may preceed by 5–30 min changes in pulse, blood pressure, pupils etc, and this is a period long enough to institute therapy.

Key Words: Pressure switch, head injury, encephalitis.

References

1. Numoto, M., Slater, J. P., Donaghy, R. M. P.: An Implantable Switch for Monitoring Intracranial Pressure. Lancet, March 5, 528 (1966).
2. Numoto, M., Slater, J. P., Donaghy, R. M. P.: An Automatic Method of Measuring and Recording Intracranial Pressure. Med. Res. Engin. 8, 38–39 (1969).

3. LUNDBERG, N., TROUPP, H., LORIN, H.: Continous Recording of the Ventricular-Fluid Pressure in Patients with Severe Acute Traumatic Brain Injury. J. Neurosurg. 22, 581–590 (1965).
4. NUMOTO, M., DONAGHY, R. M. P.: Effect of Local Pressure on Cortical Electrical Activity and Cortical Vessels in the Dog. J. Neurosurg. 33, 381-387 (1970).

Intraventricular Pressure after Severe Brain Injuries: Prognostic Value and Correlation with Blood Pressure and Jugular Venous Oxygen Tension

H. Troupp, T. Kuurne, M. Kaste, M. Vapalahti, and S. Valtonen

We have previously drawn attention to the close correlation between intraventricular pressure (IVP) and the fate of a patient with a severe brain injury [1, 2] (see also Table 1), and to the correlation between respiratory func-

Table 1

Pressure level	Intraventricular pressure correlated with the fate of the patients, January 1st, 1967 to June 30th, 1972			
	Recovered	Vegetative survival	Dead	Total
Below 15 mmHg	11	4	1	16
15–30 mmHg	14	7	2	23
31–60 mmHg	5	4	5	14
Above 60 mmHg	2	1	18	21
	32	16	26	74

tion and the fate of the patient [2, 3]. An experimental study [4, 5] showed that after a severe brain injury in rabbits the ratio of cerebral sinus pressure (CSP) to blood pressure (BP) correlated well with other important parameters; the same study also showed that sudden swings in cerebral venous oxygen tension indicated a worse prognosis. As there are still many patients with brain injuries for whom it is impossible to make an accurate prognosis at present, and as rabbits are not humans, we investigated the same parameters as in the experimental study [4, 5] in patients, assuming that cerebral sinus pressure and intraventricular pressure are identical in the rabbit [6].

Patients and Methods

Lundberg's method [7] was used to record intraventricular pressure (IVP) as described in previous reports [1, 2, 3]. For the recording of arterial blood pressure (BP) a catheter was inserted into either the superficial temporal or the radial artery, and connected to a Statham P23AA transducer. To allow measurement of jugular venous oxygen tension, the jugular vein was punctured high in the neck with a Dameco catheter, and through this an oxygen needle electrode (Metra Mess- und Frequenztechnik Radebeul) was inserted. The electrode was polarized and the signal from the electrode amplified by the M 65 F amplifier manufactured by the same firm; the output from the amplifier was further amplified in a Norma 709 amplifier and recorded with a three-channel inkwriter. The electrode was calibrated in saline or in a solution of 0.1 % β-propiolactone, by bubbling nitrogen or a known mixture of nitrogen and oxygen through it.

There were 10 patients in all. IVP and BP only were recorded continuously in 5 patients; IVP, BP and jugular venous oxygen tension ($PjvO_2$) in 4 patients, the longest recording of $PjvO_2$ being 2 h; and IVP and $PjvO_2$ were recorded in one patient.

Results

The IVP levels and the fate of the patients correlated as follows: 2 patients had an IVP of less than 15 mmHg; they recovered. 4 patients had an IVP of 15–30 mmHg; they recovered. 2 patients had an IVP of 31–60 mmHg; one recovered and one remained a vegetative wreck. 2 patients had an IVP of more than 60 mmHg; they died.

It would not have been possible to improve upon the prognostic accuracy by calculating the IVP/BP ratio. Since there was little apparent correlation between IVP and BP, the recordings were analyzed very carefully. One person assessed IVP and another BP, each without knowing what the other parameter was at that moment. The recordings were sampled at 1 h intervals, and a period of 5 min was chosen at each even hour. Changes were assessed both by *level* and by *direction*. The level was assessed as higher, the same or lower than the previous sampling; the direction as rising, even or falling within the 5-min period assessed. A change in IVP had to be at least 5 mmHg; a change in BP at least 10 mmHg.

415 observations were made of the level and direction of IVP and BP. In 206/415 instances the levels of IVP and BP in relation to the previous sampling did not follow a similar trend; for instance, there may have been a rise in BP but none in IVP. In 66/415 instances there was a discrepancy in the direction of change, if any, between IVP and BP; for instance, there may have been a rise in BP while IVP remained the same.

A rise in IVP is clinically more dangerous than a fall; consequently, we analyzed the cases in which there was a *rise* of at least 5 mmHg in IVP. There were 76 such cases; in 60 of these the rise in IVP was not reflected by a rise in BP. We also analyzed those instances in which IVP was rising during the 5-min period sampled; there were 56 such instances, and in 52 of these the rise in IVP was not reflected by a rise in BP.

A rise of 5 mmHg in IVP may be thought unimportant, and we therefore analyzed the recordings for major changes in IVP, classified into two groups: changes of 11–20 mmHg, and changes of more than 20 mmHg. We found 19 instances of a rise of 11–20 mmHg in IVP from one hour to the next; in 17 of these the higher level of IVP was not reflected in BP. We found 12 instances of a fall of 11–20 mmHg in IVP; in 10 instances, this fall was not reflected in BP.

Finally, we found 14 instances of a rise of more than 20 mmHg in IVP; in 7 of these, the higher level of IVP was not reflected in BP. There were also 12 instances of a fall of more than 20 mmHg in IVP; in 7 of these, the fall was not reflected in BP.

Figure 1 shows a 6-h recording of IVP and BP with little correlation between the two parameters.

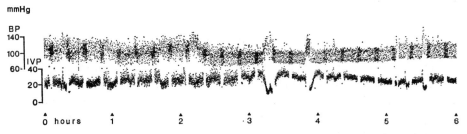

Fig. 1. Man, 24. He was involved in a car crash on Dec. 24th, 1971, and was immediately unconscious. He was admitted to the Neurosurgical Clinic; a right carotid angiogram showed no mass lesion. An intraventricular and arterial blood pressure recording was started on Dec. 26th. As the IVP was rather high, hyperventilation was started, but discontinued on the following day, when IVP stayed below 30 mmHg in general. The recording shown was obtained on Dec. 29th. The patient survived, but remained a vegetative wreck

$PjvO_2$ levels were normal in general, and they remained remarkably stable even during swings in IVP (Fig. 2). In the recordings we have made so far, the IVP has not been particularly labile, so we do not yet know how widely IVP would need to vary to lead to changes in $PjvO_2$.

Discussion

The record of the blood pressure did not materially contribute to establishing the prognosis in patients with severe brain injuries. The 2 patients who died had a high IVP, the lethal implications of which we had realized in 1967 [1]. One adult patient had a rather high IVP, which was reduced by hyperventilation and then stayed down, but he remained a vegetative wreck. In our experience this is typical for such adults, though children have responded to hyperventilation [3].

Direct and accurate recording of arterial blood pressure emphasized that, though blood pressure is still often thought to be an important factor in monitoring patients with brain injuries, *there is little correlation between IVP and BP*. Certainly there were instances when a rise in IVP coincided with a rise in BP, particularly if the rise in IVP was over 20 mmHg, but this BP response was unreliable. It has been known for many years that the Cushing response so regularly seen in animal experiments is often absent in clinical practice [8, 9], even when the method of recording BP is much more refined and accurate than the usual clinical cuff-and-stethoscope method. We think it is high time to realize the futility of trying to gauge IVP from changes in or from the level of BP.

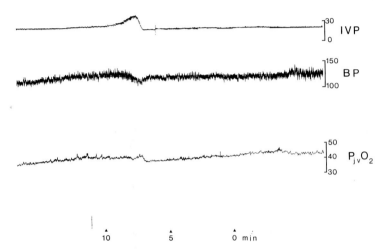

Fig. 2. This recording should be read from right to left. Pressures and tensions are given as mmHg. Man, 20. On April 11th, 1972, he crashed into a lorry with his motorcycle and was immediately unconscious. A right carotid angiogram on the day of admission showed a thin acute subdural haematoma, which was not operated upon. On April 12th an intraventricular and arterial blood pressure recording was started. The recording shown was obtained on April 12th; there was no apparent reason for the swing in IVP and BP at 7 min. The patient recovered consciousness at the beginning of May; by June 30th, he was still occasionally confused, but able to walk unaided

The recording of $PjvO_2$ has not yet contributed perceptibly to accurate prognosis. Though we intend to collect more data, we think it likely that IVP is a more sensitive indicator of the interior climate of the brain after a severe injury.

Summary

Continuous recording of the intraventricular pressure after a severe brain injury is a good guide to an accurate prognosis. An attempt was made to improve upon this by also recording blood pressure and jugular venous oxygen tension. However, neither has so far contributed to a more accurate prognosis. Blood pressure did not correlate reliably with intraventricular pressure, either in general level or in changes in any direction. Blood pressure is not an important parameter in the monitoring of a brain-injured patient; and it will usually *not* give an indication of a rise in intraventricular pressure.

Key Words : Intracranial pressure, brain injury, prognosis.

References

1. Troupp, H.: Intraventricular pressure in patients with severe brain injuries. II. J. Trauma **7**, 875–883 (1967).
2. Vapalahti, M.: Intracranial pressure, acid-base status of blood and cerebrospinal fluid, and pulmonary function in the prognosis of severe brain injury. Thesis, University of Helsinki, 1970.
3. Vapalahti, M., Troupp, H.: Prognosis for patients with severe brain injuries. Brit. med. J. **3**, 404–407 (1971).
4. Kaste, M.: Experimental brain injury. Its effects on cerebral sinus pressure, cerebral venous oxygen tension, respiration, blood pressure and acid-base balance. Thesis, University of Helsinki, 1971.
5. Kaste, M., Troupp, H.: Effect of experimental brain injury on blood pressure, cerebral sinus pressure, cerebral venous oxygen tension, respiration, and acid-base balance. J. Neurosurg. **36**, 625–633 (1972).
6. Troupp, H., Valtonen, S.: Unpublished observations.
7. Lundberg, N.: Continuous recording and control of the ventricular fluid pressure in neurosurgical practice. Acta psychiat. scand. (Suppl. 149) **36** (1960).
8. Kjällquist, Å., Lundberg, N., Pontén, U.: Respiratory and cardiovascular changes during rapid spontaneous variations of ventricular fluid pressure in patients with intracranial hypertension. Acta neurol. scand. **40**, 291–317 (1964).
9. Cooper, R., Hulme, A.: Intracranial pressure and related phenomena during sleep. J. Neurol. Neurosurg. Psychiat. **29**, 564–570 (1966).

Cardiorespiratory Changes Associated with Plateau Waves in Patients with Head Injury [1]

G. T. Tindall, C. P. McGraw, R. W. Vanderveer, and K. Iwata

Introduction

Changes in heart rate, respiration, and electroencephalogram (EEG) during spontaneous increases in intracranial pressure (ICP) in patients with intracranial lesions have been observed by other investigators [1, 2, 3, 4]. The clinical significance of these changes has not been established. The purpose of the present investigation was: 1. to evaluate the changes in heart rate, respiration and blood pressure during spontaneous fluctuations in ICP in head-injured patients, and 2. to determine their role in the initiation and termination of ICP waves.

Material and Methods

For periods ranging from 1–20 days, we have continuously recorded ICP, electrocardiogram (EKG), heart rate, and end-alveolar CO_2[2] and impedence pneumograph respirations[3] in 27 patients with acute head injuries. The recordings were made on a 12-channel Grass Polygraph[4]. At selected intervals direct arterial and jugular venous blood pressures were recorded[5], and arterial samples were withdrawn for blood gas analysis[6]. A transducer was inserted in a threaded trephine hole in each patient for continuous monitoring of subdural ICP according to a previously described technique [5].

Five ICP waves were selected for analysis and correlation with other parameters from the polygraph tracings of each patient. ICP waves were classified according to length and magnitude, as follows: 1. "pre-plateau waves" less than 5 min in duration and with a magnitude of less than 10 mmHg; and 2. "plateau waves" longer than 5 min and with a magnitude of greater than 10 mmHg.

1 This study was supported by the National Institutes of Health Research Grant NS 073705.
2 Godart Capnograph Infrared Analyzer, Utrecht, Holland.
3 Impedence Pneumograph MK IV, E. & M. Instrument Co., Inc., Houston, Texas 77017, U.S.A.
4 Grass Model 78, Grass Instrument Co., Quincy, Mass. 02170, U.S.A. All parameters except CO_2 and ICP were recorded by standard Grass transducers, amplifiers and recorders.
5 Statham P-23 Pressure Transducer, Statham Labs, Inc., Hato Rey, Puerto Rico.
6 IL pH/Gas Analyzer, Model 113, Instrumentation Laboratory Inc., Lexington, Mass. 02173, U.S.A.

Results

Cardiovascular and respiratory changes occurred in association with ICP waves in all of the 27 patients. The major determinant of the length and magnitude of the ICP waves was the control, or base line level of ICP, *i.e.*, the higher the latter, the longer and greater the magnitude of the ICP waves. If control ICP was elevated, small ICP waves usually continued to increase in magnitude and duration until a plateau wave was formed. When groups of ICP waves occurred in a patient, there was often a progressive increase in their magnitude and duration (Fig. 1)[7].

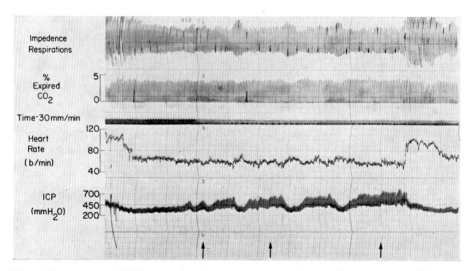

Fig. 1. Progression of ICP waves to plateau waves in a 41-year-old comatose head-injured male. Note that ICP waves become progressively longer in duration and magnitude (arrows), respirations increase in depth, expired CO_2 decreases, and heart rate increases at the termination of each ICP wave

A transient rise in expired CO_2 preceded the ICP wave in 104 of 135 (or 77%) waves analyzed. The rise began an average of 9.1 ± 2.0 sec prior to the increase in ICP and was proportional to the magnitude of the ICP wave. The increase in expired CO_2 often occurred following irregular breathing patterns (Fig. 2), but at other times was spontaneous. During the ICP waves, there was usually a decrease in respiratory rate and depth, more pronounced as the magnitude of the ICP waves increased.

There was a decrease in heart rate during an ICP wave, which became more pronounced as the magnitude of the ICP wave increased and persisted until the termination of the plateau wave (Figs. 1 and 3). Tachycardia (mean 27.3 ± 1.5 b/min), often accompanied by increased rate and depth of respiration, oc-

---

7 Figures are averages $\pm$ standard error.

curred at the crest of the ICP wave (Figs. 1 and 3). Immediately after the sudden onset of the tachycardia (mean 13.2 $\pm$ 2.8 sec) the ICP wave terminated. After the ICP returned to control level, heart rate decreased to the pre-ICP wave value. There was no consistent relationship between ICP waves and systemic arterial pressure.

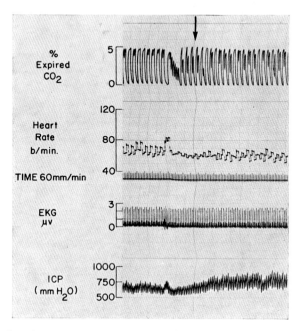

Fig. 2. Irregular breathing pattern prior to the beginning of a plateau wave in an 18-year-old patient with head injury. Note the increase in expired CO_2 after the irregular breathing pattern (arrow)

Discussion

This study has provided insight into the relationship between cardiovascular and respiratory changes on one hand and the production and termination of plateau waves on the other (Fig. 3).

Although the mechanism for formation of plateau waves is unknown, it may be that the presence of plateau waves indicates a decompensated cerebrovascular system. The same cardiorespiratory changes present at the initiation and termination of plateau waves are present in the normal individual during the small ICP waves. These small ICP waves increase in duration and magnitude with elevated ICP and may be seen to progress into the formation of plateau waves (Fig. 1). Therefore, these ICP waves may be more correctly referred to as pre-plateau waves. Plateau waves indicate that ICP is elevated significantly and that the cerebrovascular mechanisms are probably decompensating. Thus, therapeutic measures to reduce the elevated ICP should be instituted immediately in order to prevent the possibility of irreversible neuronal damage [1, 2, 6]. In our series of cases plateau waves have not necessarily been a grave prognostic indication, a finding which may reflect our policy of using mannitol (20%) to maintain the ICP below 20 mmHg (300 mm H_2O).

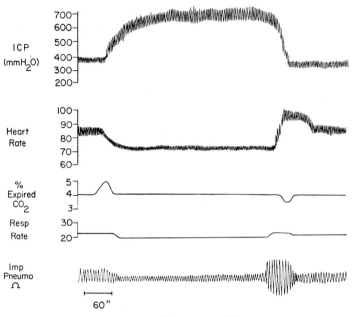

Plateau wave vs. H.R. and Resp.

Fig. 3. Diagrammatic representation of the cardiorespiratory changes occurring during a plateau wave. A transient increase in expired CO_2 precedes the increase in ICP. There is a concomitant decrease in heart rate and respiratory rate and depth as the ICP increases, which persists until the tachycardia phase at the termination. The respirations and heart rate are regular throughout the plateau wave. At the peak of ICP there is an abrupt increase in heart rate, respiratory rate and depth, above the pre-plateau levels, and a decrease in expired CO_2. Following ICP return to base line level, the heart rate and expired CO_2 also return to the pre-plateau level

Summary

Consistent cardiovascular and respiratory changes occurred in association with ICP (plateau) waves in 27 head-injured patients. Initially, a transient increase in expired CO_2 causes a gradual increase in ICP, accompanied by decreases in heart rate and respiratory rate and depth. When ICP reaches a peak, heart rate and respiratory rate and depth increase. ICP then abruptly returns to control levels, after which heart rate and respirations also return to the pre-wave levels. It is postulated that transient increases in arterial pCO_2 and subsequent cerebral vasodilation initiate plateau waves. Terminal tachycardia is a release mechanism ending the plateau wave.

Key Words: Head injury, intracranial pressure, plateau waves, heart rate, respiration.

References

1. COOPER, R., HULME, A.: Intracranial pressure and related phenomena during sleep. J. Neurol. Neurosurg. Psychiat. **29**, 564–570 (1966).
2. LUNDBERG, N.: Continuous recording and control of ventricular fluid pressure in neuro-surgical practice. Acta psychiat. scand. (Suppl. 149) **36**, 1–193 (1960).
3. COOPER, R. L., HULME, A.: Changes of the EEG, intracranial pressure and other variables during sleep in patients with intracranial lesions. Electroenceph. Clin. Neurophysiol. **27**, 12–22 (1969).
4. KJÄLLQUIST, Å., LUNDBERG, N., PONTEN, U.: Respiratory and cardiovascular changes during rapid spontaneous variations of ventricular fluid pressure in patients with intra-cranial hypertension. Acta neurol. scand. **40**, 291–317 (1964).
5. TINDALL, G., MCGRAW, C., IWATA, K.: Subdural pressure monitoring in head-injured patients. In: BROCK, M., DIETZ, H. (Eds.): Intracranial Pressure. Experimental and Clinical Aspects. pp. 9–13. Berlin-Heidelberg-New York: Springer 1972.
6. VAPALAHTI, M.: Intracranial pressure, acid-base status of blood and cerebrospinal fluid, and pulmonary function in the prognosis of severe brain injury. A prospective study in 51 brain-injured patients. Academic Dissertation, Helsinki 1970.

Correlative Study of Intracranial and Systemic Arterial Pressures in Neurosurgical Patients

J. DE ROUGEMONT, M. BARGE, and A. L. BENABID

Introduction

The simultaneous recording of intracranial pressure (ICP) and systemic arterial pressure (SAP) in neurosurgical cases seemed very important to us for two theoretical reasons:

1. ICP is influenced by the encephalic vascular pressure and thus by SAP[1];

2. Rising ICP is dangerous because of its repercussion on the cerebral blood flow (CBF). This essential value depends in part on the cerebral perfusion pressure (CPP), which is equal to SAP less ICP.

The analysis of 83 ICP and SAP recordings from 68 patients allowed us to define the relations between:

1. mean systemic arterial pressure (MSAP) and mean intracranial pressure (MICP);

2. morphology of ICP and SAP waves.

Methods

The cases recorded from were: 25 head injuries, 21 tumors, 18 cases of vascular disease, 2 of intracranial hypertension of unknown origin and 2 standard ICP cases.

ICP was recorded[2] from either the lateral ventricle (13 cases) or the epidural space (55 cases), both pressures being similar [1]. SAP was recorded from the femoral or carotid arteries. Speed of recording was 0.25 or 0.5 mm/sec for the slow wave studies, or 10 mm/sec for the fast wave analysis.

Results

1. Correlations between MICP and MSAP

The analysis of the graphs where each record is plotted according to SAP and either ICP (Fig. 1 A) or ICP/SAP (Fig. 1 B) lead us to the following observations:

---

1 We admit the relation. ICP = encephalic vascular pressure – radial component of vasomotor tonicity.

2 Thomson Telco Electromanometer (RAB) M5 amplifier, allcograph recorder.

a) There are no points above the line relating ICP to SAP, which is also the line going through ordinate ICP/SAP = 1. This shows that in our experience we never found an ICP value higher than SAP.

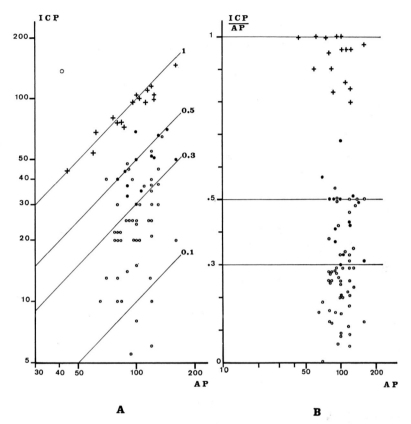

A

B

Fig. 1. crosses = encephalic death; dots = death; circles = still alive. Cases are plotted: a) according to ICP and SAP (logarithmic coordinates); b) according to ICP/SAP and SAP (logarithmic abcissa and linear ordinate). 3 boundary lines become apparent: 1. Line ICP = SAP (Fig. A) or ICP/SAP = 1 (Fig. B). There is no point above; all the cases of cerebral death are gathered just below. 2. Line ICP = 0.5 SAP (Fig. A) or ICP/SAP = 0.5 (Fig. B). Practically all the cases (except those of cerebral death) are below this line. 3. Line ICP = 0.33 SAP (Fig. A) or ICP/SAP = 0.33 (Fig. B). All the deaths are located between lines 0.5 and 0.33

b) Coming into contact with this line or just below it we found 16 cases of cerebral death; 5 cases showed a zero CPP, CPP remaining below 20 mmHg in the other cases. In all these cases, carotid arteriography revealed encephalic circulatory arrest.

c) The analysis also brought out the significance of the line going through the ordinate ICP/SAP = 0.5, representing an ICP level equal in value to half the SAP level. Most of the points are located under this line and there is a gap between this group of cases and the encephalic deaths mentioned above. More-

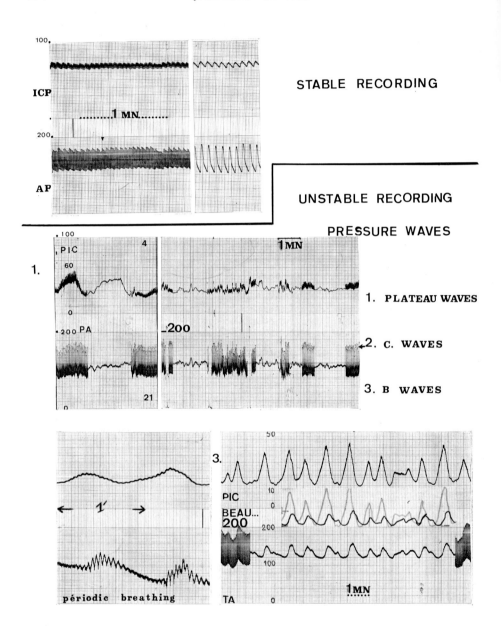

Fig. 2. *Stable recording:* recurrency of a glioma, with severe pressure signs. Note the normal appearance of the recording except for the high ICP level which is about half the SAP level. Pulse amplitude = 7 mmHg ($^1/_{10}$ of arterial pulse) respiratory waves = 2 mmHg ($^1/_4$ of SAP respiratory waves). *Unstable recording:* 1 + 2: Head injury, conscious (PaO$_2$ = 76, PaCO$_2$ = 28, pHa = 7.5). 1. Plateau-like waves without concomitant SAP oscillations. 2. 6-per-minute waves reflecting arterial vasomotor oscillations, the ratio being 0.5. 3. Glioblastoma, pressure signs, periodic breathing. Pressure waves with SAP oscillations appearing 5–8 sec later (both recordings are superposed), the amplitude ratio being about $^2/_3$

over the only cases located here developed into encephalic death, except for two who underwent prompt ventricular drainage.

d) Among the cases below this line, all those in which death occurred can be found between the ordinate ICP/SAP 0.5 and ICP/SAP 0.3. Consequently, this appears to be a decisive level, though it is not irreversible, since we found a few patients who remained between these points.

2. ICP and SAP Wave Morphology

The analysis of wave morphology points out two different groups of ICP and SAP correlative recordings (Fig. 2).

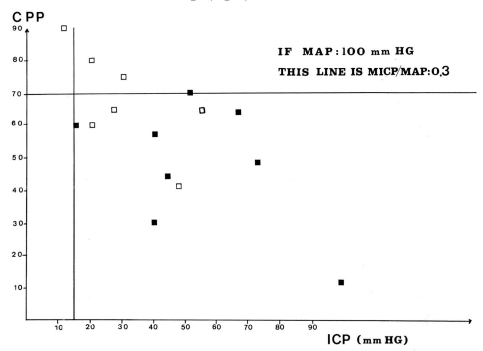

Fig. 3. Cases with 6-per-minute waves are plotted according to ICP and CPP. Dark squares = deaths, white squares = still alive

a) *Regular graphs* with no unevenness above 4 mmHg except pulse and breathing waves. ICP and SAP seem to be homogeneous and to differ from standard recordings only in the ICP level. We found this kind of recording in 23 cases and it was not possible to establish any correlation with prognosis.

b) *Irregular graphs* with spurious oscillations. It was possible to distinguish two groups of pressure waves when they were studied in connection with SAP fluctuations:

1. Waves not followed by corresponding SAP waves; these are usually plateau-like waves.

2. Waves followed by SAP waves. The mean values of both ICP and SAP seem to be similar: they are synchronous, have the same pulse rate of 5–6 per min and show no great regularity. As a rule, the morphology of such waves is anarchic. The only difference is in amplitude with a ratio of about 0.5; we observed such waves in 15 cases. Most were located in the dangerous zone mentioned above, that is to say below CPP = 70, which correlates with an ICP/SAP ratio of 0.3 [in fact most cases located there are dead (Fig. 3)].

Waves with a to 2-min rate (8 cases) often, but not always, related to periodic respiration, also seem to belong to this group, being paralleled by similar SAP waves. However, the amplitude ratio is higher in these cases, from 0.5–1, and SAP waves are not always synchronous, but often occur 5–10 sec later. Finally, we often observed different types of waves mixed. Their comparison with SAP allows a better analysis.

Discussion

Three main boundary lines emerge from these recordings and studies on the relationship between MICP and MSAP:

a) *The line ICP – SAP* where CPP = 0 and ICP/SAP = 1 ICP never goes beyond this line, above which cerebral death occurs in all cases. We imagine this pressure levelling is caused by vasomotor paralysis [2]. The loss of vasomotor tonus causes the pressure levelling and circulatory arrest. We propose that this pressure levelling be used as a test for encephalic death.

b) *The line ICP = SAP/2.* All cases above this boundary line were encephalic deaths or became such. It seemed that the regulating mechanisms of cerebral vascular resistance (CVR) were unable to ensure a sufficient CBF, until a certain reduction of CPP had taken place.

Some authors [3] report that CBF decreases as soon as CPP starts to fall, while others [4–5] find CBF remains steady as long as CPP remains above 40 mmHg. All agree, however, that when CPP is lower than 40 to 60 mmHg CBF falls rapidly. Our clinical experience bears this out: there is a fatal line beyond which CBF is jeopardized; this line corresponds to the relation ICP = SAP/2, that is, when, for example, MSAP = 100 mmHg and MICP = 50 mmHg.

c) *The line ICP/SAP = 0.3* (ICP = 30 when MSAP = 100 mmHg) should also be understood as an expression of the influence of ICP on CPP. The prognosis is such cases is difficult to estimate. ICP increases above 30 mmHg are a serious sign in cases of brain trauma [6, 7].

High intracranial pressure is not always followed by pressure waves (stable recording). However, when such waves as described by JANNY [8] and LUNDBERG [9] occur, they exhibit a very specific relationship to arterial pressure. As observed by KJALLQUIST [10] their analysis may be of importance for their pathogenic interpretation.

a) Some waves seem to be independent of SAP fluctuations. These are always plateau-like waves. Their encephalic vasomotor origin has been proven [11] and this may well explain why there is no SAP alteration in such cases [10].

b) On the other hand, the 6-per-min waves seem to be related to SAP vasomotor fluctuations [8–10]. It seems that, under these circumstances, ICP passively follows the anarchic SAP fluctuations with a ratio of $1/_2$, that is 5–10 times higher than the pulse damping. This certainly reflects a bad prognosis, as has already been noted [9] (see Fig. 3).

c) The meaning of the 1-per-min waves is less obvious. We have always observed concomitant SAP fluctuations, the ratio varying from 0.5–1. In fact, it was often noticed that such waves were not synchronous, SAP fluctuations occurring 5–10 sec later, as if ICP fluctuations were inducing SAP to follow. It is interesting that we were able to observe 1-per-min waves in patients on the respirator.

Summary

The study of simultaneous recordings of intracranial pressure and systemic arterial pressure lead the authors to the following conclusions:

1. The correlation between mean intracranial pressure and mean arterial pressure shows 3 levels of the MICP/MSAP ratio: 1, 0.5, 0.3, which seem to be significant in prognosis.

2. According to their configuration, intracranial pressure waves may be classified into regular and irregular. Pressure waves may occur with no corresponding arterial pressure changes or may be paralleled by similar waves in arterial pressure. The importance of these correlations is discussed.

Key Words : Intracranial pressure, arterial pressure.

References

1. ROUGEMONT, J. DE, BARGE, M., BENABID, A. L.: Un nouveau capteur pour la mesure de la pression intracranienne. Valeur de la dure mère en tant que membrane susceptible de transmettre les pressions. Acta neurochir. 17, 579–590 (1971).

2. LANGFITT, T. W., WEINSTEIN, J. D., KASSEL, N. F.: Cerebral vasomotor paralysis produced by intracranial hypertension. Neurology 15, 622–641 (1965).

3. MATAKAS, F., LEIPERT, M., FRANKE, J.: Cerebral blood flow during increased subarachnoid pressure. Acta neurochir. 25, 19–36 (1971).

4. JENNETT, W. B., ROWAN, J. O., HARPER, A. M., JOHNSTON, J. H., MILLER, I. H., DESHMUTH, V. D.: Perfusion pressure and cerebral blood flow. In: Ross RUSSEL R. W. (Ed.): Brain and Blood Flow, 298–300. London: Pitman 1971.

5. ZWETNOW, N., SIESJÖ, B. K., KJÄLLQVIST, A.: Cerebral blood flow during intracranial hypertension related to tissue hypoxia and acidosis. Progr. Brain Res. 30, 87–92 (1968).

6. MOODY, R. A., MULLAN, S.: Head injury monitoring: a preliminary report. J. Trauma 11, 458–462 (1971).

7. TROUPP, H.: Intraventricular pressure in patients with severe brain injuries. J. Trauma 7, 875–882 (1967).

8. GUILLAUME, J., JANNY, P.: Manométrie intracranienne continue. Intérêt de la méthode et premiers résultats. Rev. neurol. **84**, 131–142 (1951).
9. LUNDBERG, N.: Continuous recording and control of ventricular fluid pressure in neurosurgical practice. Acta psychiat. scand. (Suppl. 149) **36** (1960).
10. KJÄLLQVIST, A., LUNDBERG, N., PONTEN, V.: Respiratory and cardivascular changes during rapid spontaneous variations of ventricular fluid pressure in patients with intracranial hypertension. Acta neurol. scand. **40**, 291–317 (1964).
11. RISBERG, J., LUNDBERG, N., INGVAR, D. H.: Regional cerebral blood volume during acute transient rises of the intracranial pressure (plateau waves). J. Neurosurg. **31**, 303 (1969).

The Interdependence of Cerebrovascular Autoregulation and Intracranial Pressure[1, 2]

R. COOPER and A. HULME

Introduction

The use of chronically indwelling intracerebral electrodes and other devices for the treatment of psychiatric illness [1], investigation of epilepsy [2, and others] and management of neurosurgical patients [3, 4] permit investigation of the local and regional changes of the cerebrovascular system in man.

Material and Methods

ICP or VFP has been recorded from 80 patients admitted for investigation to the Department of Neurological Surgery, Frenchay Hospital. VFP was recorded using ventricular catheters and external pressure transducers; ICP was measured using a pressure transducer (Ferranti or Königsberg) implanted in the subdural space. Measurement of polarographic oxygen (called oxygen availability) using uncoated gold electrodes and cerebral blood flow using directly heated thermistors have been described elsewhere [5].

Results

Recordings of available oxygen and cerebral blood flow show fluctuations of amplitude that are believed to be signs of local vasomotor activity regulating the supply of oxygen to the tissue [6, 7, and others].

These apparently spontaneous fluctuations have a mean period of about 10 sec and are usually different at electrodes separated by more than a few millimeters of brain tissue (Fig. 1). Because of this independence from region to region the *local* fluctuations are not related, under normal physiological conditions, to systemic variables such as respiration, blood pressure etc. However, in abnormal or pathological conditions, the local mechanisms may be perturbed by systemic changes. For example, the fluctuations and mean level of available oxygen increase during inhalation of 100% oxygen although the flow is not changed significantly [7]. In addition, during inhalation of air enriched with CO_2 the spontaneous fluctuations of the oxygen availability disappear and there

1 With the technical assistance of Mr. W. J. WARREN.
2 With financial assistance from the Medical Research Council and the W. Clement and Jessie V. Stone Foundation.

is an increase of the mean level (Fig. 2). We believe that this loss of fluctuation is a sign of vasodilation associated with loss of autoregulation.

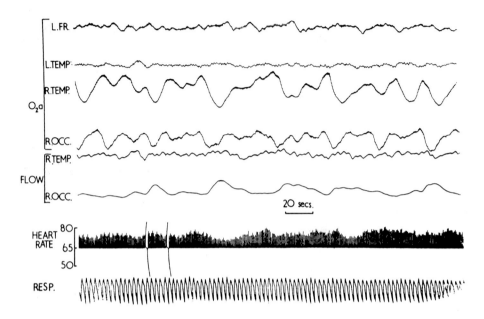

Fig. 1. Recordings of available oxygen (O_2a) and blood flow from gold electrodes and thermistors in an epileptic patient. Note independent fluctuations and lack of correlation with heart rate or respiration

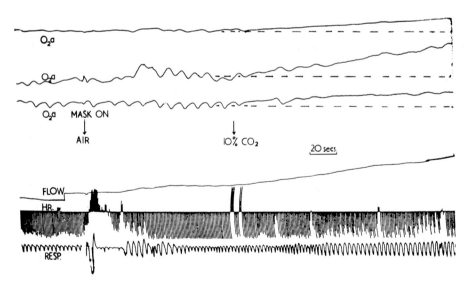

Fig. 2. Rise of mean level and loss of fluctuations of available oxygen during inhalation of 10 % CO_2 in air. The mean level of flow also rises

It is rarely possible, in man, to vary the blood pressure systematically to test the presence or lack of autoregulation but increases of intracranial pressure, and therefore a reduction of perfusion pressure, can often be observed in a variety of circumstances.

In patients with raised ICP an increase of intracranial pressure during sleep similar to the plateau waves described by LUNDBERG [8] is often seen. We have shown elsewhere [4] that these plateau waves usually occur during the rapid eye movement stage of sleep when dreaming is said to occur and when cerebral metabolism is high [9, 10]. When the intracranial pressure rises the spontaneous fluctuations of oxygen availability disappear. They return when the pressure falls (see Figs. 1 and 2 in Ref. [4]).

During induction of anaesthesia of certain neurosurgical patients the intracranial pressure often rises to high levels and the perfusion pressure can fall to very low levels. In these circumstances the spontaneous fluctuations of oxygen availability disappear and the mean level then reflects the perfusion pressure.

However, in both sleep and induction of anaesthesia there are many unknown perturbing factors such as changes of metabolism, respiration, and it is not always possible to either control or measure such changes.

In patients with intracranial hypertension injection of air or radio-opaque substances into the ventricles prior to radiography is a common diagnostic procedure. We have found that injection of small volumes of air can cause the intracranial pressure to increase to high levels with a considerable fall of perfusion pressure. In such circumstances the spontaneous fluctuations of flow and available oxygen cease and the mean levels fall. Figure 3 shows changes of ventricular fluid pressure during injection of small volumes of air and withdrawal of fluid. The upper trace shows the changes of volume imposed over a period of 30 min. The net gain was 20 ml of air injected and 17 ml of fluid removed. At each phase of the injection the VFP increased from a resting level of about 20 mmHg to values exceeding 50 mmHg; blood pressure measured intermittently using a sphygmomanometer showed smaller changes. The difference between the mean BP and mean ICP, that may be considered perfusion pressure, fell to about 50 mmHg on each of the 3 occasions when the intracranial volume was increased by 4 ml. During these periods of low perfusion pressure the spontaneous fluctuations of the oxygen availability disappeared and there was a fall of mean level. After the mean perfusion pressure was restored to levels greater than 55 mmHg the level of the oxygen availability increased and the oscillations reappeared. There were no significant changes of respiration (lowest channel) and heart rate (not shown) during the alterations of brain volume.

Discussion

The loss of autoregulation at low values of blood pressure has been well demonstrated in animals ([11] and others). Our study in man using the intra-

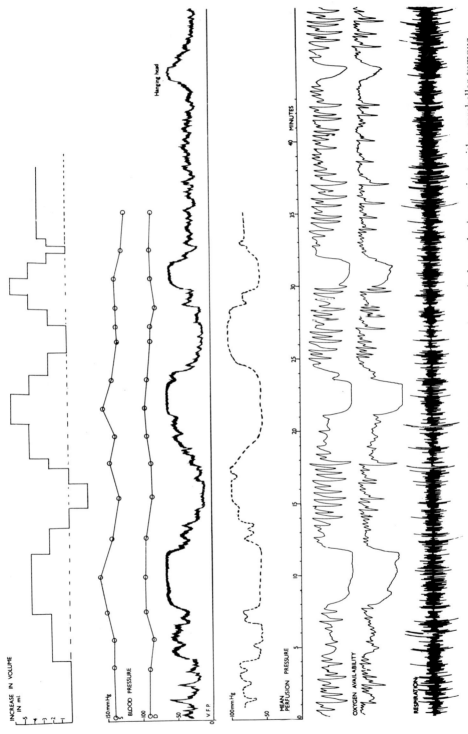

Fig. 3. Changes of mean perfusion pressure and available oxygen during air ventriculography in a patient with a cerebellar tumour

cranial pressure as a variable instead of blood pressure shows a similar loss of regulation as the pressure rises. The results in a number of patients indicate that, as in animals, there is a loss of regulation as the perfusion pressure falls below 50 mm of Hg although this value appears to vary considerably from patient to patient.

The records from some patients, for example that shown in Fig. 3, indicate that there is a sharp transition from control to loss of control at a critical intracranial pressure. The concept of a critical pressure is not new [12]; it may well be that the fall in perfusion pressure caused by a rise of ICP is not the same as the fall of blood pressure although the transmural pressure should be similar in both circumstances.

Summary

The spontaneous fluctuations of cortical oxygen availability, believed to be a sign of regulation of the cerebrovascular system, disappear as the intracranial pressure rises. This is interpreted as a loss of autoregulation when the perfusion pressure falls below a certain level between 40 and 60 mmHg.

Key Words: Oxygen availability, intracranial pressure, autoregulation.

References

1. CROW, H. J., COOPER, R., PHILLIPS, D. G.: Controlled multifocal frontal leucotomy for psychiatric illness. J. Neurol. Neurosurg. Psychiat. **24**, 353–360 (1961).
2. WALTER, W. G., CROW, H. J.: Depth recording from the human brain. Electroenceph. clin. Neurophysiol. **16**, 68–72 (1964).
3. HULME, A., COOPER, R.: A technique for the investigation of intracranial pressure in man. J. Neurol. Neurosurg. Psychiat. **29**, 154–156 (1966).
4. COOPER, R., HULME, A.: Intracranial pressure and related phenomena during sleep. J. Neurol. Neurosurg. Psychiat. **29**, 564–570 (1966).
5. COOPER, R.: Local changes of intra-cerebral blood flow and oxygen in humans. Med. biol. Engng. **1**, 529–536 (1963).
6. CLARK, L. C., MISRAHY, G., FOX, R. P.: Chronically implanted polarographic electrodes. J. appl. Physiol. **13**, 85–91 (1958).
7. COOPER, R., CROW, H. J., WALTER, W. G., WINTER, A. L.: Regional control of cerebral vascular reactivity and oxygen supply in man. Brain Res. **3**, 174–191 (1966).
8. LUNDBERG, N.: Continuous recording and control of ventricular fluid pressure in neurosurgical practice. Acta psychiat. scand. (Suppl. 149), **36** (1960).
9. BREBBIA, D. R., ALTSHULER, K. Z.: Oxygen consumption rate and electroencephalographic stage of sleep. Science **150**, 1621–1623 (1965).
10. REIVICH, M., ISAACS, G., EVARTS, E., KETY, S.: The effect of slow wave sleep and REM sleep on regional cerebral blood flow in cats. J. Neurochem. **15**, 301–306 (1968).
11. HARPER, A. M.: Autoregulation of cerebral blood flow: influence of the arterial blood pressure on the blood flow through the cerebral cortex. J. Neurol. Neurosurg. Psychiat. **29**, 398–403 (1966).
12. KETY, S. S., SHENKIN, H. A., SCHMIDT, C. F.: The effects of increased intracranial pressure on the cerebral circulatory functions in man. J. clin. Invest. **27**, 493–498 (1948).

Recurrent Hemorrhage and Hemostasis in Patients with Ruptured Intracranial Saccular Aneurysm

H. Nornes

Introduction

The purpose of this study was to gain some insight into the intracranial pressure state in patients with ruptured saccular aneurysm, with special reference to correct timing of surgical treamtent.

Material and Methods

The material consisted of 29 patients admitted with subarachnoid hemorrhage (SAH) due to a ruptured saccular aneurysm, all of whom were unfit for immediate surgery.

A miniature pressure transducer [1, 2, 3] was implanted epidurally in the fronto-parietal region for 1–29 days (average 10.9). Blood flow measurements were recorded in the internal carotid artery (ICA) on the side of the aneurysm in 2 patients selected for graded occlusion with a Selverstone clamp [4].

Results

Satisfactory recordings were obtained in all patients except one in whom the transducer broke down after 1 day. Zero-point drift within the period of implantation was usually less than $\pm$ 3 mmHg. There were no complications attributed to the implantation of the transducers.

Epidural Pressure (EDP) Pattern at Rerupture

While awaiting clinical improvement, 10 patients suffered one or more recurrent hemorrhages. The subsequent EDP course fell into two different pressure patterns. One type, seen in 8 patients (Fig. 1, upper curves), showed a steep rise in the EDP to about the same level as the actual diastolic blood pressure and a subsequent fall to considerably lower levels within minutes, giving the impression of a pressure peak. The continuous tracings showed slowly increasing EDP over the next few hours. This group is referred to as "subarachnoid hemorrhage type 1". Four of these patients died, and the autopsy revealed marked edema and minimal hematoma

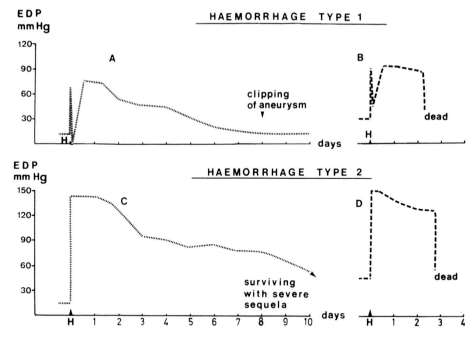

Fig. 1. *Upper curves:* Subarachnoid hemorrhage type 1. Initial pressure peak and secondary pressure increase. A. improving to stage of operability. B. Fatal outcome. *Lower curves:* Subarachnoid hemorrhage type 2. Instant increase in pressure followed by a high pressure plateau

The second type of tracing (Fig. 1, lower curves) occurred in 5 patients. The EDP instantly rose to a level between the calculated mean blood pressure and the systolic blood pressure. The EDP remained stable at this level and did not respond to hyperventilation or dehydrating agents. 4 of these patients died within a few hours or days, and the autopsy showed massive hematomas. One survived with marked sequelae.

The term "subarachnoid hemorrhage type 2" has been used for this picture.

Warning Episodes

4 patients showed a total of seven periods of transient deterioration concomitant with marked pressure peaks in the continuous EDP record. Although there was no evidence of fresh hemorrhage, 3 of these events were followed by a verified hemorrhage within 24 h and they were hence referred to as "warning episodes" [5]. An example of this pressure pattern is shown in Fig. 2.

Comment

These three EDP patterns are assumed to reflect the whole range from full spatial compensation to total decompensation. The determining factors are considered to be the volume of extravasated blood, the rate of bleeding, the vasomotor reaction, and the intracranial spatial buffering capacity.

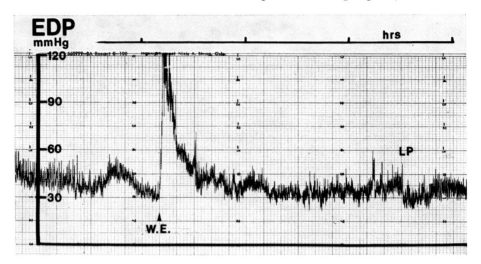

Fig. 2. Warning episode one week after initial hemorrhage. EDP rise time approximately 2 min. Peak duration 20 min. WE: warning episode. LP: lumbar puncture with no signs of SAH

EDP Level at Rupture

All 13 recorded reruptures except one occurred within 14 days after the last SAH (average 7.7 days). Ten of the reruptures occurred at or below an EDP level of 30 mmHg and only three started at higher levels. The records from patients *suffering recurrent hemorrhage* covered 62 days; pressure levels higher than 30 mmHg were recorded on 26 days and lower levels on the other 36 days. In the group of patients *without recurrent SAH* (pressure recorded for 124 days) these figures are 87 and 37 days respectively. This means that the pressure levels are generally higher than in the recurrent hemorrhage group.

Blood Flow Pattern at Rupture

One patient selected for graded occlusion of the ICA had a recurrent hemorrhage before occlusion could be accomplished. 1 h before the rerupture the EDP was 18 mmHg and the BP 140/100 mmHg. The ICA blood flow was stable at 160 ml/min. The tracings went on to show a steep rise in EDP to 136 mmHg as the patient underwent a recurrent hemorrhage and the BP measurements revealed a vasopressor response to 180/125 mmHg.

The blood flow recorded during this period of EDP elevation was steady at about 60 ml/min. Figure 3 shows the original ICA blood flow records with tracings for mean and instantaneous flow from these two sequences; the lower tracings are from the period of elevated ICP. It is seen that the flow of 60 ml/min is mainly pulsatile and that there is flow arrest during the last part of the diastole.

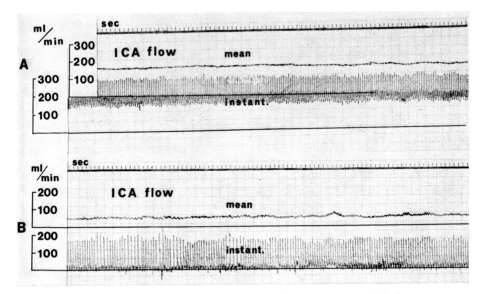

Fig. 3. Internal carotid artery blood flow, mean and instantaneous. A before rerupture. B after rerupture. Flow of about 60 ml/min of pulsatile type

The patient was deeply comatose and after 15 min with unchanged EDP and unchanged clinical condition a minor spinal tap was made. The subsequent fall in EDP to 40 mmHg caused an increase in ICA blood flow to 120 ml/min, now showing the same dynamic pattern as in Fig. 3 A.

1 h later the patient suffered another hemorrhage and died within a few minutes.

Discussion

The mechanism of arrest of hemorrhage in aneurysm rupture causing brain tamponade is easily understood: when the ICP approaches the same level as systolic BP the aneurysm leakage as well as the cerebral blood flow is arrested. This is the ultimate state in what we have designated hemorrhagic-compressive lesions seen in SAH type 2 [5].

Our data show that most subsequent hemorrhages are arrested when the EDP level is approximately the same as that of the diastolic BP. The EDP then returns to considerably lower levels within minutes. This fall in EDP has been attributed to two factors: one is the arrest of hemorrhage, and the other is the maintenance of hemostasis during a period when pressure-buffering mechanisms markedly reduce ICP. The main buffering mechanism is thought to be an outflow of CSF and blood along the craniospinal axis. This pressure pattern is typical of the so-called SAH type 1.

The pressure gradient across the aneurysm wall must be markedly reduced at the pressure peak and is presumably about zero during the last part of the diastole, so that blood flow is seriously impaired.

Two different mechanisms are generally considered important in securing cerebral blood flow: one is autoregulation, the second the vasopressor response. As the third we should include the pressure-buffering mechanism of the intracranial compartments.

The reduced pressure gradient across the aneurysm wall caused by the increased ICP at rupture may be of particular importance in the arrest of hemorrhage.

It is reasonable to assume that the hemodynamic state described, with reduced pressure gradient across the aneurysm wall and diastolic arrest of leakage, is important in the intial mooring of platelets at the site of rupture and the subsequent formation of a platelet plug.

Experimentally it has been shown that the platelet plug builds up at the site of vessel injury in 1–2 min [6]. During the next few minutes bleeding may occur through channels in the plug which gradually increases in strength as the platelets become tightly adherent to each other. Permanent hemostasis is obtained when the strength of the platelet plug and the surrounding pressure can counterbalance the forces of aneurysm blood pressure.

The data presented seem to indicate that the risk of rebleeding during the first 2 weeks after aneurysm rupture increases as the ICP returns towards normal levels. It is reasonable to believe that the relatively low frequency of recurrent hemorrhage during the first week after SAH may be due to a series of factors: 1. the strength of the hemostatic clot, 2. the presence of arterial spasms, and 3. the support provided by the increased intracranial pressure seen in most of these patients. The specific tendency for rebleeding to occur between the 7th and the 14th day after SAH may thus be due to reduced clot strength due to fibrinolysis, release of spasms in arteries, and finally the normalization of intracranial pressure.

Summary

Two different EDP patterns were found associated with verified rebleedings: one was seen with massive hematoma, the other showed cerebral edema formation and only minimal hematoma. Measurement of internal carotid blood flow during the acute stage of rebleeding shows a marked change in flow pattern. The rise in ICP and the change in blood flow pattern at rupture obviously contribute to the arrest of hemorrhage and to the maintenance of hemostasis. The observations in 29 patients at risk indicate an increasing risk of rebleeding as the EDP decreases towards the normal pressure range.

Key Words : Cerebral aneurysm, subarachnoid hemorrhage, epidural pressure, carotid artery blood flow, hemostasis.

References

1. NORNES, H., SERCK-HANSSEN, F.: Miniature transducer for intracranial pressure monitoring in man. Acta neurol. scand. **46**, 203–214 (1970).
2. NORNES, H., MAGNÆS, B.: Supratentorial epidural pressure recorded during posterior fossa surgery. J. Neurosurg. **35**, 541–549 (1971).
3. SUNDBÄRG, G., NORNES, H.: Simultaneous recording of the ventricular fluid pressure and the epidural pressure. Acta neurol. scand. **46**, 634 (1970).
4. NORNES, H.: Longterm implanted electromagnetic flow probes in man. Observations during graded occlusion for internal carotid artery aneurysms. In: CAPPELEN, CHR. (Ed.): New findings in blood flowmetry, p. 215–219. Oslo: Universitetsforlaget 1968.
5. NORNES, H., MAGNÆS, B.: Intracranial pressure in patients with ruptured saccular aneurysm. J. Neurosurg. **36**, 537–547 (1972).
6. HOVIG, T., ROWSELL, H. C., DODDS, W. J. et al.: Experimental haemostasis in normal dogs and dogs with congenital disorders of blood coagulation. Blood **30**, 636–668 (1967).

The Relationship between Ventricular Fluid Pressure and the Neuropathology of Raised Intracranial Pressure

H. Adams and D. I. Graham

Neuropathologists have always tended to equate certain macroscopic abnormalities in the fixed brain such as midline shift, and supracallosal (subfalcine), tentorial and tonsillar herniae, with raised intracranial pressure (ICP). But these features are really manifestations of distortion and displacement of the brain and, with the increasing awareness of the "period of spatial compensation" [1] during which the skull can accommodate an intracranial mass lesion without there being a significant increase in ICP, it has become pertinent to question whether distortion and herniation of the brain can in fact be equated with an increase in ICP.

For several years, therefore, we have attached considerable importance to the occurrence of foci of pressure necrosis produced by impaction of the parahippocampal gyri (Fig. 1), the cingulate gyri (Fig. 2), and the cerebellar tonsils

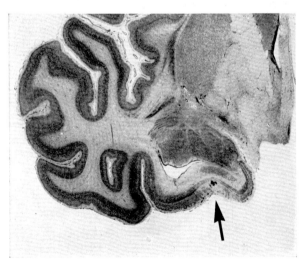

Fig. 1. Sharply defined wedge-shaped focus of necrosis (pale) with focal haemorrhage (dark) in left parahippocampal gyrus (PHG) along line of tentorial hernia. Cresyl violet X 1.6

against the tentorium, the falx, and the foramen magnum respectively, and to infarction in the medial occipital cortex (calcarine infarction) due to compression of the posterior cerebral artery, as pathological evidence of raised ICP. We thought it unlikely that ICP had been raised if none of these features were present. With the increasing use of continuous monitoring of ventricular fluid pressure (VFP), it has become possible to test this hypothesis.

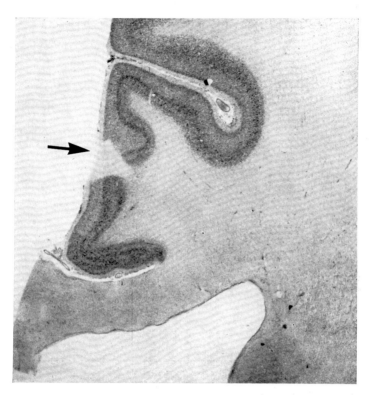

Fig. 2. Wedge-shaped focus of necrosis (pale) in right cingulate gyrus (CG) along line of supracallosal (subfalcine) hernia. Cresyl violet X 4.5

Material and Methods

35 cases (32 with head injuries and 3 with ruptured intracranial aneurysms) have so far been studied. The age range was from 1 year 6 months to 67 years, and the length of survival from the initial episode until death from 9 h to 21 months. In each case monitoring of VFP had been instituted prior to any intracranial surgery. In some cases, monitoring was continued for only 8–12 h because of the short survival of the patient, but in others it was maintained for several days. The cases were classified into 3 groups as defined by JOHNSTONE et al. [2]: in Group 1 (9 cases) the VFP was less than 20 mmHg; in Group 2 (8 cases) it lay between 20 and 40 mmHg; and in Group 3 (18 cases) it was greater than 40 mmHg. Celloidin sections (30 μ) of large bilateral blocks of brain were analysed for sharply-defined wedge-shaped foci of pressure necrosis in the parahippocampal gyri (PHG) and in the cingulate gyrus (CG) ipsilateral to

an intracranial expanding lesion, infarction in the medial occipital cortex (MOC), and necrosis in the cerebellar tonsils (CT). Infarction in the brain stem was not considered in the present study in view of the preponderance of cases of acute head injury, as it is not always possible to distinguish between primary and secondary brain stem damage post mortem in such cases [3].

Results

Group 1 : In none of the 9 cases was there microscopic evidence of pressure necrosis in PHG or CG, or of infarction in MOC. In one case there was necrosis in CT.

Group 2 : Of the 8 cases, there was pressure necrosis in PHG in 5 (all bilateral) and in CG in 2, infarction in MOC in 3 (all unilateral), and necrosis in CT in 2. In 3 cases, none of the parameters was positive.

Group 3 : Of the 18 cases, there was pressure necrosis in PHG in 18 (8 bilateral) and in CG in 5, infarction in MOC in 10 (3 bilateral), and necrosis in CT in 11.

Table 1. To show the incidence of focal pressure necrosis in parahippocampal gyrus (PHG) and in cingulate gyrus (CG), infarction in medial occipital cortex (MOC), and necrosis in cerebellar tonsils (CT) in the 3 groups of cases. The numbers in brackets refer to the number of cases where lesions in PHG and MOC were bilateral. In Group 2, all parameters were negative in the 3 cases without lesions in PHG

Group	VFP (mmHg)	No. of Cases	Microscopic abnormalities in PHG	CG	MOC	CT
1	< 20	9	0	0	0	1
2	20–40	8	5 (5)	2	3	2
3	> 40	18	18 (8)	5	10 (3)	11

Discussion

The results are very much as predicted but not quite as clearcut as we would have wished. Thus, in Group 1, there was not a single instance of pressure necrosis, as the microscopic abnormality in CT was part of an infarct affecting the territory of the posterior inferior cerebellar artery, while in Group 3 there was not a single case without either bilateral lesions in PHG or a unilateral lesion in PHG plus at least one other positive parameter. The cases in Group 2, on the other hand, appear to fall into two sub-divisions: in 5 cases the incidence of lesions was as high as in the cases in Group 3, while in the remaining 3 all of the parameters were negative.

Microscopy is a more accurate means of identifying abnormalities in PHG, CG, MOC and CT than naked eye examination of slices of brain. Thus, of the 23 cases (13 bilateral) with microscopic pressure necrosis in PHG, there were macroscopic tentorial herniae in only 15 (4 bilateral); of the 7 cases with pressure necrosis in CG, there were supracallosal herniae in 4; of the 13 cases (3 bilateral) with infarction in MOC, the abnormality was apparent to the naked eye in only 3 (1 bilateral); and of the 14 cases with necrosis in CT, there was a macroscopic tonsillar hernia in 8. On the other hand, there was naked eye evidence of tentorial herniation in 1 case, supracallosal herniation in 5, and tonsillar herniation in 3, in none of which was there any microscopic pressure necrosis.

Further cases will clearly require to be examined but it appears at this stage (a) that focal pressure necrosis in PHG is the hallmark of increased supratentorial ICP and (b) that where this is bilateral or accompanied by abnormalities of the type we have defined in CG, MOC or CT, it can be stated that VFP has been markedly increased during life. In view of the 3 cases in Group 2 where all of the parameters were negative, it is not yet clear on what post-mortem criteria one can say that VFP has not been increased.

Summary

The relationship between ventricular fluid pressure and foci of pressure necrosis in the parahippocampal gyri and in the cingulate gyrus ipsilateral to an intracranial expanding lesion, infarction in the medial occipital cortex, and necrosis in the cerebellar tonsils, was assessed in a neuropathological analysis of 35 cases. Focal pressure necrosis in the parahippocampal gyrus appears to be the hallmark of increased supratentorial intracranial pressure. When this is bilateral or accompanied by one of the other parameters studied, the ventricular fluid pressure has been markedly increased during life.

Key Words: Raised intracranial pressure, brain herniae.

References

1. LANGFITT, T. W., WEINSTEIN, J. D., KASSELL, N. F.: Cerebral vasomotor paralysis produced by intracranial hypertension. Neurology (Minneap.) **15**, 622–641 (1965).
2. JOHNSTON, I. H., JOHNSTON, J. A., JENNETT, B.: Intracranial-pressure changes following head injury. Lancet **II**, 433–436 (1970).
3. ADAMS, H., GRAHAM, D. I.: The pathology of blunt head injuries. In: CRITCHLEY, M., O'LEARY, J. L., JENNETT, B. (Eds.): The Scientific Foundations of Neurology, sect. 1 X, chap. 7. London: Heinemann (in press).

Treatment of Cerebral Edema in Man with Spirolactone[1]

P. Schmiedek, A. Baethmann, W. Brendel, E. Schneider, R. Enzenbach, and F. Marguth

Spirolactone, a competitive aldosterone blocking agent, is used as a renal diuretic, particularly in conditions where fluid retention is caused by increased aldosterone activity [1]. Our interest in the use of this compound for the control of brain edema was prompted by a study by Koczorek et al. [2], who found treatment with spirolactone relieved symptoms of increased intracranial pressure in patients with pseudotumor cerebri. It was suggested, and later partially confirmed by experimental evidence, that the action of spirolactone on the central nervous system was probably not specific but rather due to a reactive increase of aldosterone as a result of the competitive blockade of its renal site of action by the antagonist [3]. It was considered essential to the evaluation of our working hypothesis concerning the effect of spirolactone on brain edema that the effect be accurately assessed on a more objective basis than clinical impressions [4]. Therefore, in this report an attempt has been made to investigate brain tissue specimens removed from neurosurgical patients at the time of operation and to compare results of untreated patients with those of patients pretreated with spirolactone.

Material and Methods

21 patients to be operated on for brain tumor received 800–1000 mg of spirolactone[2] per day for several days before the operation. During operation tissue sampling was performed as follows: immediately after the dura had been opened, a specimen of cortex adjacent to the tumor was removed with a cryoprobe developed for this purpose in our laboratory [5] and submitted to analysis of labile metabolites, including CP, ATP, ADP, AMP, Pyr. and Lact. Two samples, one from cortex and one from underlying white matter were analyzed for enzymes (GAPDH, CE, IDH, GLDH, MDH, GOT). Water content and tissue electrolytes were measured in two additional specimens from brain compartments. For technical reasons, it was not possible to obtain a complete set of 5 tissue samples in all patients. Details of our methods of tissue

1 This study was supported by Sonderforschungsbereich 51 – Medizinische Molekularbiologie. The technical assistance of Miss A. Gruber and Mrs. R. Hoessel is gratefully acknowledged.
2 Aldactone pro injectione Boehringer Mannheim GmbH, W.-Germany.

analysis have been reported previously [6]. Spirolactone medication was continued postoperative at the same dosage for another 2–3 days. Daily measurements of serum and urine electrolytes were carried out in all patients in this group. The same parameters were investigated in a comparable group of 25 patients, the only difference being that they were not pretreated for brain edema in any way before intraoperative tissue sampling was completed.

Results

Water Content and Tissue Electrolytes. Figure 1 gives the water content and electrolyte values for the two groups. In patients pretreated with spirolactone a lower water content was found in both brain compartments. The difference is highly significant for cortex. In white matter, however, the reduction of water content was not so pronounced due to a considerably wider variation in single values. In addition, there was a concomitant decrease in the amount of sodium in cortex, seen to a more pronounced extent in white matter after pretreatment with spirolactone. Potassium, in contrast, is not noticeably affected.

Tissue Enzymes. Figure 2 shows a diagram of the tricarbonic acid cycle, indicating individual enzymatic steps axamined in this study. Relative changes of enzyme activities in the spirolactone group as compared to controls are given as percentages for cortex and white matter. It is evident that enzymes participating directly in the TCA-cycle (CE, IDH, GLDH, MDH) respond with increased levels, whereas those acting on precursor reaction steps (GAPDH, GOT) are not affected to the same extent by spirolactone.

Labile Metabolites. Neither energy-rich phosphates nor lactate showed any significant difference between spirolactone and control patients.

Urinary Excretion Studies. Figure 3 summarizes electrolyte excretion patterns. While the urinary potassium reveals only slight and inconsistent changes, the sodium diuresis is considerably increased in patients with spirolactone. The diuretic effect of the drug is also reflected in increased water excretion.

Discussion

The present study indicates that spirolactone reduces perifocal brain edema in man. This is also supported, in part, by results of similar studies reported by REULEN et al. [7, 8], who investigated and compared the effects of ethacrynic acid, spirolactone and dexamethasone on perifocal brain edema. In view of the data reported here and findings derived from exerimental studies, 3 possible mechanisms may be considered, to explain the favorable influence of spirolactone on brain edema. The water and sodium diuresis observed in patients treated with spirolactone suggests the therapeutic result is *an unspecific renal effect*. However, it seems questionable whether enhanced diuresis is the only mechanism involved. Findings concerning the metabolic activity in the cerebral

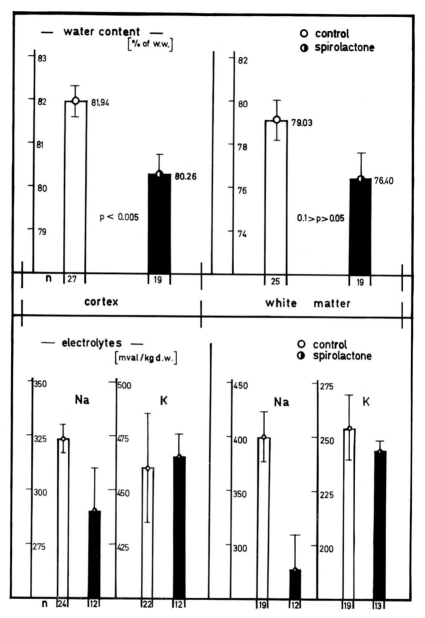

Fig. 1. Water content and tissue electrolytes in specimens from cortex and white matter of untreated and spirolactone-pretreated patients

tissue following administration of spirolactone suggest an extrarenal action of the drug on the central nervous system. Enzyme activity in the citric acid-system, which, in other target tissue e. g. the kidney [9, 10], was shown to respond to aldosterone administration, was found to be higher in brain tissue specimens from patients pretreated with spirolactone than in control specimens. This observation may lend support to the concept suggested by KOCZOREK that the edematous brain tissue does not benefit from the anti-aldosterone compound itself, but rather from the endogenous aldosterone, which is shown to increase due to spirolactone administration. This would imply a second mechanism, namely an *aldosterone-mediated effect of spirolactone* on brain tissue. Finally, recent animal experiments have yielded some evidence of a *specific cerebral effect of spirolactone*. This, at least, is our interpretation of characteristic, dose-dependent and reproducible EEG changes induced in intact but also in adrenalectomized dogs following the application of spirolactone [11]. Furthermore, studies on the blood-brain barrier permeability to a radioactive-labeled compound[3] revealed a considerable accumulation in brain tissue, suggesting a specific binding mechanism of the drug in the central nervous system [12].

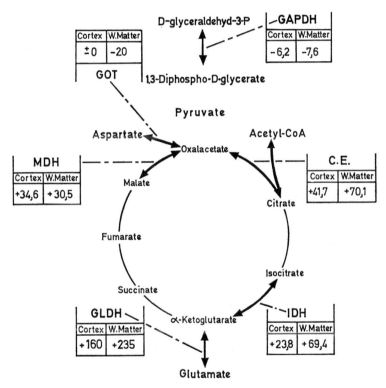

Fig. 2. Relative changes of enzyme activities in brain tissue in response to spirolactone pretreatment

In spite of the fact that we are only beginning to acquire a better insight into this approach to the treatment of brain edema, encouraging results from

---

3 SC-14266-^{3}H, G. D. SEARL + Co, Chicago, Illinois, U.S.A.

24-hours urine

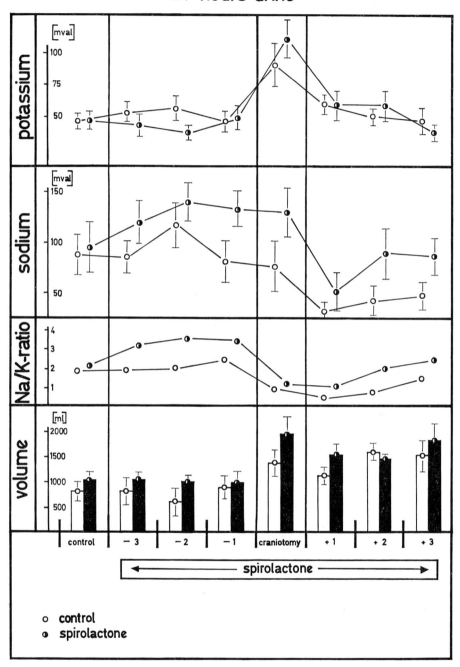

Fig. 3. Urinary excretion studies in control and spirolactone patients

a more recent series of patients pretreated with large doses of aldosterone indicate that it might be a very promising approach [13].

Summary

A reduction in the extent of perifocal brain edema was found in patients pretreated with spirolactone when compared with control subjects. Evidence is provided that the therapeutic effect of spirolactone on brain edema may be due to the following mechanisms of action: an unspecific renal effect, an aldosterone-mediated effect and/or a specific cerebral effect.

Key Words: Spirolactone, aldosterone, brain edema.

References

1. JAHRMAERKER, H.: Wann welche Diuretica? Der Internist **12**, 364–375 (1971).
2. KOCZOREK, K. R., ANGSTWURM, H., BEATHMANN, A., ENGELHARDT, R., REULEN, H. J., SCHMIEDEK, P., VOGT, W., SIMON, B., FRICK, E., BRENDEL, W.: Aldosteronausscheidung beim Pseudotumor cerebri – einer klinischen Form des Hirnödems unbekannter Ursache. In: BUECHERL, E. S., KRUECK, F., LEPPLA, W., SCHLEIER, F. (Eds.): Postoperative Störungen des Elektrolyt- und Wasserhaushaltes, S. 177–188. Stuttgart-New York: F. K. Schattauer 1968.
3. BAETHMANN, A., KOCZOREK, KH. R., REULEN, H. J., WESEMANN, W., HOFMANN, H. F., ANGSTWURM, A., BRENDEL, W.: Die Beeinflussung des traumatischen Hirnödems durch Aldosteron, Aldosteronantagonisten und Dexamethason im Tierexperiment, ibid. 168–175.
4. WESEMANN, W., PIA, H. W.: Aldadiene-Kalium in der Neurochirurgie, ibid. p. 259–270.
5. SCHMIEDEK, P., BAETHMANN, A., ENZENBACH, R.: The estimation of cerebral metabolites for the purpose of assessing the results of treatment on cerebral edema. In: Proc. Germ. Soc. f. Neurosurg. Amsterdam: Excerpta Medica 1971.
6. REULEN, H. J., MEDZIHRADSKY, F., ENZENBACH, R., MARGUTH, F.: Electrolytes, fluids and energy metabolism in human cerebral edema. Arch. Neurol. **21**, 517–544 (1969).
7. REULEN, H. J., SAMII, M., KOCZOREK, KH. R., BAETHMANN, A., SCHÜRMANN, K.: Diuretics in cerebral edema. In: THURAU, K., JAHRMAEKER, H. (Eds.): Renal Transport and Diuretics, p. 469–481. Berlin-Heidelberg-New York: Springer 1969.
8. REULEN, H. J., HADJIDIMOS, A., SCHÜRMANN, K.: The effect of dexamethasone and diuretics on water and electrolyte content, rCBF and energy metabolism in perifocal brain edema in man. Proceedings of Workshop on the Effect of Steroids on Brain Edema. June 1972. Berlin-Heidelberg-New York: Springer 1972.
9. FIMOGNARI, G. M., PORTER, G. A., EDELMAN, I.: The role of the tricarboxylic acid cycle in the action of aldosterone on sodium transport. Biochim. biophys. Acta **135**, 89 (1967).
10. KINNE, R., KIRSTEN, R.: Der Einfluß von Aldosteron auf die Aktivität mitochondrialer und cytoplasmatischer Enzyme in der Rattenniere. Pflügers Arch. ges. Physiol. **300**, 244 (1968).
11. MERTIN, J., SIMON, O., SCHMIEDEK, P.: EEG-Veränderungen unter Aldadiene-Kalium (in preparation).
12. SCHMIEDEK, P., BAETHMANN, A., SADEE, W.: Cerebral uptake of ^{3}H-spirolactone in the dog (in preparation).

13. Schmiedek, P., Baethmann, A., Schneider, E., Oettinger, W., Enzenbach, R., Marguth, F., Brendel, W.: The effect of aldosterone and an aldosterone-antagonist on the metabolism of perifocal brain edema in man. Proceedings of Workshop on the Effects of Steroids on Brain Edema. June 1972. Berlin-Heidelberg-New York: Springer 1972.

Comments to Session 7

T. W. Langfitt and J. W. F. Beks

A major issue discussed in this session was the relationship between ICP and survival in patients with acute head injuries. Several investigators have divided their patients into three groups according to the maximum level of ICP: low, medium, and high pressure. In the series reported by Donaghy and Numoto, there was not a good correlation between levels of ICP and survival. In contrast, Troupp found that the mortality rate in those patients with normal pressure was quite low whereas nearly all patients with an IVP higher than 60 mmHg died. Jennett and Langfitt commented that the mortality rate in their patients with normal or slightly elevated ICP was nearly as high as in those with elevated ICP. Thus, there is uncertainty about the correlation of ICP with neurological status and survival in acutely brain-injured patients.

Numoto demonstrated a significant difference in pressure between the supratentorial space and posterior fossa in head-injured patients. This phenomenon is now well recognized and appears to be common in these patients. Troupp described fluctuations in jugular venous PO_2 that correlated better with respiratory status than ICP. The additional important point was made during the discussion that there is no predictable correlation between cerebral venous PO_2 and the metabolic state of the brain. Therefore, cerebral and jugular venous PO_2 values cannot be used as an index of the adequacy of the cerebral circulation. Rossanda asked Troupp if the number of patients with very high levels of ICP could be explained by preoperative recording in patients with space-occupying surgical masses. Troupp replied that all the patients in his group who had space-occupying lesions were operated on prior to continuous recording of ICP.

The discussion that followed the papers presented by Tindall and de Rougemont considered the origin of pressure waves. In Tindall's studies in head injured patients he found that approximately 75% of all plateau waves were preceded by an increase in end-tidal CO_2 as a manifestation of respiratory depression. The origin of the pressure waves in the remaining patients was not determined. Cooper pointed out that pressure waves may also develop in association with accumulation of metabolic CO_2. In both instances it would appear that CO_2 accumulation is the stimulus for development of the pressure waves, but in one instance the increase in CO_2 is systemic and in the other it occurs within the brain tissue itself. There was some discussion of a possible neurogenic origin for the pressure waves, perhaps distortion of the brain stem, producing stimulation of a vasodilator center, but there was general agreement that there is no clear evidence for a cerebrovascular neurogenic origin of the pressure phenomena at present. Lundberg pointed out that pressure waves almost always develop in a "tight" situation within the intracranial space when most of the displaceable volume has been exhausted by brain swelling or expansion of a mass lesion, and the waves generally arise from an elevated base of ICP.

Cooper and Hulme described depression of rhythmic oscillations of cortical PO$_2$ during rising ICP and in other circumstances. Although they related these changes to impending loss of autoregulation, they agreed in the subsequent discussion that the rhythmic oscillations are probably a manifestation of vasomotion within the microcirculation as described by Zweifach in direct observations of brain surface. They did not test autoregulation in their patients in the conventional manner.

Nornes described a correlation between ICP and the time of re-rupture of intracranial aneurysms. Presumably as ICP falls the transmural pressure across the aneurysm increases, and bleeding is more likely. Zwetnow discussed his observations in animals following experimental lacerations of a cerebral artery. ICP rises immediately toward SAP, arresting the bleeding. ICP then falls slowly even though the volume of the hematoma remains the same due to displacement of CSF from the intracranial space. Autoregulation may remain intact and preserve CBF during a rise in ICP.

Schmiedek found a reduction in water and sodium content in biopsy specimens of cortex and white matter obtained in patients pretreated with spirolactone. There was no change in the energy state of the tissue as determined by measurements of phosphocreatine, ATP, and other metabolites. Siesjö pointed out the limitations of measuring tissue metabolites in biopsy material. As soon as the tissue is separated from its blood supply the concentration of metabolites changes rapidly, the most notable change being an immediate decline in ATP and phosphocreatine.

Session 8

Hydrocephalus
(Clinical)

Relations between Cerebrospinal Fluid Pressure (CSFP), Elasticity (E') of the Dura, and Volume of the CSF (VCSF)

R. Lorenz and E. Grote

The relations between volume and pressure within the cerebrospinal fluid system are rarely discussed, although it has been known for several decades that the laws of volume as found in the high pressure system (arterial pressure) are also applicable to the CSF-system [1]. Schaltenbrand and Wördehoff [2] tried to analyze these relations by withdrawing and replacing certain amounts of CSF. We used a modification of this method and measured CSFP during therapeutic lumbar punctures to evaluate the elasticity.

Methods

Lumbar CSF pressure was measured through a catheter or needle of 1 mm internal diameter connected to a capacity-transducer and to a conventional recorder system. The whole system complied with the known physical and physiological recommendations [3, 4, 5]. All lumba rpunctures were performed in anesthetized patients lying in the horizontal position.

In all patients arterial blood pressure, heart rate and respiratory rate were also monitored, and CSF protein and cells were measured; in some cases venous pressure was also recorded.

Material

296 examinations were performed in 158 patients. 82 curves were recorded in patients with infratentorial, 81 in patients with supratentorial space-occupying lesions. There were 35 cases of hydrocephalus, 32 of head-injury; in 67 cases curves were taken from patients with aneurysms, angiomas, and intracerebral hematomas.

Patients with manifestations of mesencephalic or bulbar herniation were excluded.

Results

1. Influence of Age

The age of patients has no bearing on the initial lumbar CSFP. In earlier investigations [6] it appeared that the pressure was higher in the first 3 decades than later. This was not confirmed; there is no clear correlation between age and the angle of decline of CSFP when CSF is removed in 5 ml fractions. This is also true of elasticity as calculated from the equation:

$$E' = \frac{P}{V}$$

The module does not depend on age, as might have been expected.

2. Influence of Time-Course, CSF Protein, Pleocytosis, and Vegetative Parmeters

Four main diagnostic groups are distinguished: supratentorial tumors, infratentorial tumors, hydrocephalus, and severe head injuries.

As shown in Fig. 1, the CSFP varies significantly according to the diagnosis and time-course. In supratentorial tumors, CSFP shows a peak in the first week after operation; in infratentorial tumors the initial CSFP is high, in hydrocephalus we find a situation similar to that in supratentorial space-occupying lesions, and in head injuries we observe a combination of both forms: initial high pressure and another peak in the second week. A normalizing trend can be seen in all groups in the second and third weeks after operation or head injury.

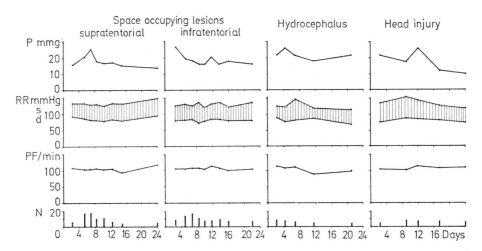

Fig. 1. Time course of the mean values of lumbar CSFP (P), arterial pressure (RR), and heart rate (PF). N = frequency of measurements

No definite correlations with systolic and diastolic blood pressure or heart rate were observed, nor was any correlation with CSF-protein or pleocytosis found. The relations are completely irregular.

3. Pressure Curve after Removal of CSF

After removal of CSF in 5 ml fractions, the decline in pressure is dependent on the initial pressure. The higher the initial pressure, the more marked the decline. At a level of 5–15 mmHg, the so-called normal range, all mean values tend to a "steady state", indicating that the resulting E′ is approximately zero (Fig. 2).

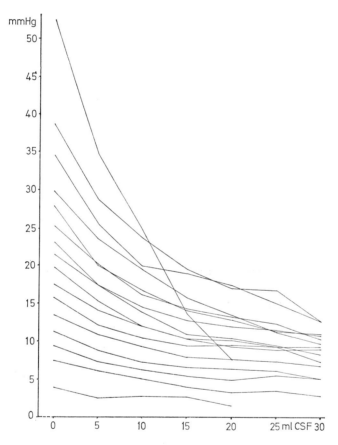

Fig. 2. Mean values of CSFP after removal of CSF in 5 ml fractions as related to the initial pressure

Depending on the time interval between operation or injury and measurement of CSFP, some patients display a steady decline in the pressure curve after removal of CSF. Nearly 50% of the patients with intracranial tumors, 10% of patients with hydrocephalus, and about 30% of patients with head injuries had so-called plateaus. This means that no fall in pressure was observed after removal of 5 ml of CSF. These plateaus usually lie within the normal range of CSFP, thus indicating that for this phase an elasticity threshold has been reached. In other words, the withdrawal of CSF is compensated. On the other hand, it seems that the plateaus are sometimes dependent upon the inital pressure (Fig. 3).

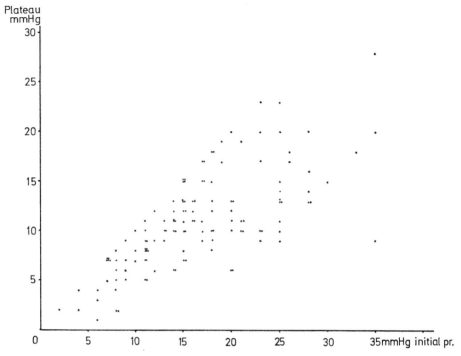

Fig. 3. Altitude of plateaus due to the initial pressure after removal of 5 ml CSF fractions

4. Influence of CSFP on Pulse Waves

The decline in CSFP leads to a decrease in pulse waves. Pulse waves also decreased in several patients whose CSFP showed no decline after removal of CSF.

Comments

Our investigations show that CSFP depends on the diagnosis and the time-interval between lumbar puncture and operation or head injury. In all groups studied CSFP was initially raised and showed some kind of peak. The CSFP curves of supra- and infratentorial tumors are significantly different. In cases of supratentorial tumors the highest CSFP-values are reached when brain edema is clinically manifestat and can thus be interpreted as a result of the edema. CSFP has a tendency to normalization. The normal range of CSFP 5–15 mmHg is reached within 14–21 days. The more marked the initial fall in CSFP after CSF removal, the more the amount of tissue seems to predominate. Curves show a more pronounced drop when the primary CSFP is high. On the other hand, in relation to the initial pressure, 10–50% of the individual curves contain a plateau where CSFP is not reduced despite removal of CSF. In hydrocephalus such plateaus are rarer than in intracranial tumors. The stimulus for CSF production may be stronger in tumors than in hydrocephalus, because in hydrocephalus one can assume a longer-lasting imbalance between CSF production and resorption resulting in a decreased production. If there is a large CSF pool, the removal of 5 ml does not play an important role; if there is predominance of tissue, the removal of 5 ml will cause a severe fall in CSFP.

The angle of decline for the mean values is dependent on the level of primary CSFP, indicating that there is an elasticity threshold, as calculated by the formula

$$E' = \frac{\Delta P}{\Delta V}.$$

This borderline lies within the normal range.

The amplitude of CSF pulse waves is known to decrease with falling CSFP. But even in cases when CSFP is constant after removal of CSF, there is some decrease in the amplitude of pulse waves. This means that the decrease in pulse waves following removal of CSF does not depend exclusively on elasticity factors.

Summary

CSFP was measured during 296 lumbar punctures, initially and after removal of CSF in 5 ml fractions. The relations between pressure and volume and the elasticity module, as calculated in form of the quotient pressure/volume, are discussed. The investigations indicate that there are significant differences in the level of CSFP, depending on the time relation between operation and puncture, and on the diagnosis. They are also correlated with the clinical manifestations of brain edema. The elasticity module gives information on the CSF volume, or the predominance of the tissue factor.

Key Words : Cerebrospinal fluid pressure (CSFP), CSF volume, brain edema.

References

1. BENDER, F.: Normaler und pathologisch veränderter Liquordruck mit Bemerkungen zur Liquordynamik. Z. ges. exp. Med. **139**, 745–752 (1965).
2. SCHALTENBRAND, G., WÖRDEHOFF, PH.: Ein einfaches Verfahren zur Bestimmung der Liquorproduktion und Liquorresorption in der Klinik. Nervenarzt **18**, 458–463 (1947).
3. FRANK, O.: Kritik der elastischen Manometer. Z. Biol. **44**, 445–613 (1903).
4. FRANK, O.: Die Elastizität der Blutgefäße. Z. Biol. **71**, 255–272 (1920).
5. WAGNER, R.: Methodik und Ergebnisse fortlaufender Blutdruckschreibung am Menschen. Leipzig: G. Thieme 1942.
6. GROTE, E., LORENZ, R.: Dynamics of CSF: relations between volume and pressure. Minerva Neurochirurgica, Milano (in press).
7. GROTE, E., LORENZ, R.: Pulse amplitudes of cerebrospinal fluid and their relation to cerebrospinal fluid pressure (in preparation).

Intracranial Volume/Pressure Relationships during Continuous Monitoring of Ventricular Fluid Pressure[1]

J. D. MILLER and J. GARIBI

Introduction

To explain the widely varying and fluctuating levels of intracranial pressure (ICP) which may be encountered in neurosurgical patients [1, 2, 3] and the differing responses of ICP in such patients to the administration of anaesthetic agents [4] the concept of a non-linear, exponential relationship between addition to the volume of the intracranial contents and ICP has been invoked. It is implicit in this type of volume/pressure relationship that as resting ICP increases, so also should the change in ICP produced by a uniform change in intracranial volume.

An exponential intracranial volume/pressure relationship was demonstrated in experimental animals by LANGFITT's group [5] and is implied in earlier clinical reports of intracranial volume/pressure relationships [6]; but the concept has yet to be tested over a wide range of levels of ICP, including the high levels now known to be present in some neurosurgical patients [1], and in patients suffering from increased ICP from a variety of causes. This was the purpose of the present study.

Patients and Methods

The investigation was carried out in 20 consecutive neurosurgical patients in whom ventricular fluid pressure (VFP) monitoring was already in progress. In all 20 patients VFP was above normal for at least part of the period of recording; 5 patients had brain tumours, 6 had head injuries, 4 hydrocephalus, 4 intracranial hemorrhage and the remaining patient had post-hypoxic brain swelling.

VFP monitoring was performed as described by LUNDBERG [1] using an externally mounted transducer[2] and slow-running chart recorder[3]. In each patient the immediate response of VFP to repeated rapid injections and/or

1 This work was supported by a grant from the Secretary of State for Scotland's Fund for Medical Research.
2 Blood pressure transducer CEC Type 4-327-L221, Devices Instruments Ltd., Welwyn Garden City, Herts., England.
3 M2 heated stylus. 2 channel chart recorder, Devices Instruments Ltd., Welwyn Garden City, Herts., England.

withdrawals of physiological saline solution to and from the ventricular catheter was studied. After a test injection/withdrawal of 0.25–0.5 ml, a constant
volume change of 1 ml was used and the results expressed as changes of VFP
in mmHg/ml. This procedure was carried out at differing levels of resting VFP
in each patient at various times during the period of VFP monitoring. All
patients were studied at the bedside and all were spontaneously breathing, un-
anaesthetised but at differing conscious levels, from alert to deeply unconscious.

Arterial blood pressure was measured by sphygomanometry repeatedly
during each study and results were rejected if there was any large fluctuation
of blood pressure. Arterial blood gases were measured by direct-reading
electrodes. 371 measurements of change of VFP per ml change in CSF volume
were made in the 20 patients.

Results

Mean arterial blood pressure in the patients at the time of study was 98.6 $\pm$
13.1 (S.D.) mmHg; arterial PCO_2 was 34.7 $\pm$ 6.4 mmHg, arterial pH was
7.41 $\pm$ 0.04 and arterial PO_2 on spontaneous air breathing was 72.4 $\pm$ 10.8
mmHg.

Changes in VFP produced by 1 ml changes in CSF volume were compared
with the resting levels of VFP and a further comparison was made between infusion and withdrawal of fluid to and from the measuring system. There was a
positive correlation between the resting VFP and the amount of increase in
VFP per ml of fluid injected (Fig. 1); 174 observations were made in 17 patients, resulting in the following regression equation:

$$y = 0.204\,x + 0.106\ (r = 0.408;\ P < 0.001)$$

where x = resting VFP, and y = change in VFP/ml. There was also a significant correlation between the resting VFP and the reduction in VFP per ml
fluid withdrawn from the measuring system (Fig. 2); 197 observations were
made in 16 patients, resulting in the regression equation:

$$y = 0.143\,x + 0.065\ (r = 0.452;\ P < 0.001).$$

The gradient of the regression line for withdrawal of fluid is less steep than
that obtained during infusion of fluid to the ventricular catheter, suggesting
that at any given level of resting VFP there will be a greater rise in VFP when
a given volume of fluid is injected than a fall in VFP when the same volume is
withdrawn. To test this impression, 56 paired observations were made in 10
patients in which 1 ml aliquots of fluid were alternately infused then withdrawn
and vice versa. Paired results were accepted for comparison only if the resting
VFP levels for each of the pair of observations were within 5 mmHg of each
other. For infusion of fluid the mean increase in VFP was 4.37 $\pm$ 0.49 (SE)

mmHg/ml. For withdrawal of fluid the decrease in VFP was 3.49 $\pm$ 0.42 (SE) mmHg/ml. This difference was significant (paired t $=3.4262$; P <0.005).

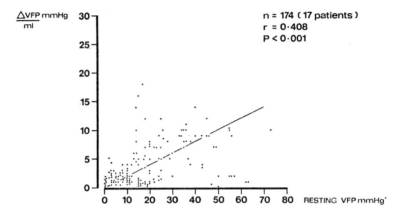

Fig. 1. Relationship between resting ventricular fluid pressure (abscissa) and the increase in VFP in mmHg per ml fluid injected into the ventricular catheter (ordinate). The regression line is shown; its equation is in the text

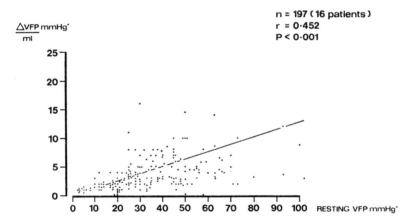

Fig. 2. Relationship between resting ventricular fluid pressure (abscissa) and the decrease in VFP in mmHg per ml fluid aspirated from the ventricular catheter (ordinate). The regression line is shown and its equation given in the text

The study demonstrated an overall adherence to the concept of an exponential intracranial volume/pressure relationship, over a wide range of resting VFP levels for both infusion (0–73 mmHg) and withdrawal (3–102 mmHg) of fluid, and in patients with several different causes for increased ICP. Analysis of the results in individual patients, however, showed enormous variations in the change in VFP per ml change in volume at any given level or resting VFP.

This is apparent from inspection of the scatter of data points in Figs. 1 and 2. For example, at a resting VFP of 15 mmHg, the increase in VFP in response to a 1 ml injection of physiological saline varied from 1.0–16.0 mmHg in different patients. These variations in response did not appear to be related to the cause of the increased ICP, since the 3 patients with the greatest pressure responses to an induced intracranial volume change were suffering from hydrocephalus, head injury and a middle cerebral artery aneurysm, following clipping. The numbers of patients in these subgroups are small, however, so that firm conclusions on this cannot yet be drawn.

Discussion

In studying only the immediate response of ICP to an induced change in CSF volume, what is being tested is the bulk compliance, or more exactly its reciprocal, the elastance, of the entire intracranial contents. It is not possible to assess by which mechanism volume compensation is being achieved, whether by shift of CSF, venous blood, or brain itself, or by alterations in CSF secretion or absorption rates. Also, when a difference in pressure response is demonstrated with infusion and withdrawal of fluid, it is possible only to suggest that the intracranial contents as a whole exhibit hysteresis, and although the hysteresis loop may be related to venous elastic tension [7] there is no way of proving this from this simple type of measurement.

Despite the limitations of these measurements, they do suggest that it is permissable to use the concept of bulk elastance of the intracranial contents in neurosurgical patients with differing brain lesions. More important, however, they are simple to perform and yield information which is helpful in the individual patient during VFP monitoring; information, moreover, which is not available by examination of the usual chart recording. It is to be hoped that this type of functional test of intracranial compensation may help in the prevention of the development of the "tight brain" by giving some advance warning of the stage at which small increases in intracranial volume cause large increases in ICP, thus enabling ICP to be held within acceptable levels.

Summary

The response of ventricular fluid pressure to 1 ml changes of CSF volume was studied in 29 patients. There is a positive correlation between the height of the resting level of VFP and the change in pressure per ml change in volume. This supports the concept of an exponential relationship between intracranial volume and pressure. Increases in volume produce a greater change in VFP than identical decreases in volume. There are large variations between patients in the response of VFP to a given change in CSF volume, even at the same resting levels of VFP. Study of the pressure response to volume changes yields valuable clinical information additional to that obtained from routine VFP monitoring.

Key Words: Intracranial volume, intracranial pressure, ventricular fluid pressure, compliance, elastance.

References

1. LUNDBERG, N.: Continuous recording and control of ventricular fluid pressure in neurosurgical practice. Acta psychiat. scand. (Suppl. 149) **36** (1960).
2. RICHARDSON, A., HIDE, T. A. H., EVERSDEN, I. D.: Long term continuous intracranial pressure monitoring by means of a modified subdural pressure transducer. Lancet **2**, 687 to 690 (1970).
3. JOHNSTON, I. H., JOHNSTON, J. A., JENNETT, W. B.: Intracranial pressure changes following head injury. Lancet **2**, 433–436 (1970).
4. JENNETT, W. B., BARKER, J., FITCH, W., McDOWALL, D. G.: Effect of anaesthesia on intracranial pressure in patients with space-occupying lesions. Lancet **1**, 61–64 (1969).
5. LANGFITT, T. W., WEINSTEIN, J. D., KASSELL, N. F.: Cerebral vasomotor paralysis produced by intracranial hypertension. Neurology (Minneap.) **15**, 622–641 (1965).
6. POLLOCK, L. J., BOSHES, B.: Cerebrospinal fluid pressure. Arch. Neurol. Psychiat. (Chic.) **36**, 931–974 (1936).
7. DAVSON, H.: Physiology of the cerebrospinal fluid, pp. 341–367. London: Churchill 1967.

Computer Modelling of CSF Pressure/Volume and its Relationship to Hydrocephalus[1]

A. Marmarou and K. Shulman

It is our contention that in the hydrocephalic infant the degree of compensation to volume disturbance within the cerebrospinal fluid (CSF) compartment is dependent upon only 2 parameters: 1. the compliance of those intracranial compartments capable of volume exchange, and 2. the resistance to CSF absorption. We reported in 1971 [1] that volume/pressure curves in hydrocephalus are not straight lines, but exponentials and that a pressure/volume index (PVI) can be established by plotting volume increments against the log of the resultant pressure. This procedure of plotting the PVI, in combination with an opening pressure represents the complete graphical description of the compliant properties of the infant. The present paper describes computer modelling based upon this concept.

Methods

1. From existing physiologic data and results of pilot experiments, a physical model was evolved which simulated in conceptual fashion the formation, storage, and absorption systems. 2. From these block diagrams a series of equations were formulated to mimic the physical model in mathematical terms. The mathematical model was then programmed on a computer. 3. Experimental tests were conducted to provide the necessary biologic data. 4. Series of controlled disturbances were then applied to both the computer model and the laboratory animal. 5. The responses of the computer and animal were then compared. 6. If the comparison between theoretical and experimental results match, then the mathematical equivalent of the system is correct and the initial physiologic statements are valid to the extent of the biological description.

Results

A. The first deals with the theoretical prediction of fluid shifts within the cranial vault in response to sudden volume disturbance. If a known volume is suddenly inserted into the CSF space, the pressure rises sharply at the moment of volume addition followed by a return to baseline. What is responsible for

1 This investigation was supported in part by a National Institute of Health Fellowship No. 5FO3GM4571002 from the Institute of General Medical Sciences.

the return of pressure to baseline? Our original thought was that the rapid
reduction in pressure is most probably due to shifts in venous blood and trans-
location of CSF with absorption of CSF playing a minor role in the rapid phase
of the volume compensatory response. The theoretical predictions from the
model show that this is not the case. According to computer studies the rapid
initial fall in pressure as well as the more gradual return is due solely to absorption of CSF. Blood volume shifts occur within seconds of the disturbance
and govern only the level of instantaneous pressure rise, while the threefold
drop in pressure occurring within a one minute period is due solely to fluid absorption. The physiologic explanation is due to 2 factors. 1. An exponential
pressure/volume curve in which at high pressure levels a small volume change
will produce a large change in pressure and 2. a higher rate of absorption at increased pressure. This occurs even though the absorption resistance is constant
in the simulated model.

Figure 1 shows the comparison between the predicted output based upon
the model equations and what was observed experimentally. The model then is
capable of predicting not only the initial rise in pressure but the actual time course
of pressure decay. It points out that compliance derived from pressure/volume
data governs the initial rise and compliance together with resistance to absorption controls the rate of decay.

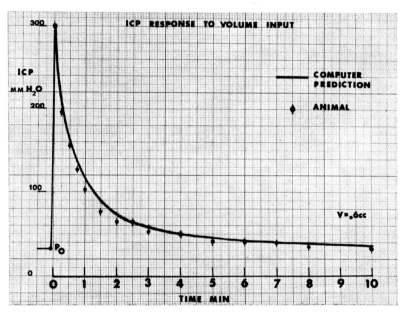

Fig. 1. Comparison of computer model prediction of pressure response and actual test data

B. The second question is what are the factors which control resting CSF
pressure? It is our concept, based on the analysis, that the resting or steady
state intracranial pressure (ICP) is governed by pressure in the dural sinus and

the product of formation rate and absorption resistance. According to the model, if dural sinus pressure and absorption resistance were held constant, a linear increase in formation rate would produce a linear or straight line increase of resting ICP. Secondly, the slope of this line would be equal to the absorption resistance. These hypotheses are depicted graphically in Fig. 2. Here we show the analytical relationship of resting ICP and formation rate. At zero formation, according to the equations, ICP equals dural sinus pressure (P_d). At normal formation rate ICP increases to opening pressure level (P_0). If formation rate were then suddenly increased to a new level and held constant, ICP would increase in rate and finally approach a steady state value (P_1). Higher steady state values of ICP would then follow a straight line as formation increased (P_2, P_3, P_4 . . .).

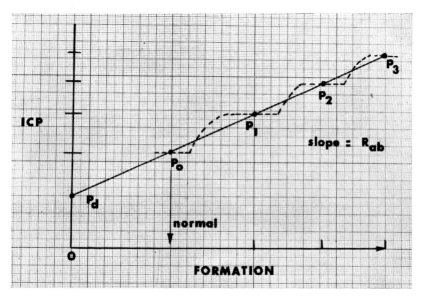

Fig. 2. Graphical description of analytical model relationship of intracranial pressure and formation. At zero formation ICP equals dural sinus pressure (P_d). At normal formation ICP equals opening pressure (P_0). As formation is increased, ICP passes through a transient phase before reaching a new steady state value (P_1). The same process occurs at higher rates of formation (P_2, P_3 . . .). The plot of the steady state values (P_1, P_2, P_3 . . .) form a straight line. The slope of this straight line is proportional to absorption resistance. This theoretical description is the first approximation to the model used in the systems analysis of ICP pressure phenomenae

We proceeded to investigate these hypotheses by implementing the following protocol. First, as a matter of procedure, the standard pressure volume data was obtained in the animal with the technique described. Second, sudden increases in formation rate were simulated by infusing saline into the cisterna magna in step wise fashion and recording the time course of pressure. No outflow was used.

The plot of steady state intracranial pressure vs inflow rate was linear. This is in contrast to the exponential rise of pressure in the pressure/volume curve. To test whether or not the slope of this straight line was equal to absorption resistance we used the following approach. We had previously determined that the transient behavior of ICP was controlled by compliance and the resistance to absorption. If this slope did in fact represent absorption resistance, then by combining the slope value with the PV data, we should be able to predict the time course of pressure in response to a step change in infusion rate. Figure 3 shows the comparison between the predicted output based upon the model equations and what was observed experimentally. The error in prediction is less than 3%.

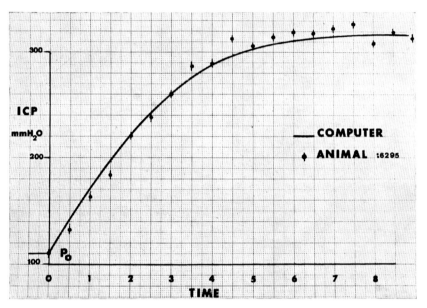

Fig. 3. Comparison of computer prediction and animal test data of pressure response to simulated formation rate increase (step change in infusion). Steady state level of 320 mm H₂O was reached in approximately 8 min

Discussion

Our main objective in this research is to use the computer to model the CSF system of the hydrocephalic infant in order to investigate a magnitude of para meters affecting intracranial pressure some of which are beyond physiological measurement. With the infant model, the flexibility in observing the effects of changes in compliance, formation and absorption is increased since the computer can be programmed to vary these parameters not only in magnitude but to follow a specific time course. The success of this approach depends upon the credibility of the model and whether or not the necessary physiologic data can be obtained. The animal studies have indicated that a reasonable approximation of the CSF system can be realized with limited information. The pressure/volume index is an example. It describes the combined effects of the compliant element and replaces the resulting exponential relationship between pressure and volume by a single number. The infusion studies have shown that a similar technique of combining individual elements can be applied to the absorptive mechanism. Future effort will concentrate on the evaluation of similar infant parameters to expand the present capability of the computer model.

Summary

A computer modelling technique has been utilized in the investigation of volume compensatory mechanisms and relationships of compliance, formation and absorption to resting levels of intracranial pressure (ICP). Pressure/volume parameters of adult cats were used to predict the transient changes of ICP. Infusion studies indicated a linear relationship between resting ICP levels and simulated increased formation rate. Computer predictions of transient ICP changes were within 5% of similar animal responses.

Key Words : Cerebrospinal fluid pressure–volume compensation, computer analysis, ICP–compliance, pressure/volume index.

References

1. SHULMAN, K., MARMAROU, A.: Pressure-volume considerations in infantile hydrocephalus. Develop. Med. Child Neurol. (Suppl. 25) **13**, 90–95 (1971).
2. MARMAROU, A.: A mathematical model of the CSF system: PhD Thesis (in press).

Long Term Measurement of Extradural Pressure in "Low Pressure" Hydrocephalus[1]

L. Symon, N. W. C. Dorsch, and R. J. Stephens

The differential diagnosis of communicating hydrocephalus remains uncertain. The development of effective shunt systems for the treatment of hydrocephalus [1, 2] and the enthusiastic report of Adams et al. [3] led to an increase in the number of referrals of these potentially surgically suitable patients to neurosurgical services. Our own experience with shunt systems in low pressure hydrocephalus [4] were not altogether happy, however, the complication rate of the procedure in such patients being so appreciable that a further attempt to fractionate communicating hydrocephalus from atrophy seemed vital.

Our experience of proven communicating hydrocephalus had shown us that pressure might be on one day normal and on the next considerably raised. It therefore seemed to us that the development of continuous measurement techniques to observe the pressure profile in such patients over a period of some days might indicate patients in whom the pressure was raised at some time, and who might therefore be expected to benefit from shunting from those in whom the pressure was never raised.

Material and Methods

The requirements for an ideal intracranial pressure transducer have been stated by the National Academy of Engineering Sub-Committee on Technology and Systems Transfer, 1971, to be: 1. Extradural; 2. No risk of infection and low discomfort; 3. Implantable, preferably wire-less; 4. Small physical size in mass; 5. Calibration capacity from outside; 6. Stable; 7. Minimal temperature sensitivity; 8. Impervious to environment; 9. Extended use availability 7–30 days; 10. Sensitivity less than 1 mm of mercury relative to atmospheric; 11. Not too expensive.

These have been modified, in our own device, under 6 headings:
1. Accurate in the appropriate pressure range
2. Stable
3. Calibration availability in situ
4. Minimal risk
5. Minimal discomfort
6. Low cost.

1 This work was supported by the Medical Research Council.

The device used is an implantable transducer in which strain gauges (either semi-conductor or in more recent instances, metal foil), are attached to either side of one arm of a U-shaped metal strip, and the assembly mounted within a chamber in a disc of epoxy resin. A small polyethylene tube connects to atmosphere, and in transducers for human use the leads from the strain gauges are taken out through a stainless steel tube which acts as a handle when the device is implanted. The detailed construction of the device has been described [5]. The gauges are postponed so that pressure applied to the face of the transducer will compress one gauge and stretch the other. Use of 2 gauges greatly reduces temperature drift. Recent transducers have been constructed using 4 gauges with a complete bridge in 2 halves on the transducer arm, thus further minimising temperature drift. The operating characteristics of this new device are summarised in Fig. 1.

The transducer is implanted extradurally through a burrhole under general anaesthetic, usually in the post-frontal pre-coronal region parasagitally. A symmetrical burrhole for ventricular tapping and checking of ventricular pressure measurement is made at the same time on the other side, over the non-dominant hemisphere.

Seventeen studies have been carried out on 16 patients, one patient being studied twice with an interval of nearly two years separating the two recordings. The majority were referred for exclusion of communicating hydrocephalus as a cause of their advancing intellectual deterioration. All had had pneumo-encephalographic studies, and many had had RISA-encephalography. Communicating hydrocephalus following subarachnoid hemorrhage did not form the major portion of our study, since the diagnosis in these circumstances was usually obvious and the justification for transducer studies less clear.

Results

Of the 16 patients studied, nine showed unequivocal A waves occurring through the night and in most instances generally a much more active trace than the remainder of the patients. The pressure waves which we have regarded as A waves are different from those described by LUNDBERG [6] in high pressure cases in that though they are sustained rises of pressure, they seldom reach the heights obtained in other conditions (Fig. 2). The A waves described by us have lasted up to 40 min but more generally have been from 10–15 min in length. They are characterised by an increase in amplitude of the recording as well as an increase in pressure. The maximum height reached by one of our patients with communicating hydrocephalus under a basically normal pressue through-out the day was 44 mmHg on an A wave at night. Several other patients reached levels of 30–35 mmHg. Baseline pressures were not significantly different in the group who showed A waves from the group who did not. However, the group who showed A waves had a generally more active trace with more fre-

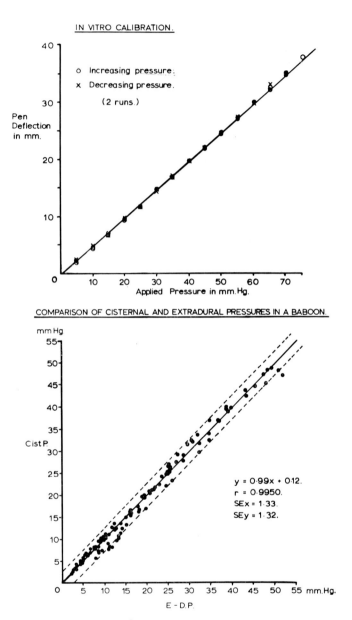

Full Bridge Foil Gauge. Gauge resistance – 120 Ω. Gauge factor – 2.1. Frequency response – Flat to 60 Hz. Resonant Frequency – > 80 Hz. Sensitivity – 4.8 μV/mmHg. at 1.15 V bridge excitation. Drift. Spontaneous – Zero. With Temperature: – 0–0.2 mmHg/C°. Sensitivity change – 0.3%/C°.

Fig. 1. Characteristics of a full bridge foil gauge made in our laboratory

quent B waves. The presence of B waves themselves was no guarantee that long lasting rises in pressure would occur at any time. All the patients who showed A waves have been shunted, with the exception of one who showed an A wave in the night following an air ventriculogram. This man's pressure trace had otherwise been quiet and we therefore did not proceed.

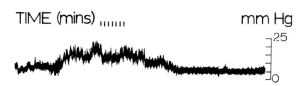

Fig. 2. A characteristic plateau wave such as occurs in patients with communicating hydro-cephalus. Extradural pressure recording

Those nine patients were submitted to a shunt and were in the majority of instances followed for some days after the shunt procedure. Invariably the pressure trace became much quieter, there were many fewer irregularities of pressure, and in most instances pressure became negative at some time during the day. In one man who was shunted with an anti-siphon valve the pressure was negative for most of the 24 h, only appearing positive on the trace during the night (Fig. 3).

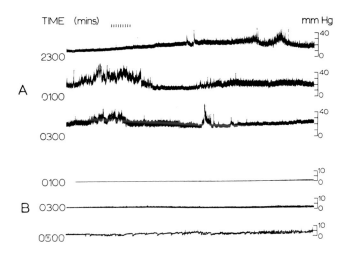

Fig. 3. Portions of overnight recording from a patient with communicating hydrocephalus before and after the insertion of a ventriculo-atrial shunt. The inactivity of the pressure trace after shunting and the fact that the pressure is for some of the time below zero are evident

Discussion

The available methods for differential diagnosis for communicating hydro-cephalus had, up to this time, been air encephalography and isotope encephalo-graphy, introduced by Bannister, Guilford and Kocen in 1967. It has been our experience that in a typical case these investigations give the same answers, isotope or air retained in the ventricles, but no dispersal of isotope or air over the cortical surface. On numerous occasions equivocal results appear in both. From our previous observations of the varying pressure in communicating hydrocephalus, and from the work of Hussey and his colleagues [7] and Lorenzo et al. [8], it seems that communicating hydrocephalus might depend upon an imbalance between production and absorptive mechanisms in such patients, so that the patients were permanently at an unstable part of the pres-sure/volume curve.

Our studies have shown that in a proportion of cases referred with a clini-cal diagnosis of communicating hydrocephalus, episodic rises of pressure occur, principally during sleep, and that these may be differentiated by detailed nursing records from artifacts produced by the patient turning in his sleep coughing, sneezing, or R.E.M. sleep. The majority of these patients who, show episodic A wave type rises, show traces of an activity entirely different from the relatively inactive pressure trace of the demented patient, suggesting that this group of patients has indeed a critically balanced production absorption CSF. capacity leading to disturbances of intracranial pressure with slight in-creases in intracranial volume, perhaps on a vascular basis, occurring principally during sleep. The exact mechanism of such disturbances is of great interest. Lundberg [6] has already shown that pCO_2 changes do not occur at any rate in the rising phase of A waves, nor have bedside recordings shown arterial pressure change at such times.

In the dement, intraventricular measurement or measurement of pressure in the lumbar subarachnoid space by fluid-conducting systems are unsatisfactory, the patients are almost always uncooperative and the risks of infection are great. In the ventricle also ventricular irritation may be provoked by the catheter, thereby making subsequent shunting virtually impossible. Subdural monitoring has been tried in our clinic and in others but the great difficulty of maintenance of a fluid-tight transducer in the subdural space has up to this time precluded its routine use. We were fortunate in having available the original cat transducer described by Corne et al. [9] which was modified for use in baboons by Corne, Stephens, and Symon [10] and further modified for man and animals as later described [5]. The device has been implanted and shown to function continuously for periods of up to 9 months in animals, and it has been implanted extradurally in patients for over 3 weeks now without problem. The capacity for external zero-reference in measuring systems as at present existing is absolutely essential. This necessitates some connection of the machine to the exterior, usually a method for membrane inflation such as we have adopted, and it does not therefore seem justified to consider the additional electronic complexity of an entirely implantable machine.

Summary

Extradural monitoring of intracranial pressure is safe and satisfactory for long-term use. Some patients, at least, with dilated ventricles and probable communicating hydrocephalus show A waves, which we suspect to be a manifestation of disordered CSF. absorptive capacity. The presence of B waves does not appear significant, especially if they are few. Extradural recording has been carried out satisfactorily in demented patients, and although it involves small surgical operations for the insertion and removal of the transducer, is substantially without risk of infection, and we believe, therefore, that it can be applied as a diagnostic test in communicating hydrocephalus.

Key Words : Extradural pressure, communicating hydrocephalus.

References

1. NULSEN, F. E., SPITZ, B. B.: Treatment of hydrocephalus by direct shunt from ventricle to jugular vein. Surg. Forum. **2**, 399–403 (1951).
2. PUDENZ, R. H., RUSSELL, F. E., HURD, A. H. et al.: Ventriculoauriculostomy – a technique for shunting cerebrospinal fluid into the right auricle. Preliminary Report, J. Neurosurg. **14**, 171–179 (1957).
3. ADAMS, R. D., FISHER, C. M., HAKIM, S., OJEMANN, R. G., SWEET, W. H.: Symptomatic occult hydrocephalus with "normal" cerebrospinal-fluid pressure. A treatable syndrome, New Engl. J. Med. **273**, 117–126 (1965).
4. ILLINGWORTH, R. D., LOGUE, V., SYMON, L., UEMURA, K.: The ventriculo-caval shunt in the treatment of adult hydrocephalus. Results and complications in 101 patients. J. Neurosurg. **35**, 681–685 (1971).
5. DORSCH, N. W. C., STEPHENS, R. J., SYMON, L.: An intracranial pressure transducer. Biomed. Engng. **6**, 452–457 (1971).
6. LUNDBERG, N.: Continuous recording and control of ventricular fluid pressure in neurosurgical practice. Acta. psychiat. scand. (Suppl. 149) **36**, 1–193 (1960).
7. HUSSEY, F., SCHANZER, B., KATZMAN, R.: A simple constant infusion manometric test for measurement of C.S.F. absorption. II Clinical studies. Neurology **20**, 665–680 (1970).
8. LORENZO, A. V., PAGE, L. K., WATTERS, G. V.: Relationship between cerebrospinal fluid formation, absorption and pressure in human hydrocephalus. Brain **93**, 679–692 (1970).
9. CORNE, S. J., STEPHENS, R. J.: Periarterial and extradural devices for measuring changes of blood pressure and intracranial pressure in conscious animals. J. Physiol. (Lond.) **188**, 9–10 P (1966).
10. CORNE, S. J., STEPHENS, E. J., SYMON, L.: The effect of drugs on the intracranial pressure of baboons. Brit. J. Pharmacol. **34**, 212 P (1968).

Ultrastructure of Cortical Capillaries and Cerebral Blood Flow in Low Pressure Hydrocephalus

J. H. SALMON

Cerebral blood flow is controlled by three variables: perfusion pressure, viscosity of the blood and the diameter of the vessels. Cerebral blood flow (CBF) is decreased in patients with low pressure hydrocephalus and this blood flow is increased following therapeutic intracranial hypotension [1, 2]. BROCK [3] has demonstrated that the increase in CBF is a result of an increase in the gradient between the tissue perfusion pressure and the venous pressure. The venous pressure varies with intracranial pressure. As the perfusion pressure and the intracranial pressure are ordinarily normal in patients with low pressure hydrocephalus, the decrease in CBF in these patients must be the result of an abnormality of the capillary. This report attempts to define this capillary abnormality, using electron microscopy, and its relationship to the decreased CBF.

Material and Methods

Cortical biopsy was performed on seventeen patients with low pressure hydrocephalus at the time of the shunt operation. A one centimeter square core of gray and superficial white matter was removed and a one millimeter slice immediately placed in buffered glutaraldehyde. The tissue was then fixed and prepared for examination with the electron microscope. Photographs were obtained at a standard magnification and the image was enlarged exactly 4X during printing. All capillaries were photographed.

Using a compensating polar planimeter, the area of the capillary was measured using the outer margin of the basal lamina as the extreme limit of the capillary. In addition, the area of the basal lamina, nucleus and the lumen was measured. The remainder of the area represented the cytoplasm. The exact area of the capillary and its components in square microns was then calculated.

Control cortical biopsies were obtained from rat brain, dog brain, and from two patients who were undergoing cortical excision for treatment of epilepsy.

Cerebral blood flow was studied by injecting the inert gas ^{133}Xe via the internal carotid artery and monitoring the radioactivity with a single, large probe collimated to cover the estimated area of one cerebral hemisphere. Compartmental analysis was done. All values were corrected to a standard a pCO_2 of 40 mmHg.

Results

The endothelial nucleus was swollen (Fig. 1) and frequently compromised the lumen. The chromatin appeared to be of normal amount but seemed to be dispersed about the margins of the nuclear envelope. The karyoplasm was very pale in the central portion of the nucleus. The size of the lumen was variably decreased but in many capillaries was slit-like.

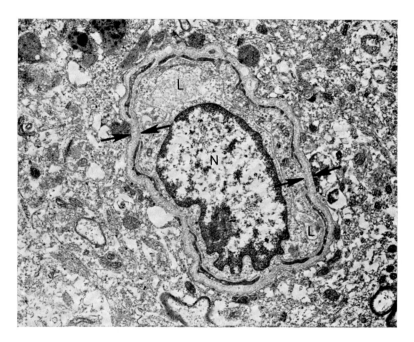

Fig. 1. The swollen endothelial nucleus (N) bulges into the slit-like lumen (L) of the capillary. The basal lamina (arrows) measures 4700 Å, (A) normal is 1300 Å. 4000 ×

The basal lamina was grossly widened in many of the capillaries, appearing amorphous with loss of the characteristic lamination. The basal lamina width was measured at representative places and was found to vary from 3600 Angströms (Å) to 7200 Å with a mean thickness of 4900 Å. For comparison, a normal appearing capillary basement membrane (basal lamina) varied from 670 to 1900 Å with a mean of 1300 Å. The thickness of the basal lamina normally varies with the degree of distension of the capillary and the proximity of the nucleus. Capillaries were largest when the cross section included a major portion of the endothelial nucleus and the lumen was filled with a red blood cell (45 micron^2). The normal basal lamina occupies approximately 2 micron^2 or 5% of the area of the capillary. In the abnormal capillaries, the area of the basal lamina was two to three times greater and, with a grossly thickened basal lamina, occupied an area seven micron^2 or 28% of the entire capillary area.

In these chronically ill patients, the endothelial cytoplasm did not appear swollen or edematous. The foot plates of the perivascular astrocytes were swollen, but this is an expected artefact in biopsy material fixed by immersion.

Many normal appearing capillaries were immediately adjacent to the abnormal capillaries described above. This would seem to indicate that the lesions were not artefactual.

Table 1. The cerebral vascular resistance (CVR) was increased, the cortical blood flow (CBF$_G$) decreased and the metabolic gray matter (W$_G$) decreased in hydrocephalics. Cortical biopsy revealed thickening of the basal lamina and narrowing of the capillary lumen

		Hydrocephalus	Normal
Area of	Basal Lamina	10–25 %	5 %
	Nucleus	30 %	20 %
	Lumen	5–50 %	60 %
	CVR	2.2	1.2
	CBF$_G$	45 ml	80 ml
	W$_G$	28 %	50 %

The cerbral blood flow of the gray matter (CBF$_G$) in these patients varied from 33 to 66 ml/100 g/min. The mean flow was 45 ml (Table 1). The relative weight of the gray matter (W$_G$) varied from 17–43% with a mean of 28%. The cerebrovascular resistance, calculated from the CBF$_G$ and mean internal carotid artery pressure varied from 1.4 through 3.3 with a mean of 2.2. The expected normal in our laboratory is 1.2.

Discussion

DONAHUE and PAPPAS [4] have demonstrated that the basal lamina of the cerebral capillaries of the rat becomes thicker with maturity. FLORA et al. [5] carried out an electron microscopic study of human intracranial vessels at various decades of life. They suggested a significant and possibly primary role of abnormalities of the basal lamina ground substance in the development of degenerative cerebrovascular disease. YODAIKEN et al. [6] showed a significant difference in the mean thickness of the basal lamina of capillaries in skeletal muscle of diabetic patients (average 2857 Å) and normal controls where the average thickness was 1898 Å. All subjects with a basal lamina thickness of less than 1800 Å were non diabetics and all with a basal lamina thickness of more than 2800 Å were diabetic.

The patients who had abnormal capillaries also had an abnormally low CBF. This is not surprising, as the inert gas technique is dependent on the rapid exchange of Xenon across the capillary into the cerebral substance. The increased CVR is also consistent with the histological finding of narrowing of the capillary lumen.

It has been postulated that the force on the ventricular wall is the primary factor causing cerebral dysfunction in patients with low pressure hydrocephalus. Our findings would indicate that the abnormality of the microvasculature is the more likely cause.

Summary

Cerebral blood flow studies and cortical biopsies were done in patients with low pressure hydrocephalus. When studied with the electron microscope, the cortical capillaries showed narrowing of the lumen and thickening of the basal lamina. The capillary abnormalities were associated with an increase in cerebrovascular resistance and a decrease in cerebral blood flow. It is believed that abnormal neurological function in these patients is the result of abnormalities of the microvasculature.

Key Words: Low pressure hydrocephalus, cerebral capillaries, cerebral blood flow, capillary ultrastructure.

References

1. GREITZ, T. V. B., GREPE, A. O. L., KALMER, M. S. F., LOPEZ, J.: Pre- and postoperative evaluation of cerebral blood flow in low-pressure hydrocephalus. J. Neurosurg. **31**, 644 651 (1969).
2. SALMON, J. H., TIMPERMAN, A. L.: Effect of intracranial hypotension on cerebral blood flow. J. Neurol. Neurosurg. Psychiat. **34**, 687–692 (1971).
3. BROCK, M., HADJIDIMOS, A. A., DERUAZ, J. P. et al: The effects of hyperventilation on regional cerebral blood flow. On the role of changes in intracranial pressure for shifts in rCBF distribution. In: TOOLE, J. F., MOOSSY, J., JANEWAY, R., (Eds.): Cerebral Vascular Diseases, p. 114–123. New York: Grune & Stratton 1971.
4. DONAHUE, S., PAPPAS, G. D.: The fine structure of capillaries in the cerebral cortex of the rat at various stages of development. Amer. J. Anat. **108**, 331–347 (1961).
5. FLORA, G., DAHL, E., NELSON, E.: Electron microscopic observations on human intracranial arteries. Changes seen with aging and atherosclerosis. Arch. Neurol. **17**, 162–173 (1967).
6. YODAIKEN, R. E., SEFTEL, H. C., KEW, M. C., LILLENSTEIN, M., IPP, E.: Ultrastructure of Capillaries in South African Diabetics. Diabetes **18**, 164–175 (1969).

Comments to Session 8

K. SHULMAN and R. HEMMER

The observations made in this session dealt with infantile and adult hydrocephalus and attempted to apply data obtained in hydrocephalus to a fuller understanding of other states of ICP. The major theme was the relation of ICP to changes in intracranial volume. The contribution of LORENZ and GROTE included 35 adults and children with hydrocephalus, who were studied by means of lumbar spinal tap and fluid withdrawal; final pressure was then related to initial pressure. These authors described a plateau in the withdrawal curve, which is a region of the pressure/volume curve in which similar volume withdrawal produces only a minimal pressure change. The pulse-pressure changes described have been discussed by many authors in the past. No new hypotheses resulted from their attempt to define an elasticity coefficient.

More refined attempts at pressure/volume determinations and at an understanding of intracranial elasticity and capacitance (the reciprocal of elasticity) were made by MILLER and his group and by MARMAROU and SHULMAN. MILLER's technique of single bolus injections of saline into the ventricle and single withdrawals of known volumes of fluid allowed him to demonstrate a statistically significant relationship of pressure to volume as an exponential function by grouping all patients. This allows the potential of comparing the patient's response at different times in assessing degrees of compensation available, i.e. "the tight brain".

MARMAROU and SHULMAN described the relationship of pressure and volume in 1971 (Developmental Medicine and Child Neurology, Vol. 13, Suppl. 25, p. 90). Continuation of this work has redefined the pressure/volume index (PVI) and the use of the PVI and opening pressure to characterize the capacitance of the cranial cavity. A systems-analysis approach presented, using computer modelling of the CSF system to validate MARMAROU's mathematical equations. Comparison of physiologic data with computer-generated curves showed the equations to be valid. This technique offers considerable promise in dissecting the mechanisms underlying phenomena associated with increased ICP, such as the plateau waves, etc.

The discussion of these three papers essentially lent support to the exponential relationship of pressure to volume, although no participant commented on the fact that the pressure/volume relationship in hydrocephalus does not seem to differ from that of the patient with head injury. OMMAYA asked that additional data be obtained on the high and low range of pressure and the Chairman suggested that all pressure changes be induced by instantaneous volume addition rather than slow infusions, to obviate absorptions through normal mechanisms during introduction of the fluid.

That patients with so-called "low-pressure hydrocephalus" do have periods of pressure elevation above 10 mmHg is clear if continous ICP recordings are performed, particularly during sleep. SYMON's data, confirmed by those of HULME and TROUPP, show modest elevations of up to 25 mmHg and some sustained plateau elevations in this range. The return to normal or subnormal pressures after placement of a shunt is also clear. It was not, however, made clear that all patients who have increased pressure do in fact improve after the shunt and that long-term ICP measurement will always select the right patients for shunting.

The evidence of changes in capillary structure given by SALMON suggests a continuation of the acute changes described, initially by HEMMER (1964) and subsequently by others, in the hydrocephalic cortex, namely an increase in extracellular fluid space and disruption of the neuropil of the cortex. If these capillary changes are longstanding in dementia and are not reversible, the usefulness of a shunt in such patients is questionable.

Session 9

Drugs and Anesthetic Agents
(Clinical)

Intracranial Pressure during Anesthesia with Ketamine

W. J. Bock, W. Gobiet, J. Liesegang, and W. Grote

The anesthetic "Ketamine" has been widely used since its introduction. It has specific anesthetic and analgetic properties and can be administered both i. m. and i. v. When given by intravenous injection its effect starts within 20 sec, following intramuscular injection after some minutes.

During the anesthetic phase there is heavy analgesia, which outlasts the anesthetic stage. The side-effects observed so far are mainly related to cardiac activity and to circulation: temporary rises in blood pressure and pulse rate. The effect of Ketamnest is probably due to disruption of associative connections in the brain. Due to its advantages it has gained wide application in the field of neuroradiology. In view of the nature of neurologic and neurosurgical patients, it is essential to understand the changes in ICP following administration of Ketamine. The few reports published on this subject describe an increase in CSFP following the application of Ketamine.

17 neurosurgical patients in whom VFP was measured during the post-operative course were studied. All patients were conscious and none was under the influence of other anesthetics.

VFP was measured by means of a pressure transducer (Statham) connected to a catheter in the frontal horn of the side not operated upon. Arterial pressure, pulse rate, central venous pressure, and blood gases ware also studied. We administered 2 mg/kg Ketamine i. v. within 30 sec. No atropine was used.

Following the injection of Ketamine a distinct CSFP increase was observed in all patients.

The average CSFP increase was from $19,95 \pm 2,8$ mmHg to $48,30 \pm 4,3$ mmHg, with an average difference in pressure of $28,35 \pm 4,9$ mmHg. Statistical analysis by the Students'-test showed this difference was highly significant $(P > 0.001)$. The extent of the CSFP increase is shown in Figure 1.

In 3 cases a pressue increase of more than 60 mmHg was observed.

As shown in Figure 2, the mean CSFP values tend to rise steeply following the injection of Ketamine (Fig. 2). After a period of 4 min a pressure peak is attained. Even after 15 min a pressure increase of 50% persists. The initial values are not reattained after 20 min.

No significant changes were observed in arterial pressure, pulse rate, central venous pressure or blood gases.

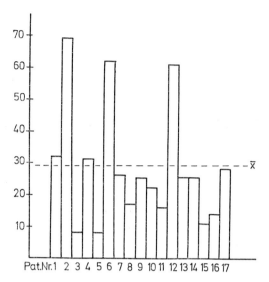

Fig. 1. Overall increase in ICP in our series

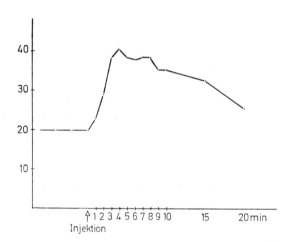

Fig. 2. ICP increase in time course

The ICP increase following the administration of Ketamine raises the question as to its indication in patients with intracranial masses.

We consider it advisable not to use Ketamine anesthesia in patients in whom an ICP increase is suspected.

Effects of Some Anesthetic Drugs on the Ventricular Fluid Pressure and on the Systemic Blood Pressure Both Arterial and Venous

J. ZATTONI and C. SIANI

Introduction

The effects of general anesthetic drugs on intracranial pressure has been a frequent subject of research for some years, beginning with the pilot research by WORINGER et al. [1, 2]. However, basic knowledge of their mechanism has only recently been obtained. Especially important are the data of McDOWALL and coworkers [3, 4, 5] on the direct vasodilatatory action of the volatile anesthetics on the cerebral circulation.

We have studied the effects of thiopental, propanidid and halothane on ventricular fluid pressure (VFP). The data obtained in a first series of investigations [6, 7, 8, 9] indicated that these drugs can produce very rapid changes in the VFP, the mechanism of which can only be supposed to reside in primary or secondary changes in the intracranial circulation [6, 9]. In later experiments the VFP was recorded simultaneously with the systemic arterial (ABP) and venous (VBP) blood pressures. In this way the behaviour of two of the three vascular factors (ABP, VBP and cerebral blood flow) capable of producing rapid VFP changes [10] were checked.

Material and Methods

40 neurosurgical patients affected by different types of cerebral lesions (9 normotensive and 7 hypertensive patients with hydrocephalus, 3 aneurysms and/or angiomas, 11 supra- and 7 sub-tentorial tumors, 3 cases presenting with other cerebral diseases) were examined under typical conditions of clinical anesthesia. 30–40 min before recording was started, the patients were premedicated with 0.5 mg atropine, usually combined with 5–12.5 mg droperidol, more rarely with 10 mg morphine.

VFP was recorded through a catheter inserted into the frontal horn of the lateral ventricles of the brain. ABP and VBP were recorded in 15 patients through catheters inserted into the femoral artery (in one case the superficial temporal artery was used for control) and in the subclavian or superior caval veins. All pressure functions were recorded by means of electromanometric units (Statham P23AC pressure transducers and Grass polygraph model 5D) and their average value calculated; VBP was also measured at the extreme points of its oscillations. Pneumogram (PNG), electrocardiogram (ECG) and, in three cases, electroencephalogram (EEG) were simultaneously recorded.

Thiopental (38 i. v. injections in 26 patients in a dose of 0.10–0.40 mg) and propanidid (21 i. v. injections in 17 patients in a dose of 0.10–0.50 mg) were injected to induce general anesthesia in conscious patients under spontaneous ventilation (SpV) or to deepen it in patients under spontaneous or controlled ventilation (CoV). Halothane (49 administrations of 0.5–2%, generally 1–1.5%, Fluotec) was administered only in patients in CoV during thiopental-nitrous oxide-oxygen anesthesia. The real value of the alveolar ventilation during CoV was calculated by means of the Herzog-Engström nomogram.

Results

1. Thiopental injection was always followed by a fast fall of the VFP (Fig. 1), the absolute value of which was strictly related to the basal VFP value. In cases under SpV, the VFP began to rise within 2–3 min, showing a strong

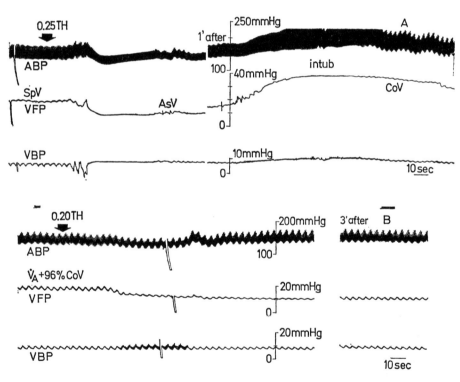

Fig. 1. Patient with acqueductal stenosis due to a tumor of the brain stem. A injection of thiopental (0.25 mg) to induce general anesthesia: parallel changes occur in the VFP and ABP. B deepening of anesthesia in the same subject under controlled hyperventilation: ABP returns to its initial value while the hypotensive intracranial effect remains

hypertensive reaction after the third minute (Fig. 1 A). In cases under CoV the decrease in VFP showed a tendency to stabilize or to revert very slowly (Fig. 1 B): it could still be present after 9 min.

ABP had a similar course to VFP during the phase of intracranial hypotension; it might show a strong increase above its initial value, or remain lower during the phase of intracranial hypertension. ABP rebounds were never observed in patients under CoV; often ABP returned to its initial value very early. VFP began to decline on average 8 sec earlier than ABP; this difference was not confirmed when the superficial temporal artery was used instead of the femoral.

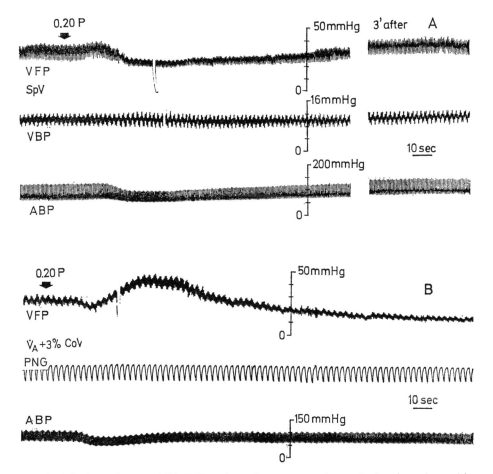

Fig. 2. Injection of propanidid (0.20 mg) to deepen general anesthesia. A patient with brain tumor: parallel decrease of the VFP and ABP. B another patient with brain tumor: opposite changes in VFP and ABP

VBP did not change in patients under CoV; in the other cases it showed fast respiratory oscillations during polypnoic reaction, and sometimes slight and slow increases during the intracranial hypertensive phase.

2. Propanidid injection was always followed by changes in VFP in all patients under SpV; patients under CoV were often unaffected. Frequency, direction, amplitude and sequence of the VFP changes varied widely from case to case. However, two patterns were frequently recorded both in subjects under CoV and in those under SpV: a fast decrease in VFP (Fig. 2A), similar to the effect typical of thiopental, or a rapid increase (Fig. 2B). All changes disappeared within 4–6 min.

ABP always decreased with a tendency to normalization. VBP behaved as in point 1.

3. In most cases halothane produced an increase in VFP (Fig. 3). This effect always disappeared when administration was discontinued. Both the increase and the decrease in VFP began after an average of 60 sec. In 4 of the 10 cases in which the same concentration of halothane was given more than once at intervals of 10–60 min, the hypertensive effect was not reproducible within 4–6 min (2 normotensive and 1 hypertensive patient with hydrocephalus, 1 patient with cerebral tumor; respective basal VFP values were 14.6, 18.4, 4.2 and 13.8 mmHg.

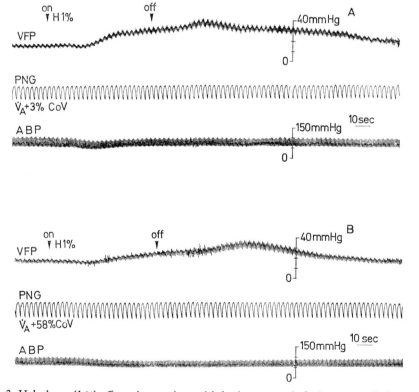

Fig. 3. Halothane (1 %) effects in a patient with brain tumor. A during controlled normo-ventilation. B during controlled hyperventilation. Note the more marked effect on the VFP and on ABP in A

ABP decreased in all cases, while VBP remained almost steady. Apart from the cases without hypertensive effects, the increases in VFP observed after 3 min of administration were usually higher

a) when basal VFP was superior to 16 mmHg;
b) in presence of space-occupying lesions;
c) hyperventilated in patients and
d) when the mean of ABP fell by more than 8 mmHg (Fig. 2, compare A and B). These differences were not statistically significant.

Comments

1. The VFP decrease always produced by thiopental (Fig. 1) and sometimes by propanidid (Fig. 2 A) is probably due to the fall in ABP, which induces a reduction in cerebral blood flow. This fall in APB is too fast to be counterbalanced by the autoregulation of the cerebral circulation [10].

2. The long-lasting intracranial hypotensive effect of thiopental by injection in patients under CoV (Fig. 1 B) cannot be attributed, as in point 1, to the behavior of ABP. It may be at least partially due to a cerebral vasoconstriction with reduction of the cerebral blood flow due to depressed oxygen uptake in the brain [9].

3. The VFP increase observed immediately after propanidid injection (Fig. 2 A) is in contrast with that described under 1. The effect is qualitatively different from the latter and can be interpreted only as a consequence of an increase in cerebral blood flow due to a local vasodilator action.

4. The intracranial hypertensive reaction occurring only in patients under SpV in the late phase of the effects of thiopental (Fig. 1 A) (and sometimes of propanidid) may be easily related to the respiratory depression induced by such drugs and to the associated hypercapnia. However, the marked and rapid increase in ABP occurring in this phase (probably also due to hypercapnia) may contribute [9] to the increase in VFP by means of a further increase of the cerebral blood flow.

5. Our data on halothane confirm the results of McDowall and coworkers, and show that the VFP response to this anesthetic drug may present very large quantitative differences from patient to patient (and sometimes even be absent) and at different periods in the same patient. The simplest assumption is that the cerebral vascular reactivity responsible for the intracranial hypertensive effect may vary within very large limits in neurosurgical patients and during general anesthesia.

Summary

The effects of thiopental, propanidid and halothane on the intracranial, arterial and venous blood pressures were studied in neurosurgical patients under typical clinical conditions. Indirect evidence was obtained that even non-volatile anesthetic drugs can modify intracranial pressure by acting directly on the cerebral blood flow.

References

1. Woringer, E. A., Brogly, G., Schneider, J.: Etude de l'action des anesthésiques généraux usuels sur la pression du liquide céphalorachidien. Anesth. Analg. 8, 649–661 (1951).
2. Woringer, E. A., Brogly, G., Dorgler, R.: Données nouvelles sur les mecanismes des variations des pressions veineuse et céphalo-rachidienne sous l'influence des certains anesthésiques généraux. Ibid. 17, 18–33 (1954).
3. McDowall, D. G., Barker, J., Jennett, W. B.: Cerebrospinal fluid pressure measurements during anesthesia. Anaesthesia 21, 189 (1966).
4. McDowall, D. G.: The effects of clinical concentrations of halothane on the blood flow and oxygen uptake of the cerebral cortex. Brit. J. Anaesth. 39, 186–196 (1967).
5. Jennett, W. B., Barker, J., Fitch, W., McDowall, D. G.: Effects of anaesthesia on intracranial pressure in patients with intracranial space-occupying lesions. Lancet II, 61–64 (1969).
6. Zattoni, J., Siani, C.: Effetto bifasico sulla pressione endocranica di dosi cliniche di tiopentone. Minerva anest. 35, 1251–1260 (1969).
7. Zattoni, J., Siani, C.: Studio dell'azione ipertensiva endocranica dell'alotano in malati neurochirurgici in ventilazione controllata. Arch. ital. Otol. 57, 351–358 (1969).
8. Zattoni, J., Siani, C., Giasotto, G., Libonati, P.: Effetti della propanidide sulla pressione endocranica dell'uomo. Rass. Med. sper. 16, 303–307 (1969).
9. Siani, C., Zattoni, J.: Effetti di un tiobarbiturico sulle pressioni endocranica, arteriosa sistemica e venosa sistemica dell'uomo. Boll. Soc. ital. Biol. sper. 45, 1475–1477 (1969).
10. McDowall, D. G.: Fluid dynamics of the cerebral circulation. In: Heinemann, W.: Scientific foundations of anaesthesia, p. 106–112. Med. Books (1970).
11. McDowall, D. G.: The effects of general anaesthetics on cerebral blood flow and cerebral metabolism. Brit. J. Anaesth. 37, 236–245 (1965).

Stabilization and Disturbance of Osmoregulation in the Cerebrospinal Fluid[1]

A. Prill, E. Volles, and W. Dahlmann

Introduction

This review reports studies on osmolality regulation between arterial blood and lumbar cerebrospinal fluid (CSF). In the case of an acute or subacute brain lesion the patient's life is not endangered by the intracranial space-occupying process or cerebral ischemia so much as by the reactive cerebral edema and disturbances of water regulation in the central nervous system (CNS). The conditions affecting water regulation in the CNS and CSF are therefore considered.

Material and Methods

The studies were performed in patients under physiological conditions and in pathological states with brain lesions. Lumbar CSF was continuously recorded by means of an electromanometer. Osmolality was ascertained in mosm/kg water (freezing-point method). Electrolytes were determined by flame photometry. The results were subjected to statistical analysis.

Results and Discussion

Sodium ions are decisive in stabilizing osmoregulation outside the central nervous system. Study of the osmolalities in arterial blood and lumbar fluid demonstrates that the mean values in CSF are 3–4 mosm/kg H_2O higher than those in blood. The absolute values in CSF are within the range of 285–287 mosm/kg H_2O. Under physiological acid-base conditions and normal electrolyte regulation between blood and CSF the mean values are m = 284.835 ± 5.799 standard deviation (s) for the blood and m = 285.466 ± 4.723 (s) for the CSF (n = 73). In pathological states the values are comparable: metabolic acidosis: (n = 34) m = 284.234 ± 7.949 (s) for blood, and m = 287.000 ± 7.114 (s) for CSF; metabolic alkalosis: (n = 11) m = 285.909 ± 6.348 (s) for blood, and m = 287.455 ± 6.297 (s) for CSF (4). Furthermore, our observations have shown a close correlation between the osmolalities in the CSF (y) and in the blood (x). The correlation coefficient is r = 0.885 (p < 0.001) for the normal range of the acid-base status in the blood (n = 73).

1 Supported by Grant of the „Stiftung Volkswagenwerk" Hannover, W.-Germany. Project: Biomedical engineering; Section: Function of the blood-brain barrier.

Accordingly, there is a very strong mutual dependence, with a regression line of y = 0.720x + 81.298. In decompensated metabolic acidosis (n = 34) the values are r = 0.970 (p < 0,001) and y = 0.868x + 40.093; for compensated and decompensated metabolic alkalosis in the blood (n = 11) r = 0.964 (p < 0.001) and y = 0.956x + 14.125. (4). This result raises the question of whether the sodium ion concentration has a similar importance for the water- and osmoregulation in the CSF.

Surprisingly, we have found that in the steady state, the correlation between osmolality and sodium concentration in CSF, with a coefficient of —0.187, is only insufficient, even if significant (Fig. 1). It follows that with a regression coefficient of 0,182 the mutual dependence of these parameters is very weak. This is valid, although the CSF/blood distribution for sodium shows a constant value of 100–103% [1, 3]. Therefore it appears incorrect to assume, for the steady state in CSF under physiological conditions, that it is only the sodium ion concentration which stabilizes the water equilibrium. It appears decisive that, of the free ions, sodium with approximately 150 meq/kg H_2O constitutes only half of the total osmolality.

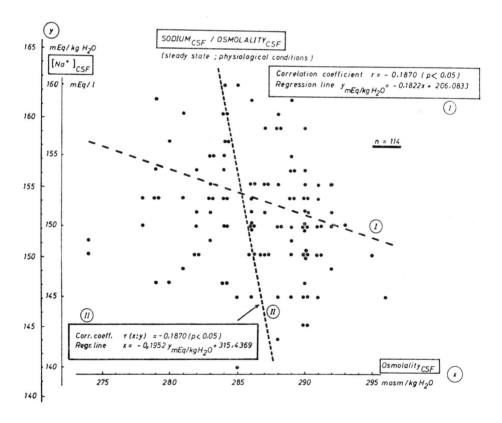

Fig. 1. Correlation and regression between sodium ions and osmolality in the CSF

When the equilibrium in the water regulation is disturbed, however, it can be shown that the sodium ions stabilize the water regulation between the extraneural space and the CSF.

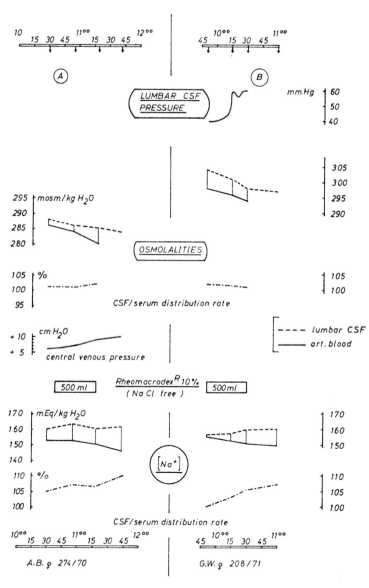

Fig. 2. Osmoregulation in the CSF after infusion of salt-free Dextran solution. Water passes from the extraneural distribution space into the CSF; the CSF pressure rises. As opposed to what happens in blood, there is no decrease of sodium ion concentration by dilution in CSF, but an increase of the electrolyte content. An active discharge from the blood to the CSF appears to take place in order to stabilize the osmolality in an adequate relation to that of the blood

In chronic pathological states, for example in renal insufficiency, a compensatory increase of the sodium exchange with the CSF sets in to stabilize the water balance [4]. This is necessary because the rate of exchange for urea from the blood to the CSF is only about 85–90 % [1, 3]. Consequently, the blood becomes hyperosmolar with respect to the CSF. A water flow from CSF to the extraneural distribution space would be the consequence. This is counterbalanced by the compensatory increase in exchange of sodium ions from the blood to the CSF.

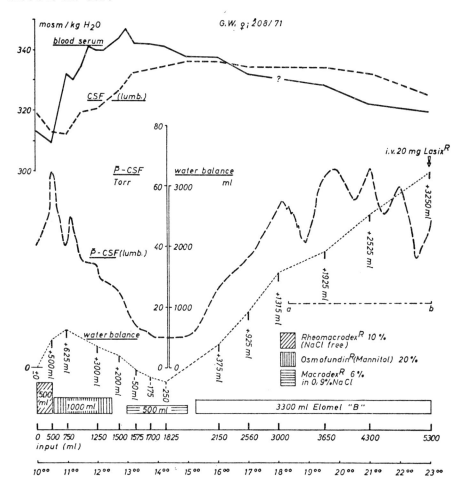

Fig. 3. Infusion of water of low electrolyte content after reducing the CSF pressure by means of mannitol. In this case of hypotonic hyperhydration with positive water balance the CSF pressure is elevated by the fluid increase in the CSF space unless the osmolality is decreased

However, it is possible to influence this regulation either by different concentrations of substances effective in osmoregulation between the CSF and the blood, or by disturbances in the water distribution. A difference of more than

10 mosm/kg H_2O in CSF/blood osmolality leads to an increased CSF pressure due to water exchange from the extraneural distribution space to the CSF [2, 3, 4]. This is the case in the cerebral dysequilibrium syndrome. When, however, a large quantity of water is quickly administered without ions or molecules effective in osmotic regulation, water passes from the extraneural distribution space to the CSF (Fig. 2A). This can be experimentally achieved by rapid infusion of salt-free dextran solution. Dextran, with an average molecular weight of 40,000, causes an increase in oncotic but not in osmotic pressure. Consequently, only a part of the dextran solution water is bound. This part of the relatively free water passes from the extraneural space into the CSF. This shift of water gives rise to dilution of the fluid in the CSF space. Accordingly, not only the osmolality in the blood, but also that in the CSF falls as dilution continues. This is also shown in Fig. 2B, where CSF pressure rises with increased fluid volume. A noteworthy feature of this process is the fact that the CSF sodium concentration does not diminish parallel to the CSF dilution. In contrast, the decrease in blood sodium concentration is accompanied by a relative or sometimes even an absolute increase of sodium in the CSF. Hence, there is every reason to believe that an increased amount of sodium ions is actively discharged from the blood to the CSF for stabilization of osmolality in an adequate relation to the blood. The divergent behavior of increasing sodium concentration and decreasing osmolality is surprising. The divergence may be explained by the diluting effect of the water on nondissociated but osmotically active substances such as urea.

It is apparent, however, that the spinal fluid pressure does not only depend on the osmolality gradient between CSF and the extraneural water distribution space. When, as seen in Fig. 3, the lumbar CSF pressure is markedly reduced after infusion of mannitol, a subsequent infusion of water of low electrolyte content does not only lead to an increasing positive water balance but also to a rise in CSF pressure [5], although the osmolality in the cerebrospinal fluid remains constant. Hyperhydration of the body with expansion of the extraneural water distribution space and simultaneous positive water balance leads to a definite increase in the spinal fluid pressure. This pressure increase is not only reduced by urea or mannitol but also easily reduced by diuretics.

Summary

Under physiological conditions and in steady state there is a close correlation and a strong mutual dependence between the osmolality in the blood and in the CSF. However, the regulation of the water balance in the CSF is not regulated solely by sodium ions. In pathological states and exchange of sodium from the blood to the CSF sets in to stabilize the water balance. This regulation can be disturbed in hypotonic hyperhydration.

Key Words: Blood/CSF water regulation, CSF/blood osmolality.

References

1. Davson, H.: Physiology of the cerebrospinal fluid. London: Churchill 1967.
2. Pappius, H.: The effects of rapid hemodialysis on brain tissues and cerebrospinal fluid of dogs. Canad. J. Physiol. Pharmacol. 45, 129–145 (1967).
3. Prill, A.: Die neurologische Symptomatologie der Niereninsuffizienz. Berlin-Heidelberg-New York: Springer 1969.
4. Prill, A.: Osmoregulation and disturbances of the water balance in the cerebrospinal fluid and the central nervous system. Triangle (Basel) 10, 157–168 (1972).
5. Volles, E., Prill, A., Dahlmann, W.: Results of continuous spinal fluid pressure measurements for testing the intracranial water regulation. Proc. Germ. Soc. Neurosurg. Amsterdam: Excerpta Medica 1972 (in press).

The Alleviation of Increased Intracranial Pressure by the Chronic Administration of Osmotic Agents

D. P. BECKER and J. K. VRIES

Introduction

The chronic administration of osmotic agents might be an effective way to treat elevated intracranial pressure (ICP) if the systemic effects of water and electrolyte depletion could be avoided. ICP reduction is not dependent upon diuresis or water and electrolyte depletion. It is primarily a function of the osmotic gradient between brain and plasma created by the osmotic agent. We therefore felt that replacement of the output from diuresis would not affect ICP reduction and might permit us to use osmotic agents over a prolonged period of time.

Material and Methods

18 patients from the neurosurgical service were selected for treatment with osmotic agents. Patients had ICP recordings by the LUNDBERG technique [1] and fulfilled the following criteria: 1. no evidence of a focal mass lesion or hydrocephalus by contrast studies; 2. mean ICP of 25 mmHg or greater after treatment with steroids and controlled ventilation; 3. deeply comatose (one or both pupils dilated and fixed and/or decerebrate or flaccid motor response); 4. rapidly deteriorating neurological condition. Subdural hematomas had been evacuated, and patients deteriorating after this had repeat contrast studies.

Each patient received 1 g/kg of Mannitol or isosorbide to begin therapy. Thereafter each received intermittent doses (every 2–3 h) or a continuous infusion sufficient to maintain ICP below 25 mmHg.

Each patient had hourly recordings of vital signs, central venous pressure (CVP), and intake and output. Weights were obtained daily. Each patient had the following laboratory studies determined at the beginning of therapy and every 4 h: 1. hematocrit and hemoglobin; 2. serum electrolytes; 3. blood urea nitrogen and glucose; 4. serum osmolarity; 5. urinary sodium and potassium. Serum creatinine, calcium and magnesium were determined once daily.

Fluid replacement was managed by matching the urinary output with a solution containing the estimated losses of sodium, potassium, calcium, and magnesium[1]. Adjustments were made as necessary to maintain normal CVP and normal serum electrolytes.

Results

Overall results are presented in Table 1. ICP was reduced below 25 mmHg in all 18 patients, and maintained at this level with repeated (every 2–3 h) or continuous infusions. The patients can be divided into two groups depending on the serum osmolarity at the time of initial ICP control (ICP below 25 mmHg). Group 1 consists of patients requiring osmolarities of 310 mosm/l or less to control ICP. In group 1 it was possible to wean all patients off osmotic agents at the end of therapy with maintenance of normal ICP. Group 1 patients survived the early effects of their brain insults and 5 of 9 made functional recoveries. There were no complications of osmotic therapy in group 1. The results with Mannitol and isosorbide appeared comparable. The higher peak osmolarities noted in the patients treated with isosorbide were felt to reflect the dehydration which occurred in these patients because of our earlier fluid replacement regimen.

In group 2 a very high serum osmolarity (over 320 mosm/l) was required to reduce ICP below 25 mmHg. All but one patient in group 2 died. There were 3 cases of renal failure and 5 cases of systemic acidosis. The main cause of death in these patients was increased ICP when osmotic therapy could not be continued because of complications.

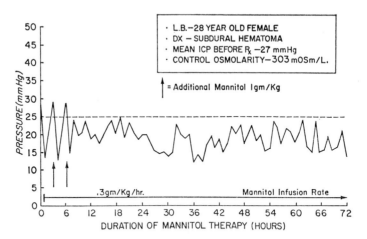

Fig. 1. 72 h ICP record of patient 2 beginning at the start of Mannitol therapy. Duration of therapy was 9 days. ICP was controlled during this period with osmolarities less than 310 mosm/l. Patient made a full recovery without complications of therapy and returned to her former employment

---

1 The patients treated with isosorbide earlier in the series had dehydration because fluid replacement was not strictly matched to urine output.

The record of a patient from group 1 is shown in Fig. 1. Following eva-
cuation of a subdural hematoma which resulted from a closed head injury the
patient developed a dilated fixed left pupil and right sided decerebrate posturing. An angiogram showed no evidence of a focal mass lesion. Treatment with
Mannitol reduced her mean ICP from 27 mmHg to less than 25 mmHg at an
osmolarity of 303 mosm/l. Her pupil became reactive and her decerebrate posturing disappeared. She was continued on Mannitol for 9 days and ultimately
made a full recovery and returned to work.

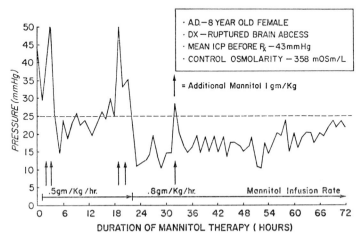

Fig. 2. 72 h ICP record of patient 10 beginning at the start of mannitol therapy. Duration of
therapy was 13 days. ICP was controlled until the final day with high osmolarities (358 to
475 mosm/l). Death occurred from increased ICP when renal failure and systemic acidosis
forced discontinuation of mannitol therapy

The record of a patient from group 2 is shown in Fig. 2. This patient
had a brain abcess which ruptured into the ventricle. She presented with fixed
dilated pupils, flaccid motor response, and failing respirations. After ventricular
drainage and aspiration of the abcess cavity the patient was unchanged. ICP
at his point was 43 mmHg. Treatment with Mannitol brought her ICP below
25 mmHg but a rate of infusion of .8 g/kg/h and multiple supplemental doses
of 1 g/kg were required to maintain this. The initial osmolarity at ICP control
was 358 mosm/l. Following ICP reduction the patient's pupils became reactive,
her respirations improved, and she began showing decerebrate posturing. Subsequently, during treatment, her osmolarity steadily rose. All attempts to cut
back the infusion rate caused prompt neurolgical deterioration. The patient
ultimately reached a serum osmolarity of 475 on the 13th day of therapy and
died of increased ICP when complications forced discontinuation of the infusion. During the final phase of her course she developed systemic acidosis and
renal failure. Neurologically she was maintaining her improvement up to the
final rise in ICP.

Table 1. Control osmolarity is that level at which ICP was reduced below 25 mmHg. Patients with a diagnosis of subdural hematoma had the clot evacuated and follow-up contrast studies revealed no recurrence

Patient	Age Sex	Diagnosis	Initial ICP (mmHg)	Control Osmolarity (mosm/l)	Peak Osmolarity (mosm/l)	Complications of Therapy	Lenght of Rx (Days)	Outcome
				Group 1				
1. J.M.	43 M	gunshot wound	30	301	321	–	9	Survived at vegetative level
2. L.B.	28 F	subdural hematoma	27	303	303	–	9	full functional recovery
3. G.J.	35 M	cerebrovascular occlusion	26	301	305	–	7	alert, residual hemiparesis
4. M.W.	17 M	cerebral contusion	44	290	321	–	6	vegetative level × 2 weeks, died of unrelated problem
5. T.R.	32 M	subdural hematoma	25	306	342	–	2	functional recovery, residual hemiparesis
6. T.C.[a]	49 M	ruptured aneurysm	25	310	332	–	3	alert, residual hemiparesis
7. W.B.[a]	55 M	astrocytoma, post-op. edema	28	305	441	–	4	full functional recovery
8. R.P.[a]	31 M	cerebral contusion	30	303	312	–	4	full functional recovery
9. E.N.[a]	39 F	cerebral contusion	26	310	420		5	full functional recovery

Group 2

10.	A.D.	7 F	ruptured brain abcess	43	358	475	systemic acidosis and renal failure	13	died
11.	T.R.	10 F	cerebral contusion	25	324	405	systemic acidosis	6	died
12.	J.B.	5 M	cerebral contusion	45	320	374	systemic acidosis	5	died
13.	D.H.	33 F	ruptured aneurysm	41	325	400	renal failure	8	died
14.	D.O.[a]	32 M	subdural hematoma	30	355	431	systemic acidosis	3	died
15.	S.L.[a]	65 M	cerebral contusion	26	–	439	–	4	died
16.	G.C.[a]	22 M	cerebral contusion	37	345	420	renal failure	3	died
17.	G.H.[a]	62 F	subdural hematoma	26	353	434	systemic acidosis	3	died
18.	B.D.[a]	17 F	ruptured aneurysm	40	337	392	–	1	was recovering, died 10 days later of rebleed

[a] isosorbide

Discussion

The type of patient defined in this paper has rarely survived in the past. Treatment with osmotic agents in our small series of 18 patients has resulted in 10 survivors. Further analysis of the results reveals an important relationship between the osmolarity necessary to achieve initial control of ICP and final outcome. All patients controlled below 310 mosm/l survived without complications. Patients controlled above this level approached a 100% complication and mortality rate.

Several animal studies suggest the reasons for this relationship. Stuart and co-workers [2] have measured the degree of brain dehydration in dogs given mannitol infusions to the point of death (average 437 mosm/l). The average degree of dehydration was 20%. On a human scale this would be comparable to a 250 cc loss of brain volume. In theory, then, if one raised the serum osmolarity to 437 mosm/l, one could compensate for a 250 cc mass effect. However, there are 3 limiting factors: 1. at a serum osmolarity above 375 intracellular dehydration becomes severe enough to disrupt cellular metabolism. This eventually leads to systemic acidosis [3]; 2. at serum osmolarities above 350 progressive renal failure occurs [2], possibly related to intracellular dehydration of kidney cells; 3. at osmolarities of 300–310 mosm/l the threshold for the blood brain barrier to mannitol is exceeded, and mannitol progressively accumulates in the cerebrospinal fluid [4]. This lowers the gradient between brain and plasma. To maintain constant brain volume reduction, the plasma mannitol concentration must progressively rise. Patients in group 1 probably have a small enough mass lesion effect that ICP control can be achieved at osmolarity levels which are tolerated on a long term basis (310 mosm/l or less). This is not the case for patients in group 2. Initial ICP reduction can be achieved at high osmolarities in these patients, but progressive amounts of osmotic agents are required to maintain this reduction. This ultimately leads to renal failure and systemic acidosis.

Summary

A method for the chronic control of elevated ICP by repeated (every 2–3 h) or continuous administration of osmotic agents has been described. Overall success depends on initial ICP control with serum osmolarity levels at 310 mosm/l or less. If satisfactory ICP reduction requires serum osmolarity levels above this, progressively larger infusions of the osmotic agent will be necessary to maintain control. This will lead ultimately to renal failure and systemic acidosis, and other forms of therapy should be considered.

Key Words: Mannitol, intracranial pressure, hypertonic solutions, brain edema.

References

1. Lundberg, N.: Continuous recording and control of ventricular fluid pressure in neurological practice. Acta psychiat. scand. (Suppl. 149) **36** (1960).

2. STUART, F. P., TORRES, E., FLETCHER, D., Moore, F. D.: Effects of repeated and massive mannitol infusion in the dog: structural and functional changes in kidney and brain. Ann. Surg. **172,** 190–204 (1970).
3. SOTOS, J. F., DODGE, P. R., MEARA, P., TALBOT, N. B.: Studies in experimental hypertonicity. Pediatrics **26,** 925–938 (1960).
4. SILBER, S. J., THOMPSON, N.: Mannitol-induced central nervous system toxicity in renal failure. Invest. Urol. **9,** 310–312 (1972).

The Role of Vascular and Hemodynamic Factors in the Pathogenesis of Intracranial Hypertension Caused by Focal Lesions of the Brain

Y. A. Zozulia and A. P. Romodanov

Introduction

Increase of intracranial pressure due to intracranial space-occupying lesions and, in particular, to tumors, constitutes a stimulus for the development of certain compensation mechanisms initially creating a balanced intracranial pressure. At a certain stage of tumor growth, compensation of the rising intracranial pressure becomes inadequate and CSFP increases, leading to clinical signs and symptoms of the so-called hypertensive syndrome. As is known, intracranial hypertension develops as a result of various factors, such as increase in tumor size, increase in brain volume due to edema, disturbances in CSF circulation and in CBF. The proportion of each of these components varies with tumors of different locations and biological properties and at different phases of the tumor development. Nevertheless, more than one of these components is always involved in the genesis of intracranial hypertension.

The purpose of this communication is to report the results of a study on the vascular and hemodynamic factors involved in the pathogenesis of intracranial hypertension. During recent years this problem has been investigated by several authors [1–8].

Material and Methods

CBF was studied in 68 patients with tumors of the cerebral hemispheres. Along with CSFP recordings, quantitative CBF measurements – global and regional (in 5–6 regions of the cerebral hemisphere involved) – were made by means of radioactive ^{133}Xe injected into the internal carotid artery. Mean regional cerebral blood flow as well as blood flow in the cortex and white matter were calculated by graphic analysis of the isotope clearance curves. Regional reactivity of the cerebral vessels was studied using different functional tests: inhalation of 7 and 9% CO_2, inhalation of pure oxygen, hyperventilation. Autoregulation was investigated by means of transitory arterial hyper- and hypotension. The same studies were carried out in the course of reduction of the intracranial pressure by strong dehydrating agents (hypertensive solutions of urea and Mannitol). Arterial pH and pCO_2, the content and ratios of lactate and pyruvate in the blood and cerebrospinal fluid were also determined.

In experiments on 15 dogs, a gradual increase in ICP was produced by the technique of VIROZUB and SERGIYENKO [9]. A special cannula was placed in the parietal or parieto-occipital region close to the sagittal line. A mass for compression of the brain was introduced into the receiver of the cannula (from 0.2–0.3 ml to 2 ml with an interval of 3–5 days) permitting variation in the rate of ICP increase. Before the introduction of each mass the increase of CSFP in the cisterna magna was measured. CBF was examined by serial angiography and by oxyhemographic registration of the passage time of an indifferent dye through the cerebral blood vessels. CBF was recorded continuously by means of thermistors. Injection of the blood vessels with India ink and caliber studies of the circle of WILLIS and small cerebral vessels were also performed, and the degree of edema of the brain was assessed.

Results

The development of intracranial hypertension shows several stages: a) stage of compensation, when the increase in CSFP following introduction of a compressing mass is rather rapid, and clinical manifestations of hypertension are absent; b) stage of subcompensation, when an increase of the compressing mass is accompanied by a delayed and incomplete rise of the cerebrospinal fluid pressure; focal symptoms of cerebral involvement begin to appear; c) stage of decompensation, when a marked CSFP increase is associated with displacement and herniation of different parts of the brain. This stage passes to the terminal period which is characterized by fatal disorders due to compression of the medulla oblongata. In the presence of intracranial space-occupying lesions, total CBF does not change during the stage of compensation, although a perifocal rCBF increase is observed. The reactivity and tone of the cerebral blood vessels rises or remains unchanged. Autoregulation is not impaired.

With experimental increase in size of the compressing focus and in ICP (stage of subcompensation) cerebral transit time was longer (up to 10.25–11.75 sec as against 6–7 sec under normal conditions), while global CBF was reduced.

Around the lesion, a period of increased rCBF was followed by a decrease. Intravital injections revealed impaired filling of the capillaries and small blood vessels, especially in the zone of compression. The diameter of the main arteries diminished to three-quarters to one-half of the initial values. Cerebrovascular resistance increased. Studies of the regional reactivity revealed a reduced or distorted response of cerebral vessels to CO_2 and impaired autoregulation around the lesion. In regions distant from the compressing focus these hemodynamic parameters were less disturbed.

In the stage of decompensation cerebral transit time was markedly protracted (up to 17–21 sec), CBF was significantly diminished and cerebrovascular resistance increased. The caliber of the main arteries was reduced to one-third of the initial value. Response of the blood vessels to CO_2 was reduced or absent. Autoregulation was notably impaired or failed completely, and changes in systemic arterial blood pressure were followed by passive changes in CBF. Regional CBF reduction around the compression was overlapped by a marked CBF reduction in both the involved and the contralateral cerebral hemispheres. In addition to an elevation of CSFP to 30–35 mmHg and a reduction of CBF to 18–21 ml/100 g/min there was an accumulation of lactate and pyruvate and an increase of the lactate/pyruvate ratio in the blood and cerebrospinal fluid, as well as a reduction of arterial pCO_2. Changes in reactivity of the cerebral arteries to CO_2 did not always occur simultaneously to impairment of autoregulation.

Hemodynamic studies in patients with tumors of the cerebral hemispheres indicate that the more marked the rise in ICP the more significant the reduction in CBF and the increase in cerebrovascular resistance. In instances of pronounced intracranial hypertension mean CBF decreased to values as low as 22 ml/100 g/min.

As ICP increases, ischemia in the cerebral cortex appears earlier, is more pronounced and shows a greater progression than in the white matter. The more or less marked general CBF reduction in most patients with brain tumors is associated with different degrees of interregional rCBF variation in the involved hemisphere. This variation usually exceeds 15–20%, not infrequently reaches 70–80% and sometimes 100% and more.

Conclusion

Our results suggest the following pathogenic mechanism for intracranial hypertension due to space-occupying lesions: initially compensation is preserved by active changes in the diameter of cerebral vessels; exhaustion of these reserves results in distortion and subsequent loss of reactivity of the cerebral arteries to CO_2. Autoregulation is impaired. These initially local perifocal changes spread to the entire brain in a vicious circle: reduction of cerebral blood flow – hypoxia – acidosis – perifocal hyperemia – cerebral edema – advance of intracranial hypertension – brain compression – further reduction of the cerebral blood flow and metabolism.

Key Words: Intracranial hypertension, cerebrospinal fluid pressure, regional cerebral blood flow, reactivity of cerebral blood vessels, autoregulation of the cerebral blood flow.

References

1. SERGIYENKO, T. M., KOVALENKO, N. A.: Functional state of the cerebral blood vessels and cerebral hemodynamics in patients with tumors of the cerebral hemispheres. In: Voprosy neiroonkologii, Kiev, 6–8 (1968).

2. BROCK, M.: Regional cerebral blood flow changes following local brain compression in the cat. Scand. J. clin. Lab. Invest. (Suppl. 102) (1968).

3. FIESCHI, C.: Regional CBF in acute apoplexy including pharmacodynamic studies. Scand. J. clin. Lab. Invest. (Suppl. 102) (1968).

4. ZWETNOW, N.: CBF autoregulation to blood pressure and intracranial pressure variations. Scand. J. clin. Lab. Invest. (Suppl. 102) (1968).

5. ZWETNOW, N.: Effect of increased CSF pressure on the blood flow and on the energy metabolism of the brain. An experimental study. Lund, 1970.

6. MEYER, J. S. et al.: Effects of cerebral compression by a mass lesion on regional cerebral blood flow. Panminerva med. **13**, 195–196 (1971).

7. NAGAI, H.: Effect of increased intracranial pressure on cerebral hemodynamics. Panminerva med. **13**, 192–193 (1971).

8. JOHNSTON, J. H. et al.: Cerebral blood flow in experimental intracranial hypertension. Panminerva med. **13**, 193 (1971).

9. VIROZUB, I. D., SERGIENKO, T. M.: A technique of gradual increase of the intracranial pressure in the chronic experiment in animals. Vop. Neĭrokhir. **6**, 36–40 (1952). (In Russian.)

Halothane, Hypocapnia and Cerebrospinal Fluid Pressure in Neurosurgery[1]

R. W. Adams, G. A. Gronert, T. M. Sundt, and J. D. Michenfelder

Introduction

Recent studies by McDowall, Jennett, Barker, and Fitch [1–4] demonstrated that halothane may increase intracranial pressure, especially in patients with intracranial space-occupying lesions, and suggested that hypocapnia may not prevent such increases. A subsequent editorial [5] concluded that halothane is relatively contraindicated for intracranial surgery. The validity of this conclusion may be questioned because in the patients studied by the McDowall group, the levels of hypocapnia were inconstant, awake cerebrospinal fluid pressure (CSFP) was not measured, and the effect of halothane was observed for only 10 min. The present study was designed to examine the effect of continuous administration of halothane on CSFP at a constant level of hypocapnia induced either before or together with the introduction of halothane. In addition, the combined effect of droperidol, fentanyl, nitrous oxide, and hypocapnia on CSFP was examined.

Materials and Methods

In 48 patients undergoing craniotomy for tumor or vascular lesions, cerebrospinal fluid pressure was continuously measured from prior to induction of anesthesia through removal of the bone flap. A malleable needle was placed in the lumbar subarachnoid space and attached via a saline filled system to a Statham strain gauge whose zero point was adjusted to a mid-cranium level and which was connected to a Sanborn direct writer. Great care was taken to prevent any loss of CSF. The patency of the CSF system between the head and the lumbar subarachnoid space was confirmed at the start of each case by observing the expected increase in CSFP in response to passive elevation of the head and was reconfirmed at the end of the recording period by observing the pressure increase in response to digital pressure on the dura. Induction of anesthesia was accomplished with thiopental 200–500 mg followed by succinylcholine 100 mg and intubation. Following intubation, all patients were paralyzed with gallamine 140–200 mg and hyperventilated by Bird ventilator to $PaCO_2$ levels less than 30

1 This investigation was supported in part by Research Grant NS-7507, from the National Institutes of Health, Public Health Service.

torr as determined by an IR blood gas analyer. Arterial pressure and central venous pressure were also measured continuously using indwelling catheters and Statham strain gauges. The patients were divided into 3 groups based on the random selection of 1 of 3 possible anesthetic-maintenance regimens. In group 1 (21 patients) halothane (0.5–1.0% inspired) was administered immediately after endotracheal intubation simultaneous with the onset of hyperventilation. In group 2, (17 patients) halothane (0.5–1.0% inspired) was administered 10 min after endotracheal intubation and the onset of hyperventilation, when $PaCO_2$ levels of 20–30 torr had been established. Group 3 (10 patients) received no halothane but was maintained with an initial intravenous injection of Innovar (1 ml/20–25 pounds) and intermittent supplemental injections of fentanyl (1 ml every 15–45 min).

Results

The awake mean CSFP was similar in all three groups and was essentially unchanged immediately following induction, intubation, and the onset of mechanical ventilation. Thereafter, the response varied in each of the 3 groups.

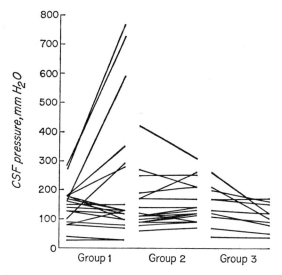

Fig. 1. Maximal changes in CSFP following halothane or Innovar. Group 1: Halothane and hyperventilation begun simultaneously. Group 2: Halothane after 10 min hyperventilation. Group 3: Innovar with hyperventilation

Figure 1: In group 1 with simultaneous onset of halothane and hyperventilation: CSFP increased in 7 patients over a range of 50–500 mm H_2O (3.7–36.9 mmHg). In group 2 with delayed administration of halothane (following 10 min of hyperventilation) a small increase in CSFP occurred in 10 patients over a range of 10–90 mm H_2O (0.7–6.6 mmHg). In group 3 no increase in CSFP occurred following Innovar and in 8 of 10 patients, a small decrease was observed.

Table 1: The mean CSFP increase compared to post-induction levels in those 7 cases in group 1 was 260 mm H_2O (19.2 mmHg) compared to 26 mm H_2O (1.9 mmHg) in the 10 cases in group 2 when hypocapnia was established before the administration of halothane. The degree of hypocapnia achieved was similar in each group, and none of the CSFP changes could be related to changes in central venous pressure or mean arterial pressure.

Table 1. Cerebrospinal fluid pressure increase. Compared to post-induction level

| | | Increased, mmHg | |
Group	N	Mean ± SD	Range
1	7	19.2 ± 13.3	3.7–36.9
2	10	1.9 ± 1.6	0.7– 6.6

* P < 0.01.

Figure 2: Represented here are the courses of CSFP of one case from each group, those from groups 1 and 2 being the studies that demonstrated the greatest CSFP increases in their groups. The effects of induction and intubation on CSFP shown here were frequent findings in our patients, i.e., a slight rise in pressure following application of the oxygen mask, the transient fall in pressure after the administration of pentothal, and the marked rise and fall in pressure with laryngoscopy, intubation, and the beginning of ventilation. Not all patients had large rises associated with intubation. This response varied with degree of narcosis, muscle relaxation, and difficulty of intubation.

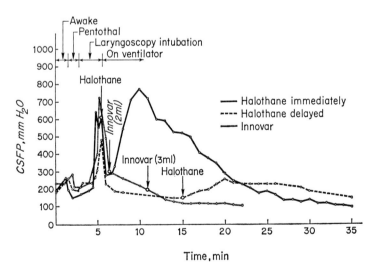

Fig. 2. CSFP course of one case from each group

In addition to the difference in magnitude of rise seen with halothane started immediately and that given after hyperventilation, the pressure increases were limited in duration in spite of the continuing administration of halothane. This was seen in all 17 cases. The average interval between onset of halothane and the start of the pressure rise was $2^1/_2$ min, peak pressure at 7 min, and return to prerise levels in 21 min. The course shown for the patient receiving Innovar was the most consistently seen pattern in group 3.

Discussion

Alterations in intracranial pressure are due to change in volume of one or more of the 3 cerebral tissue compartments: cerebrospinal fluid, brain parenchyma, and intravascular volume. Under normal conditions, increases in volume in one compartment are compensated for by decreases in other compartments. This accounts for normal CSFP in many patients with space-occupying lesions. Once the capacity for compensation is exhausted, further increase in volume will result in sharp increases in pressure. If this occurs during an operative procedure before the skull is opened, pressure gradients can develop between brain compartments resulting in herniation or fall in perfusion pressure causing hypoxia or infarction. Rapid changes in volume occur only in the vascular compartment, and it is here that the agents and techniques of anesthesia have their effect. Deterioration of neurosurgical patients under general anesthesia is a long-recognized problem which was earlier attributed to poor anesthetic technique, i.e., obstruction of airway, light anesthesia, inadequate relaxation, poor position for cerebral venous drainage, hypoventilation and accumulation of carbon dioxide, all known to increase venous pressure or dilate cerebral vasculature with secondary increase in intracranial pressure. More recently the effects of anesthetic agents themselves have been indicated as a factor in increasing pressure. Experimental evidence has shown halothane and other volatile agents to have cerebral vasodilating effects at normocapnia with resultant increase in cerebral blood flow and cerebral blood volume [6,7], and it is this response that is probably the cause of increased intracranial pressure in the post-induction period [8,9,10]. It was originally thought that intracranial pressure would remain elevated as long as the patient was receiving halothane, but investigations in the dog [1] in addition to this study, show the pressure increase to be of limited duration. McDowALL suggests that this is probably best explained by an additional vascular adjustment since the dogs showed a simultaneous fall in cerebral blood flow and cerebral venous pressure, something that would not result from compensation of volume in another tissue compartment.

It has been shown that the cerebral vasculature remains responsive to changes in carbon dioxide tension during halothane anesthesia [11]. In contrast to our results, however, the JENNETT group reported that prior induction of hypocapnia did not consistently prevent halothane-induced CSFP increases [4]. The basis for such divergent results is not entirely clear. However, comparison of our protocol of study with that of JENNETT and associates' study reveals one difference. JENNETT intended to produce $PaCO_2$ levels of 35–45 torr. Inadvertent hypothermia (commonly below 35° C) required correction of their blood gas measurements such that, in many instances, corrected $PaCO_2$ values were below 35 torr and hence hypocapnic. However, at temperatures other than 37° C "normal" $PaCO_2$ is not known and therefore the CO_2 tension at which cerebral vascular resistance is "normal" is not known. It is possible, therefore, that those patients of JENNETT and associates' study considered to be hypocapnic because of hypothermia were not in fact hypocapnic as regards the response of the cerebral vessels.

In previously reported similar studies [1–4] using normocarbia, all patients had a rise in CSFP with halothane. In our studies utilizing hyperventilation in all cases, fewer than half the patients had increases in CSFP and when hyperventilation was established prior to the introduction of halothane, the degree of rise of CSFP, when any rise occurred, was decreased by 85–90% for mean values.

It is concluded from this study that, in addition to droperidol-fentanyl, halothane can be safely administered to neurosurgical patients providing that its administration is preceded by a period of hyperventilation to $PaCO_2$ less than 30 torr.

Summary

The effect of halothane and hypocapnia on cerebrospinal fluid pressure (CSFP) was examined in 48 patients undergoing craniotomy. All patients were hyperventilated to $PaCO_2$ levels less than 30 torr; 21 patients (group 1) received halothane (0.5–1.0%) simultaneously with the onset of hyperventilation, and 17 patients (group 2) received halothane (0.5–1.0%) after hyperventilation had been established for 10 min. Large increases in CSFP occurred only in group 1 (7 patients). A third group (10 patients) was given Innovar in the absence of halothane, and no increase in CSFP occurred. We conclude that halothane is capable of increasing CSFP in patients with intracranial disease, but these increases are transient and can be minimized or abolished by the prior induction of hypocapnia.

Key Words: Halothane, CSF pressure, hypocapnia.

References

1. McDOWALL, D. G., BARKER, J., JENNETT, W. B.: Cerebrospinal Fluid Pressure Measurements During Anaesthesia. Anaesthesia **21**, 189–201 (1966).
2. McDOWALL, D. G., BARKER, J., JENNETT, W. B.: Cerebrospinal Fluid Pressure Measurements During Anaesthesia. Anaesthesia **21**, 98–99 (1966).
3. JENNETT, W. B., McDOWALL, D. G., BARKER, J.: The Effect of Halothane on Intracranial Pressure in Cerebral Tumors. J. Neurosurg. **26**, 270–274 (1967).

4. JENNETT, W. B., FITCH, W., McDOWALL, D. G., BARKER, J.: Effect of Anaesthesia on Intracranial Pressure in Patients with Space-Occupying Lesions. The Lancet 1, 61–64, Jan. 11, 1969.
5. Editorial, Brit. J. Anaesth. 41, 277–278, April 1969.
6. WOLLMAN, H., ALEXANDER, S. C., COHEN, P. J., CHASE, P. E., MELMAN, E., BEHAR, M. G.: Cerebral Circulation of Man During Halothane Anesthesia. Anesthesiology 25, 180–184 (1964).
7. CHRISTENSEN, J. S., HØEDT-RASMUSSEN, K., LASSEN, N. A.: Cerebral Vasodilation by Halothane Anaesthesia in Man and its Potentiation by Hypotension and Hypercapnia. Brit. J. Anaesth. 38, 927–934 (1967).
8. RICH, M., SCHEINBERG, P., BELLE, M. S.: Relationship Between Cerebrospinal Fluid Pressure Changes and Cerebral Blood Flow. Circulat. Res. 1, 389–395 (1953).
9. RISBERG, J., LUNDBERG, N., INGVAR, D. H.: Regional Cerebral Blood Volume During Acute Transient Rises of the Intracranial Pressure (Plateau Waves). J. Neurosurg. 31, 303–310 (1969).
10. SMITH, A. L., NEUFELD, G. R., OMINSKY. A. J., WOLLMAN, H.: Effect of Arterial CO_2 Tension on Cerebral Blood Flow, Mean Transit Time, and Vascular Volume. J. appl. Physiol. 31, 701–707 (1971).
11. ALEXANDER, S. C., WOLLMAN, H., COHEN, P. J., CHASE, P. E., BEHAR, M. G.: Cerebrovascular Response to $PaCO_2$ During Halothane Anesthesia in Man. J. appl. Physiol. 19 (4), 561–565 (1964).

Comments to Session 9

G. McDowall and R. Wüllenweber

This session is best discussed in 2 parts. The first contains 2 papers dealing with osmolality of cerebrospinal fluid and the control of intracranial pressure by use of hyperosmolar agents, while the second part consists of three papers on anesthetic drugs.

Part 1

The finding of Prill et al. that no correlation existed between CSF sodium concentration and CSF osmolality was questioned by Siesjö, who stated that these two factors should be related since although only half CSF ions are sodium, almost all the rest are anions in balance with the sodium. All Prill's measurements were made on lumbar CSF, but no one present was able to say what delay was involved in the transmission of a change in ventricular fluid osmolality to lumbar CSF.

Shulman asked how Becker knew the quantity of fluid removed from the brain at different blood osmolalities. Becker replied that his comments in this area were based on extrapolation from results in animals. The chairman suggested that since a ventricular catheter was present it might have been valuable to measure CSF osmolality in addition to blood osmolality, particularly in view of Prill's comment that fluid was removed from the brain when a difference of 10 mosmols/kg H_2O existed between blood and CSF. Such measurements of CSF osmolality would be especially valuable if chronic administration of mannitol is to be employed clinically, since CSF mannitol concentration will rise progressively under these circumstances. Becker replied that he and his colleagues were reluctant to remove ventricular fluid in these patients.

Part 2

In the discussion on ketamine all discussants agreed that intracranial pressure increased with this drug. Kreuscher stated that he had measured CBF in dogs given ketamine and been unable to detect an increase in CBF. He believed that the ICP increase resulted from an increase in central venous pressure which he had observed. It was pointed out, however, that Takeshita and colleagues [4] have published results of CBF in man showing an increase with this drug, and Dawson and Michenfelder [1] reported similar increases in CBF in the dog. The recent editorial in *Anesthesiology* [5], which states that ketamine is a cerebral stimulant, could lead to the interpretation that increased cerebral metabolism produces increased CBF and so a rise in CSFP.

SHULMAN asked if these results meant that one should not use this drug in neuroradiology in young children, which would (he felt) be unfortunate, since the drug is so useful for such cases. Others agreed with the usefulness of the drug in these circumstances, but it was felt that caution was obviously indicated when the drug was so employed.

KREUSCHER asked ADAMS if the hyperventilation employed in his study had led to a change in the lactate: pyruvate ratio in CSF, which might indicate hypocapnic cerebral ischaemia. ADAMS replied that he and his colleagues had not made such measurements, but he doubted whether the degree of hypocapnia employed could have produced cerebral ischaemia. SIESJÖ commented that in his recent work he had found that rats tolerate hyperventilation to $PaCO_2$ values of under 20 mmHg without significant shifts in the lactate: pyruvate ratio.

HULME showed a slide in which cerebral oxygen availability was shown to fall during intubation, in line with the major increases in ICP that are known to occur at this time.

McDOWALL said he viewed the results presented by ADAMS as being in agreement with those of JENNETT et al. [3] in that: 1. ADAMS had confirmed that some patients with space-occupying lesions had major increases in ICP with halothane, and 2. that neuroleptanalgesic drugs did not elevate ICP. ADAMS' finding that halothane-induced increases in ICP were transient did not, he felt, exclude the possibility that the ICP hypertension lasted long enough to be capable of producing detrimental effects mainly by means of exaggeration of ICP gradients and brain shift [2].

The observations of ADAMS et al. are important in that they may indicate that halothane can be safely used in neurosurgery, providing hyperventilation is employed prior to halothane administration, and that this hyperventilation has been successful in reducing $PaCO_2$ below 30 mmHg.

References

1. DAWSON, B., MICHENFELDER, J. D., THEYE, R. A.: Effects of ketamine on canine cerebral blood flow and metabolism: modification by prior administration of thiopentone. Curr. Res. Anesth. **50**, 443–447 (1971).
2. FITCH, W., McDOWALL, D. G.: Effect of halothane on intracranial pressure gradients in the presence of space-occupying lesions. Brit. J. Anaesth. **43**, 904 (1971).
3. JENNETT, W. B., BARKER, J., FITCH, W., McDOWALL, D. G.: Effect of anaesthesia on intracranial pressure in patients with space-occupying lesions. Lancet **1**, 61–64 (1969).
4. TAKESHITA, H., OKUDA, Y., SARI, A.: The effects of ketamine on cerebral circulation and metabolism in man. Anesthesiology **36**, 69 (1972).
5. WINTERS, W. D.: Epilepsy or anaesthesia with ketamine. Anesthesiology **36**, 309 (1972).

Session 10

Miscellaneous
(Clinical)

Concentration of Acid Monoamine Metabolites in Ventricular CSF of Patients with Posterior Fossa Tumors[1]

K. A. West, L. Edvinsson, K. C. Nielsen, and B.-E. Roos

It is now generally accepted that brain monoamines act as neurotransmitters [1, 2, 3, 4]. In certain pathological conditions, such as Parkinson's disease [5, 6, 7], dementia and depression [8, 9], the concentrations of the acid monoamine metabolites in the cerebrospinal fluid (CSF) and brain are markedly reduced. In animal experiments it has been shown that the brain monoamine neurons are affected by intracranial hypertension, and that the neuronal sensitivity to the increased ventricular fluid pressure (VFP) is related to the topography of the neuronal systems in relation to the ventricles [10, 11, 12, 13]. Thus, the neurons containing dopamine are the most sensitive to increased VFP, the noradrenaline neurons next, whereas the nerves containing serotonin (5-hydroxytryptamine, 5-HT) are least sensitive. The CSF concentrations of homovanillic acid (HVA), which is the final metabolite of dopamine, and of 5-hydroxyindoleacetic acid (5-HIAA), which is the final metabolite of 5-HT, have been shown to be increased in hydrocephalic infants [14, 15] and animals [13, 16]. This increase is considered to be due to impaired absorption of the metabolites from the CSF. The present report deals with the variations in acid monoamine metabolite concentration in ventricular CSF as related to the level of the VFP and to some other clinical data in patients with posterior fossa tumors.

Material and Methods

The material comprises 18 patients (mean age 38,3 years) with tumors in the posterior fossa and 7 non-tumor patients (mean age 47,3 years) (Tables 1 and 2). The VFP was recorded according to LUNDBERG [17]. The tip of the ventricular catheter was placed in the right or the left frontal horn. The recordings were performed for about 30 min in the control cases and 2 h to 2 days in the tumor patients. The pressure values were expressed as mean values relative to atmospheric pressure at frontal skin surface. The ventricular CSF was obtained in the control patients immediately before the performance of air-ventriculography during the stereotaxic operation for pain or compulsive neurosis. The

1 Supported by grant No. B73–04X–732–07 from the Swedish Medical Research Council.

operation was done under neuroleptanalgesia in control patients 4, 5, 6 and 7 (Table 1). In the tumor patients the ventricular CSF was withdrawn during ventriculography. The VFP recording and the withdrawal of CSF were performed under halothane anesthesia in cases 6, 8, 10 and 14 (Table 2). Part of the CSF

Table 1. Clinical data and the levels of ventricular HVA and 5-HIAA in the 7 control cases

Case	Age (Years)	Sex	VFP (mmHg)	Ventri- cular size	HVA (μg/ml)	5-HIAA (μg/ml)	Diagnosis
1	68	F	5	Norm.	0.192		Pain following a burn
2	55	F	3	Slightly enl.	0.175	0.086	Facial pain
3	72	F	10	Slightly enl.	0.248	0.125	Suspected cerebellar metastasis
4	32	F	1	Norm.	0.327	0.086	Compulsive neurosis
5	37	F	7	Norm.	0.106	0.062	Compulsive neurosis
6	40	F	8	Norm.	0.376	0.062	Compulsive neurosis
7	27	F	-2	Norm.	0.197	0.068	Compulsive neurosis

Mean $\pm$ S.E.M.
47.3 $\pm$ 6.7   5.1 $\pm$ 1.3   0.232 $\pm$ 0.035   0.082 $\pm$ 0.010

sample was immediately placed in a refrigerator (0 to $+ 4°$ C) and was frozen to $-30°$ C within 4 h. The rest was sent for cytological analysis and determination of the total protein content. There were no signs of inflammatory changes in the CSF of any of the patients. Salicylates were avoided for several days prior to withdrawal of the CSF samples. Samples for determination of HVA and 5-HIAA were kept in the frozen state until analyzed. The level of HVA was determined fluorometrically by the method of ANDÉN et al. [18] and concentration of 5-HIAA according to a slightly modified version of the fluorometric method of ASHCROFT and SHARMAN [14]. Other clinical data, such as the extent of the papilledema or the size of the ventricular system, were assessed by ophthalmologists or radiologists.

Results

The mean values ($\pm$ standard error of the mean) for the concentrations of HVA and 5-HIAA in the ventricular CSF of the control patients were 0.232 $\pm$ 0.035 μg/ml and 0.082 $\pm$ 0.010 μg/ml respectively (Table 1). The mean

VFP in the same patients was 5.1 $\pm$ 1.3 mmHg. The size of the lateral ventricles was within normal limits in all but two of these cases. The concentrations of HVA and 5-HIAA were significantly higher in the group with posterior fossa tumors than in the control group (Student's-test $0.001 < p < 0.01$) (Table 2).

A significant increase ($0.001 < p < 0.01$) in both metabolites was also found when the tumor patients with increased intracranial pressure and/or papilledema were compared with the tumor patients where these parameters were normal or absent (Table 3). The ventricular size was normal in 2 of the patients with tumors in the posterior fossa. In 5 of the tumor patients the lateral ventricles were highly dilated and in the remaining 11 patients only slightly or moderately dilated. Increased levels of acid metabolites in CSF were found in 3 of the tumor patients with moderately or highly enlarged lateral ventricles but normal VFP (cases 5, 7, and 11, Table 2). In these 3 patients no air was found intracranially after pneumoencephalography and/or no air was shown to pass out from the ventricular system during air ventriculography. The VFP was, furthermore, normal or almost normal in 5 other tumor cases (cases 3, 9, 13, 15 and 16, Table 2), but their lateral ventricles were assessed as normal or only slightly enlarged, and no blockade to the passage of air was found during pneumoencephalography or ventriculography. In these latter 5 cases the levels of ventricular HVA and 5-HIAA were only slightly, not significantly, increased ($p > 0.05$).

Discussion

The mechanisms controlling the transfer of acid monoamine metabolites to the CSF as well as their absorption from the CSF are essentially unknown. It is generally believed that the metabolites are released into the ventricular CSF rather than into the subarachnoidal CSF over the brain convexity. Absorption of the acid monoamine metabolites is considered to take place in the region of the fourth ventricle [19]. It can therefore be expected that a blockage of the CSF outflow will be accompanied by increased levels of the monoamine metabolites in the ventricular CSF. This is in keeping with the results obtained in the present investigation and with other results in humans and in animals [14, 15].

An increase in the acid metabolites during hydrocephalic conditions may, however, indicate an altered amine metabolism in the brain tissue. Recent experimental findings [10, 11, 13] support this view. Further, there was evidence for a disturbed relation between the acid metabolite concentrations in the brain and in the ventricular CSF, probably as a result of neuron damage, together with the altered mechanisms responsible for the transfer of acid metabolites from brain to CSF [10, 11, 13]. It is reasonable to believe that similar changes in amine metabolism may take place during intracranial hypertension also in the human brain. Judging from observations on experimental animals it can be expected that the levels of catecholamines and 5-HT are either normal or

Table 2. Clinical data and acid monoamine metabolite levels in the ventricular CSF of the 18 tumor patients

Case	Age (Years)	Sex	VFP (mmHg)	Papill-edema (dioptr.)	Ventricular size	HVA (µg/ml)	5-HIAA (µg/ml)	Diagnosis
1	41	F	20	3	Moderately enl.	0.240	0.180	Tentorial meningeoma
2	51	M	25	0	Highly enl.		0.170	Cerebell. metast. tumour
3	33	F	15	4	Norm.	0.026	0.080	Acoustic neurinoma
4	7	F	45	4	Highly enl.	0.660	0.169	Pontine glioma
5	51	M	8	0	Highly enl.	0.137	0.177	Pontine glioma
6	9	F	40	3	Moderately enl.	0.514	0.094	Cerebell. astrocytoma
7	47	M	3	0	Highly enl.	0.609	0.056	IV-ventr. ependymoma
8	3	F	20	1	Slightly enl.	0.516	0.218	Cerebell. astrocytoma
9	55	M	5	3	Slightly enl.	0.526	0.230	Cerebell. metast. tumour
10	6	M	35	1	Moderately enl.	0.291	0.109	Cerebell. astrocytoma
11	53	M	10	3	Moderately enl.	0.256	0.109	Cerebell. haemangioma
12	62	F	20	3	Moderately enl.	0.423	0.254	Cerebell. astrocytoma
13	45	F	15	1	Slightly enl.	0.529	0.048	Acoustic neurinoma
14	11	M	30	2	Highly enl.	0.447	0.097	Cerebell. astrocytoma
15	52	M	5	0	Normal	0.262	0.121	IV-ventr. ependynoma
16	65	M	10	1	Slightly enl.	0.314	0.131	Cerebell. metast. tumour
17	54	F	25	2	Moderately enl.	0.516	0.170	Acoustic neurinoma
18	45	F	20	2	Moderately enl.	0.460		Cerebell. astrocytoma
Mean ± S.E.M.	38.3 ± 5.0		19.5 ± 2.9	1.8 ± 0.3		0.396 ± 0.042	0.142 ± 0.015	

Table 3. The mean levels ($\pm$ S.E.M.) of HVA and 5-HIAA in the ventricular CSF in controls related to the degree of papilledema and mean VFP in cases with tumors in the posterior fossa. Significant differences between the acid monoamine metabolite levels in controls and tumor cases: [a] $= 0.001 < p < 0.01$. Number of cases in parenthesis

Acid monoamine metabolites	Metabolite levels in the controls	Metabolite levels in the tumor cases		VFP	
		Papilledema None	Present	Normal	Increased
HVA μg/ml	0.232 $\pm$ 0.035 (7)	0.336 $\pm$ 0.141 (3)	0.408 $\pm$ 0.044 (14)[a]	0.332 $\pm$ 0.073 (8)	0.452 $\pm$ 0.042 (9)[a]
5-HIAA μg/ml	0=082 $\pm$ 0.010 (6)	0.131 $\pm$ 0.028 (4)	0.145 $\pm$ 0.018 (13)[a]	0.119 $\pm$ 0.022 (8)	0.162 $\pm$ 0.018 (9)[a]

reduced in the brain tissue during intracranial hypertension in man. Thus, it can be assumed that the increased levels of the acid metabolites in CSF in the present material are associated both with a decrease in brain catecholamines and 5-HT and a decrease in the levels of their acid metabolites in brain tissue.

The level of HVA in the ventricular CSF in the present material differed greatly from the values of the control group reported by GULDBERG et al. [20]. The different criteria used in the selection of the control groups from the 2 patient materials may account for the observed differences in mean concentrations. The normal level of the VFP in man in the recumbent position is considered to be 0–11 mmHg [17, 21]. The mean VFP in the present control material was 5.1 mmHg and thus falls within the accepted range of normal values.

Summary

The concentrations of the acid monoamine metabolites HVA and 5-HIAA were measured in the ventricular CSF of 18 children and adults with posterior fossa tumors and of 7 adult non-tumor control patients. Significantly higher concentrations of the metabolites were found in the tumor patients than in the controls. This increase was particularly evident in the tumor patients with signs of increased VFP or blockade of the ventricular CSF-outflow pathways with associated internal or obstructive hydrocephalus. The changes in the concentrations of the metabolites in ventricular CSF are discussed with reference to previously presented data on monoamine and metabolite concentrations in the brain of experimental animals.

Key Words: Acid monoamine metabolites, cerebrospinal fluid, intracranial pressure.

References

1. CARLSSON, A., FALCK, B., HILLARP, N.-Å.: Cellular localization of brain monoamines. Acta physiol. scand. (Suppl. 196) 56, 1–28 (1962).
2. PORTIG, P. J., VOGT, M.: Release into the cerebral ventricles of substances with possible transmitter function in the caudate nucleus. J. Physiol. 204, 687–715 (1969).
3. BANERJEE, U., BURKS, T. F., FELDBERG, W., GOORICH, C. A.: Temperature responses and other effects of 5-hydroxytryptophan and 5-hydroxytryptamine when acting from the liquor space in unanaesthetized rabbits. Brit. J. Pharmacol. 38, 688–701 (1970).
4. COUCH, J. R.: Responses of neurons in the raphe nuclei to serotonin, norepinephrine and acetylcholine and their correlation with an excitatory synaptic input. Brain Res. 19, 137 to 150 (1970).
5. EHRINGER, H., HORNYKIEWICZ, O., Verteilung von Noradrenalin und Dopamin (3-Hydroxytyramin) im Gehirn des Menschen und ihr Verhalten bei Erkrankungen des extrapyramidalen Systems. Klin. Wschr. 38, 1236–1239 (1960).
6. JOHANSSON, B., ROOS, B.-E.: Acid monoamine metabolites in the cerebrospinal fluid of patients with Parkinson's syndrome. Proc. 8th Int. Congr. Neurol. Vol. IV/1, 141–144, Vienna 1965.

7. WEST, K. A., ROOS, B.-E.: The ventricular fluid pressure and the concentrations of homovanillic acid in different compartments of the cerebrospinal fluid in patients with Parkinson's disease. Exc. Med. Inter. Congr. Ser. No. 217 (1970).

8. DENCKER, S. J., MALM, U., ROOS, B.-E., WERDINIUS, B.: Acid monoamine metabolites of cerebrospinal fluid in mental depression and mania. J. Neurochem. 13, 1545–1548 (1966).

9. GOTTFRIES, C. G., GOTTFRIES, I., ROOS, B.-E.: Homovanillic acid and 5-hydroxyindole-acetic acid in the cerebrospinal fluid of patients with senile dementia, presenile dementia and parkinsonism. J. Neurochem. 16, 1341–1345 (1969).

10. EDVINSSON, L., OWMAN, CH., ROSENGREN, E., WEST, K. A.: Brain concentrations of dopamine, noradrenaline, 5-hydroxytryptamine, and homovanillic acid during intracranial hypertension following traumatic brain injury in rabbit. Acta neurol. scand. 47, 458–463 (1971).

11. OWMAN, CH., ROSENGREN, E., WEST, K. A.: Influence of various intracranial pressure levels on the concentration of certain arylethyl-amines in rabbit brain. Experientia 27, 1036–1037 (1971).

12. WEST, K. A.: Sympathetic influence on intracranial pressure. Comm. Dept. of Anatomy, Univ. Lund, Sweden, No. 9 (1971).

13. EDVINSSON, L., NIELSEN, K. C., OWMAN, CH., ROSENGREN, E., WEST, K. A.: Concomitant fall in brain dopamine and homovanillic acid in hydrocephalic rabbits. Exp. Neurol. (1972) (in press).

14. ASHCROFT, G. W., SHARMAN, D. F.: 5-hydroxyinoles in human cerebrospinal fluid. Nature 186, 1050–1051 (1960).

15. ANDERSSON, H., ROOS, B.-E.: Increased level of 5-hydroxyindoleacetic acid in cerebrospinal fluid from infantile hydrocephalus. Experientia 22, 539–541 (1966).

16. ANDERSSON, H.: Acid monoamine metabolites in experimental hydrocephalus. Develop. Med. Child Neurol. (Suppl. 15), 58–61 (1968).

17. LUNDBERG, N.: Continous recording and control of ventricular fluid pressure in neurosurgical practice. Acta psychiat. scand. (Suppl. 149) 36, 1–193 (1960).

18. ANDÉN, N. E., ROOS, B.-E., WERDINIUS, B.: On the occurence of homovanillic acid in brain and cerebrospinal fluid and its determination by a fluorimetric method. Life Sci. 2, 448–458 (1963).

19. ASHCROFT, G. W., DOW, R. C., MOIR, A. T. B.: The active transport of 5-hydroxyindol-3-ylacetic acid 3-methoxy-4-hydroxyphenylacetic acid from a recirculatory perfusion system of the cerebral ventricles of the unanaesthetized dog. J. Physiol. (Lond.) 199, 397–425 (1968).

20. GULDBERG, H. C., ASHCROFT, G. W., TURNER, J. W., HANEIK, A.: The use of cerebrospinal fluid in the study of dopamine and 5-hydroxytryptamine metabolism in parkinsonism. In: GILLINGHAM, F. J., DONALDSON, I. M. L. (Eds.): Third Symp. on Parkinson's Disease., 50–54. Edinburgh: E. and S. Livingstone Ltd. 1969.

21. BRADLEY, K. C.: Cerebrospinal fluid pressure. J. Neurol. Neurosurg. Psychiat. 33, 387 to 397 (1970).

The Valvular Action of the Arnold-Chiari Malformation[1]

B. WILLIAMS

Introduction

Hernias within the craniospinal axis, as elsewhere, are caused by pressure differences. When such a hernia is tightly impacted there are pressure gradients across it, but during its development such pressure differences may be temporary. The Arnold-Chiari Malformation (ACM) is a herniation of the hind brain, downwards through the foramen magnum, which is moulded to form a close fitting plug with a potentially valve like action. The effects of pulsation upon this and on lesser degrees of cerebellar herniation are of interest.

The pressure within the intracranial and intraspinal contents is subject to continuous pulsation. The arterial and capillary vessels transmit the "arterial" pulse, and the venous channels, including the epidural veins of the spine, transmit "venous" pulses from the thoracoabdominal cavity during respiration, straining, coughing and so on. These pulsations pass as waves through the cerebrospinal fluid (CSF) and cause movement of that fluid.

GARDNER [1] has suggested that "arterial" pulsation is responsible for filling of the syrinx in communicating syringomyelia, but since "venous" pulsations are of greater amplitude they are more likely to produce destruction of tissue [2].

The present work on the nature of propagation of CSF pressure pulses during coughing and straining was intended to clarify the role of pulsatile factors in pathological conditions as well as normal transmission of CSFP [3].

Material and Methods

Pressure recordings have been carried out in conscious patients, 32 adults and 11 babies, with suspected obstruction of the CSF pathway in the cervical spine or at the foramen magnum. Recordings were taken simultaneously from the lumbar region and from above the suspected blockage, either the cisterna magna or the ventricles. Adults were in the sitting position with the transducers calibrated to zero and levelled at the thoracic inlet. Traces were made during sharp, single coughs and forced expiration.

1 Financial support has been provided by Reckitt & Coleman Ltd. and by the Hull branch of the Association for Spina Bifida and Hydrocephalus.
2 A Statham P23H differential transducer was used with a Devices M19 recording system.

Babies with hydrocephalus and spina bifida were studied lying in the lateral position with the transducers levelled at the midline. Recordings were taken before and after the closure of the spinal defect during rest, crying and during compression of the meningocele sac and the head.

In adults the mean or baseline pressures were always initially equal.

After a cough the initial rise in CSF pressure took place first in the lumbar region and was followed not less than 0.04 sec later by a rise in the cistern or ventricle. The lumbar pressure rose to a higher level and usually faster than the upper pressure. Then the lumbar pressure almost invariably fell sooner, more rapidly and further than the upper. Any obstruction of the pathways diminished the amplitude and the rate of rise of the upper pressure. In patients with a partial blockage the baseline of the lumbar pressure fell below the previous resting level after each cough impulse and this effect was sometimes summative (Fig. 1). This may be termed "pressure dissociation" and both cisterno-lumbar pressure dissociation (CLD) and ventriculo-lumbar pressure dissociation (VLD) were also produced by forced expiration (Fig. 2).

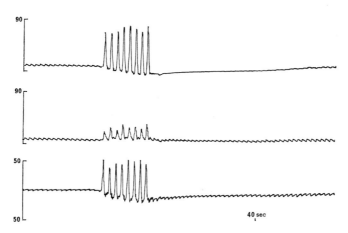

Fig. 1. Cisterno-lumbar pressure dissociation (CLD) after eight coughs. Patient with cervical spondylosis. Note the feeble amplitude of the cisternal cough impulse and abolition of the "arterial" pulse while the lumbar pressure is low. The top trace is lumbar, the middle trace is cisternal and the bottom (differential) trace is lumbar *minus* cisternal, pressures in mmHg

Figure 2 shows a recording from a 30 year old patient with syringomyelia in whom lumbar pneumoencephalography showed tonsillar herniation and failure of air to enter the ventricles. Ventriculography proved the communication from the fourth ventricle to a typically lobulated syringomyelia cavity. Studies showed that a VLD of 25 mmHg could be produced by blowing. This lasted for several seconds but equalized suddenly. At operation the tonsils were decompressed and partially removed with good clinical improvement; further studies performed a month after surgery showed no VLD.

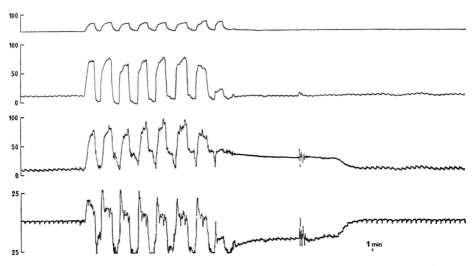

Fig. 2. Ventriculo-lumbar pressure dissociation after eight forced expirations. Case of communicating syringomyelia in which after operation the lumbar and cisternal pressures could not be significantly separated. Top trace is expiration pressure, second trace is lumbar pressure, third trace is ventricular pressure and the bottom (differential) trace is lumbar *minus* cisternal, pressures in mmHg

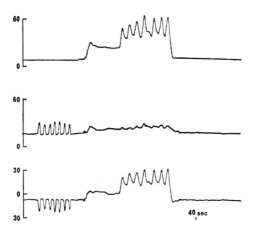

Fig. 3. Recordings from a baby with myelomeningocele and established VLD at birth. The head was compressed seven times, then the abdomen squeezed, then the meningocele compressed seven times. Intraspinal pressure affects intracranial but not vice versa. Lumbar trace on top, ventricular in the middle and lumbar *minus* cisternal (differential) below, pressures in mmHg

In the babies, pressure in all the meningoceles was atmospheric, tense meningoceles are exceptional. The intraspinal pressure was that of the sac. At the time of the pre-operative studies in some babies the intraventricular pressure was raised, VLD was therefore established at the outset. Compression of the head sometimes produced a rise in intraspinal pressure as well as intracranial pressure but commonly it did not (Fig. 3). Compression of saccular meningoceles conversely *always* produced a rise of intracranial pressure.

Some babies had developing VLD which only showed after drying. Pressure traces in these children showed that elevation of lumbar and intraventricular pressures tended to occur in parallel but that as the lumbar pressure fell the ventricular pressure remained high. After cessation of a period of crying the ventricular pressure gradually fell to approach that in the spinal theca suggesting a valve at the foramen magnum. Such babies have always developed progressive hydrocephalus, accompanied by established VLD.

Babies in which there was an initially raised intracranial pressure with low lumbar pressure always developed progressive hydrocephalus. VLD always disappeared after the insertion of a shunt and in one baby after decompression of the foramen magnum.

Those babies observed to have equal pressures in the spine and the head after spinal closure have not developed progressive hydrocephalus.

Discussion

When the intracranial and intraspinal compartments are in free communication the lumbar and upper traces are similar, any difference is caused by energy loss attenuation of pulses may be proportional to any obstruction present [4].

The pattern of CSF pressure waves in response to changes in thoraco-abdominal pressure means that there is an ebb and flow of the CSF particularly through the cervical regions and the foramen magnum.

Pressure dissociation is caused by fluid which has moved upwards being prevented from dropping downwards. The finding of pressure dissociation, however, does not prove the presence of a valve since none could be shown in the cases of cervical spondylosis (Fig. 1).

The valvular mechanism suggested [2] for communicating syringomyelia is strongly supported by the pressure traces of Figure 2. The sudden equalization of pressure after a period of VLD in the pre-operative trace would be explained by the "valve" becoming unseated as the tonsils disengage from the foramen magnum.

The valvular action of the fully developed Arnold-Chiari malformation found in spina bifida cases seems clear. Pressure studies support the clinical observations of VAN HOUWENINGE GRAFTDIJK [5]. It seems that once "developing" VLD is present, and there is a tendency for the pressure to remain active across the ACM for some minutes after crying, progression to "established" VLD with hydrocephalus is usual. Illustrative traces have been published elsewhere [6]. If the pressure makes the hind brain move it can presumably cause repeated temporary impaction of the ACM and eventually cause permanent impaction with established VLD and blockage of the outlets of the fourth ventricle. Hydrocephalus has been correlated with VLD closely in this small series.

The concept of low intraspinal pressure explains the aggravation of hydrocephalus after birth by exposure of the meningocele to lower than intrauterine pressure. Also important is the onset of crying. The occasional aggravation of hydrocephalus after removal of a meningocele may occur because the sac acts as a vent and keeps the lumbar pressure close to atmospheric. Once this is removed a low intraspinal pressure state can be developed by crying which pumps fluid from the spine up into the head.

Summary

Differential pressure manometry above and below cervical or foramen magnum obstruction shows that following upward pulses of CSF there may be dissociation between the pressures to either side of the block, the spinal pressure being the lower. Impaction of the hind brain produces a superadded valvular effect. This may contribute to filling of a syrinx in communicating syringomyelia and impaction of the hind brain in the foramen magnum in the Arnold-Chiari malformation.

Key Words: Syringomyelia, Arnold-Chiari malformation, electromanometrics, meningomyelocele, cervical spondylosis.

References

1. Gardner, W. J.: Hydrodynamic mechanisms of syringomyelia: its relationship to myelocele. J. Neurol. Neurosurg. Psychiat. 28, 247–259 (1965).
2. Williams, B.: Current concepts of syringomyelia. Brit. Jour. Hosp. Med., 4, 331–342 (1970).
3. O'Connell, J. E. A.: Cerebrospinal fluid mechanics. Proc. roy. Soc. Med. 63, 507–518 (1970).
4. Williams, B.: Combined cisternal and lumbar pressure recordings in the sitting position using differential manometry. J. Neurol. Neurosurg. Psychiat. 35, 142–143 (1972).
5. Van Houweninge Graftdijk, C. J.: Over hydrocephalus. Thesis, University of Leiden (1932).
6. Williams, B.: Further thoughts on the Valvular Action of the Arnold-Chiari malformation. Develop. Med. Child. Neurol. Supp. 25, 105–112 (1971).

Variations of Intraventricular and Local Brain Pressures during Neurosurgical Procedures

C. RIVANO, G. F. ROSSI, and J. ZATTONI

Introduction

The purpose of the present research was to provide objective data on the pressure forces to which the brain is subjected during endocranial neurosurgical procedures. On the basis of previous personal experience [1, 2, 3, 4], it was thought advisable to approach the problem along two main lines of investigation: 1. by considering the pressure changes affecting the whole or most of the brain, as might be indicated by recording the ventricular pressure; 2. by considering the pressure undergone by limited brain regions directly subjected to neurosurgical manipulations, as revealed, for instance, by recording the pressure exerted by the retracting spatula on the underlying cerebral tissue.

Material and Methods

1. Recording of the ventricular pressure (VFP): 25 patients were examined, operated upon for endocranial tumors (13 supratentorial and 7 subtentorial cases), aneurysms or angiomas (4 cases), or epilepsy (1 case). VFP was recorded through a catheter inserted into the frontal horn of the ventricle contralateral to the side of craniotomy and connected to an electromanometric recording unit (Statham P23AC pressure transducer and Grass polygraph mod. 5D.).

2. Recording of the local pressure (LBP): 25 patients operated upon for endocranial tumors (14 cases), intracerebral hematoma (7 cases) and trigeminal neuralgia (4 cases) were utilized. LBP was recorded by the technique developed in our laboratory [2, 3 and 4] (a flat oval plastic bag fixed to the "active" surface of the retracting spatula and connected to the electromanometric unit). This technique provided an accurate measurement of the pressure exerted by the manually operated spatula on the underlying brain tissue.

Pneumogram, electrocardiogram and, in many cases, systemic arterial and venous blood pressures were recorded to study possible relations between VFP and respiratory or circulatory events.

In all patients but one (operated upon for epilepsy) surgery was performed under general anesthesia and controlled ventilation.

Results

1. Changes in VFP

1. *Controls.* The increase in VFP is directly related to the pressure applied extradurally or directly to the brain. This was shown by intentional application of progressively increasing pressure, from 8.4–60 mmHg.

The degree of VFP increase was also related to the initial value of VFP itself, being higher when basal VFP was high and vice versa. When basal VFP was between 8.6 and 20 mmHg (average 15 mmHg: 8 cases) the ratio between force applied and VFP increase was 0.22–0.32 (average 0.27). When the basal VFP ranged between 1.9 and 6.1 mmHg (average 3.1 mmHg: 9 cases) this ratio fell to 0.13–0.15 (average: 0.14).

2. *Surgical Manipulations.* 2 main types of changes in VFP were found.

a) *Long-lasting changes,* i.e. VFP changes outlasting the surgical procedures producing them.

Removal of the osteoplastic flap and opening of the dura were always followed by long-lasting VFP changes (Fig. 1). Decrease as well as increases in VFP were observed, according to the values recorded for VFP prior to the operation; 1. VFP always fell when the basal pressure was higher than 4–5 mmHg (Fig. 1A, 1B), the degree of fall in VFP being related to the value

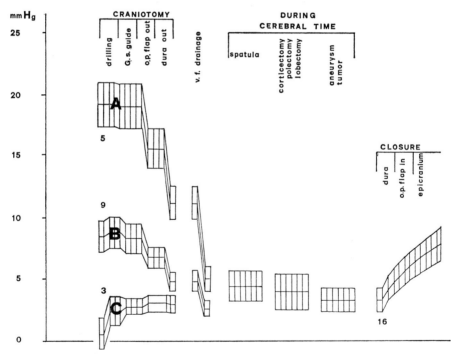

Fig. 1. "Long-lasting" changes of VFP following craniotomy, ventricular drainage, closure of the dura and repositioning of the osteoplastic flap. The mean values obtained in several patients are given. Basal VFP was high in A; middle in B and low in C

of the basal pressure (compare Fig. 1A, 1B). Similar results were observed following ventricular drainage or surgical opening of ventricular or cisternal spaces (Fig. 1). 2. VFP increase was recorded when the basal pressure was lower [1].

Closure of the dura and replacement of the osteoplastic flap were always followed by a slight increase in VFP (Fig. 1).

b) *Short-lasting changes*, i.e. reversible VFP changes lasting as long as the neurosurgical manipulation responsible for them (Fig. 2).

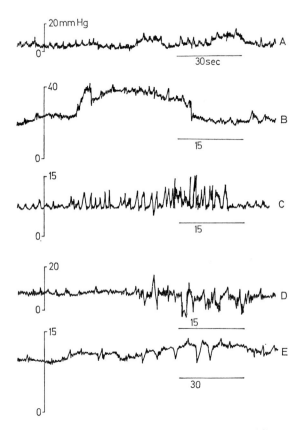

Fig. 2. "Short-lasting" changes of VFP during: A Drilling. B Gigli saw guide. C Application of the rongeur. D Digital isolation of tumor. E Application of the spatula

VFP increase was recorded during skull drilling (about 4 mmHg), insertion of the Gigli saw guide (maximum 32 mmHg), enlargement of craniotomy by rongeur (maximum 10 mmHg), brain retraction by spatula (maximum 4.3 mmHg), digital deep intracerebral tumor isolation (one case; 7.5 mmHg). Repositioning of the osteoplastic flap was accompanied by VFP increase in only one case.

2. Changes in LBP

Local pressure exerted on the underlying brain by the manually operated retracting spatula varied according to the type of operation performed (Fig. 3). The pressures most frequently recorded ranged between 1.5 and 18.4 mmHg for periods of 1–8 min. The maximum LBP value (46–110 mmHg, for repeated periods of 1–3 min) was found in a case of parasagittal meningioma;

LR

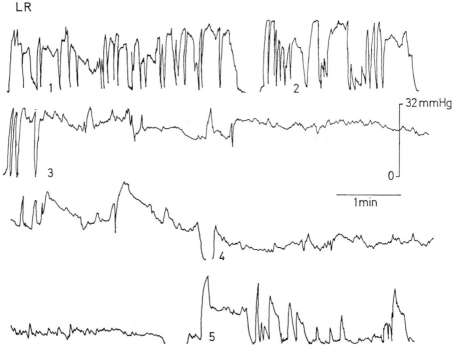

Fig. 3. Local pressure exerted on the underlying brain by the retracting spatula in a case operated upon for deep interhemispheric tumor: 1–2 progress of the spatula down the scissure; 3–4 partial removal of the tumor; 5-hemostasis and final control

high pressures were applied in a case of occipital paramedian tumor (22 mmHg for 10 min) and during retrogasserian rhizotomy (10–25 mmHg for repeated periods of 4–15 min). It is important that in the above cases, i.e. when pressures above 20 mmHg were repeatedly recorded, transitory neurological deficit appeared.

Comments

The findings reported above appear to raise the following points of practical neurosurgical interest.

1. The pressure changes undergone by the whole brain during endocranial neurosurgical procedures – as revealed by direct monitoring of VFP – reach their maximum values following manipulations of a) osteo-dural covers and

b) cerebro-spinal fluid spaces. Direct brain manipulation has only a very slight effect on VFP. Introduction of the Gigli saw guide alone into the extradural space is followed by a VFP increase much higher than that produced by digital isolation of an intracerebral tumor.

2. The extent, and in some surgical procedures, even the occurrence, of these changes is strictly related to the basal VFP.

3. The local pressure exerted by the retracting spatula on the underlying brain tissue does not appear to be related to the simultaneous effect on VFP.

4. The local effect of the retracting spatula may be followed by local brain damage in relation to the degree of pressure exerted and to its duration.

Summary

Two main types of changes in ventricular pressure were found: a) long-lasting changes, which followed large craniotomy and opening of cisternal or ventricular system; b) short-lasting changes, produced by skull drilling, introduction of Gigli saw, use of the spatula, digital isolation of deep tumor.

Local pressure exerted by the spatula on the brain changed according to the type of operation performed.

References

1. ROSSI, G. F., ZATTONI, J.: Variazioni della pressione endoventricolare da manualità neurochirurgiche in corso di interventi sopratentoriali. Minerva neurochir. **13**, 79–83 (1969).
2. SIANI, C., ZATTONI, J.: Registrazione della pressione endocranica dallo spazio epidurale. Nota tecnica e dati clinici. Rassegna Med. sper. **16**, 277–283 (1969).
3. ZATTONI, J., SIANI, C., SEMINO, L.: Fattori tecnici che influenzano la pressione intracranica epidurale quando registrato con dispositivi occupanti spazio. Boll. Soc. ital. Biol. sper. (in press).
4. BORZONE, M., DAVINI, V., RIVANO, C., SILVESTRO, C., TERCERO, E., SIANI, C., ZATTONI, J.: Wakefulness of the monitoring local brain pressure by spatula (in press).

Complications Due to Prolonged Ventricular Fluid Pressure Recording in Clinical Practice

G. Sundbärg, Å. Kjällquist, N. Lundberg, and U. Pontén

An essential condition for the use of continuous recording of the ventricular fluid pressure (VFP) in clinical work is an acceptably low rate of complications. In the departments of neurosurgery in Lund such recording has been used routinely since 1956 in about 1000 patients. The entire material has been reviewed with regard to acute complications. The occurrence of late-appearing sequelae has not been investigated but we have no reason to believe that the rate of e. g. epilepsy has increased due to the recording procedure [1].

Material and Methods

The original technique [1] has been modified several times but its essential features are unchanged. For technical details see [1]. To prevent and control infection the following routine is practiced. All tubing and connections are autoclaved and kept as disposable sets ready for immediate use. The transducers are sterilized with 25% glutaraldehyde. Connection of the ventricular catheter to the transducer, filling of the system with fluid and all other preparations for ventricular puncture are performed under strict aseptic conditions in the operating theatre. During recording, all measures that require opening of the closed fluid system e. g. calibration, sampling of CSF, insufflation of air for pneumography, are carried out with strict adherence to aseptic technique. Drainage of CSF, intermittently or continuously, is done within the closed system. Samples of CSF for cell-counts and cultures are taken immediately after insertion of the ventricular catheter and every second or third day during recording. The CSF is withdrawn from the "head-cock". On removal, the tip of the catheter and the rubber plug are cultured separately as well as the CSF. No antibiotics are given prophylactically. However, a great number of patients are treated with antibiotics during the period of recording for other reasons, such as pulmonary or urinary tract infections.

At the end of 1971 we had performed 997 recordings in 938 patients (Fig. 1) and during the first half of 1972 another 64 recordings were completed. Nine of these 997 recordings were total failures, as it was impossible to establish any lasting connection with the ventricular system. All the remaining recordings lasted between a few hours and 69 days, with an average of eight days. Air studies were performed in about 65% of all the patients, and about 75% of

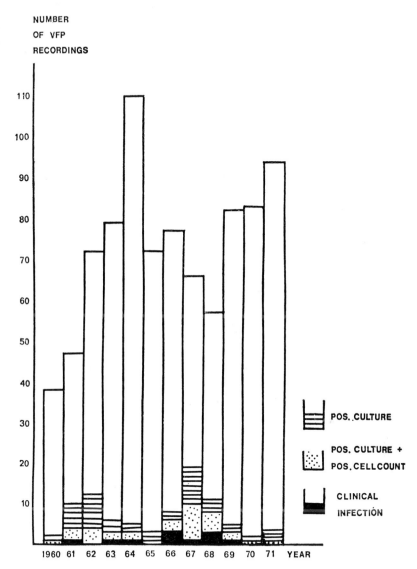

Fig. 1. Number of positive cultures, pathological cell counts and clinical infections as compared to total number of VFP recordings during the period 1960–1971. The cultured samples of CSF and the samples for cell counts were withdrawn from the ventricles during recording and when the ventricular catheter was removed at the end of recording

the patients underwent intracranial operations. The frequency of such measures did not differ to any extent from one year to another.

Results

Minor complications, mainly of a mechanical nature, occasionally occurred, such as leaking stop-cocks disconnection of tubing by restless patients, breakdown of transducers etc.

One case of intracerebral hematoma caused by the ventricular puncture was recorded. The patient, a 34-year old woman, was admitted in 1965 because of papilledema. The final diagnosis was pseudotumor cerebri. The VFP was moderately elevated. An oxygen ventriculography the day after ventricular puncture showed an expansive lesion in the frontal lobe. The ventricular catheter was then removed. Because of increasing symptoms of raised intracranial pressure the patient was operated on five days later and an intracerebral hematoma was evacuated. The patient was examined as an out-patient in July 1972 and proved to be symptom-free apart from occasional epileptic seizures and slight secondary atrophy of the papillae.

In two cases of subarachnoid hemorrhage, routine air studies for diagnosis of ventricular dilatation revealed filling defects in the lateral ventricle in the vicinity of the catheter tip. In one case this defect was suspected to be a tumor; it was punctured with stereotactic technique and proved to be a clot. In both cases the filling defects gradually and uneventfully disappeared. No other hemorrhagic complications have been recorded in our series.

Table 1. The table shows the frequency of different types of bacteria during different periods. The material is divided into definite infections (def.), suspected infections (susp.) and cases judged to be secondarily contaminated (cont.). In several patients there was a combination of two types of bacteria, which explains the discrepancy between the totals in the table and the number of cases in Fig. 1

Period		Staph. albus	Staph. aureus	Pseudo- monas	Coli	Water sapro- phytes, e.g. Sarcina	Other or non class.	Total
1956–1965	cont.	16	1		2	5	10	34
	susp.	9	1	1			4	15
	def.	1	1			1		3
1966–1968	cont.	8		2	1	3	2	16
	susp.	6		1		3	7	17
	def.	1	3	2	1		1	8
1969–1971	cont.	7						7
	susp.	4					1	5
	def.	1						1
1956–1971	cont.	31	1	2	3	8	12	57
	susp.	19	1	2		3	12	37
	def.	3	4	2	1	1	1	12

Infectious complications offer a constant challenge in usage of the method. Eleven patients (1.1%) had positive signs of intracranial infection i.e. clinical symptoms, growth of bacteria in the ventricular fluid and pathological cell-counts. Two of these patients were severely ill, the causative agents being pseudomonas and staphylococcus aureus respectively, but all 11 patients recovered. In 35 cases (3.5%) infection was suspected because of positive cultures and cell-counts, but none of these patients showed any evident signs of intracranial infection due to the pressure recording and only some were treated with antibiotics. In 51 cases (5.1%) positive cultures occurred but cell-counts were not significantly pathological and there were no other signs of infection. None of these patients received treatment (see Fig. 1). 91% of the patients with certain and 87% of those with suspected infections had been subjected to ventriculography as compared to the overall rate of 53% ventriculographies in the whole series. All the patients who definitely had infections had undergone intracranial operations, two of them twice and one even three times. There was no correlation at all between the duration of recording of the VFP and the rate of infection. The majority of patients with definite or suspected infections developed complications within a few days after the ventricular puncture, ventriculography or operation. The bacteria cultured are presented in the Table.

In a large number of patients ventricular fluid was drained intermittently or continuosly, in some cases for several weeks. There was no evidence that drainage increased the risk of infection.

Discussion

The only significant risk with an indwelling catheter in the ventricle is infectious complication. The alarming increase of suspected and definite infections during the period 1966–68, as shown in Figure 1, necessitated revision of the technique and there was some doubt as to the advisability of continuous recording of the VFP as a routine aid in clinical work. The technique was modified in several ways, such as substitution of the sterilization fluid, exclusive use of autoclavable catheters and tubing, ensurance of a strictly closed fluid system, and intensification of the supervision of asepsis and sterility. The ensuing improvement may be a result of these modifications but other factors such as the "bacteriological environment" of the hospital or department may also be responsible. In any case, no conclusion is possible regarding the cause of the accumulation of infections in 1966–68.

The favorable trend during the last three years (Figs. 1 and 2) shows that the risk of infection can be satisfactorily controlled, and, thus, we consider the present technique sufficiently safe to permit routine use in cases in which control of the intracranial pressure is important.

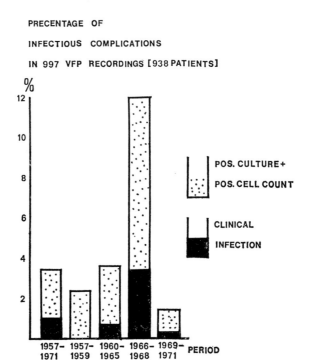

Fig. 2. Frequency of positive cultures/pathological cell-counts and clinical infections in percent of total number of recordings during 1956–1971 (997 recordings in 938 patients). A total of 11 patients (1.1%) had clinical signs of meningitis. There were no deaths or sequelae ascribable to infectious complications

Summary

During the period 1956–71, 997 continuous recordings of the VFP were carried out in a total of 938 patients. Ventricular fluid was sampled for cell-counts and bacterial cultures at regular intervals. No antibiotics were given prophylactically. One case of intracerebral hematoma, eleven cases with definite (1.1%) and 35 with suspected CSF-infections (3.5%) were recorded. The majority of infections occurred during one 3-year period (1966–68). During 1969 to 1971 there was only one definite infection in 283 cases (0.4%). There was no mortality. Air studies and operations increased the risk of infection; prolonged recording or drainage of CSF did not.

Key Words: Ventricular fluid pressure, complications, infections.

References

1. Lundberg, N.: Continuous recording and control of ventricular fluid pressure in neurosurgical practice. Acta psych. scand. (Suppl. 149) 1–193 (1960).

The Uses of Intracranial Pressure Monitoring in Clinical Management

B. Jennett and I. H. Johnston

Enthusiasm for a new method of clinical measurement must be tempered with a critical evaluation of its usefulness and hazards. However, such an evaluation cannot be undertaken until considerable experience has been gained with the method. Hitherto most reports of continuous intracranial pressure (ICP) measurements in various clinical circumstances have been concerned with demonstrating technical feasibility, and with describing phenomena observed in different clinical conditions [1, 2, 3, 4, 5, 6]. The single most important observation to emerge from these reports is that pressure increases are frequently episodic, so that isolated measurements (e. g. during ventricular tapping or at lumbar puncture) may be misleading. The clinical state of the patient has also been shown to be an unreliable guide to ICP changes.

Considering the importance ascribed to raised ICP, as a potentially harmful component of a wide range of clinical conditions, it might seem obvious that a reliable and safe method of measuring ICP would be widely adopted – yet no attempt has so far been made to define the range of clinical application in actual practice. This paper describes the uses which have been made of continuous monitoring in one clinic, using one established method (LUNDBERG's ventricular catheter). It is not concerned with technical details or difficulties of the method, nor with pathophysiological explanations, nor with hypotheses; short term monitoring during anaesthesia and surgery, or during cerebral blood flow measurements, are not discussed.

In the last 4 years some 200 patients have been monitored continuously at the bedside. Most cases have been measured for 48–96 h, although technical difficulties or suspicion of infection have sometimes led to premature discontinuation; only one patient developed serious ventriculitis and he recovered. Initially the method was applied to 2 main groups of patients. All severe head injuries had monitoring set up as soon after admission as possible (usually within 24 h of injury), whether or not there was clinical suspicion of raised pressure or deterioration; and patients who had undergone open surgery for ruptured aneurysm had an intraventricular catheter placed before leaving the operating theatre. Later a variety of patients with other conditions were monitored.

Information about the ICP may affect management decisions in three different circumstances:

1. In diagnosis, either of the nature of the disease process as a whole or of changes in that state.

2. In treatment, by indicating when measures to reduce ICP should be applied, and also by monitoring the efficacy of such treatment.

3. In prognosis.

Diagnosis

The recognition that ICP is not unduly high, in clinical circumstances suggestive of raised pressure, has been the most useful single application. Amongst 72 monitored patients who had recently sustained a severe head injury there were many with severe brain stem dysfunction which might equally well be ascribed to primary injury or to secondary compression – and in the first 24 h after injury it can be difficult to be certain whether this clinical state has been present from the onset or has developed secondarily. In such circumstances the finding of normal (or only moderately raised) pressure is helpful because it may obviate the need for further neuroradiological investigations, for exploratory burr holes or for the administration of chemical agents to reduce ICP which is presumed to be high. In this series there were also 5 patients who showed definite clinical deterioration which would normally have led to active measures being taken; but ICP recordings showed that there had been no rise in pressure. There were also 2 patients in whom angiography showed considerable temporal lobe swelling, with shift of midline structures, but in whom the pressure proved normal; whether or not such patients require surgical intervention might depend on where on the pressure/volume curve they proved to be, as described in another paper from the Glasgow team [7].

After intracranial surgery anxiety about possible development of intracranial hematoma may be allayed by ICP monitoring; clinical deterioration is likely to result in the patient's being taken back to theatre as the safest way of excluding this complication; in 2 of 7 deteriorating patients after aneurysm surgery monitoring showed the pressure to be normal and an unneccessary second operation was avoided.

In patients with papilloedema and no localising signs, benign intracranial hypertension (pseudo-tumor) may be suspected. ICP monitoring may indicate that the pressure is not raised; this proved to be the case in 5 out of 24 such patients; the final diagnosis was pseudo-papilloedema, confirmed in 4 cases by fluorescein angiography.

The Discovery of Raised Intracranial Pressure Which is Not Suspected Clinically

This is clearly restricted to patients undergoing routine ICP monitoring – in our clinic for severe head injuries and post-operative aneurysm cases. Only occasionally did steadily increasing ICP indicate the development of a mass lesion which had not been suspected clinically. However, with controlled ventilation increasingly advocated for head injuries associated with major chest injuries, and also for those thought likely to benefit from hyperventilation, it is of considerable value to be able to monitor the pressure in such circumstances: because when the patient is paralysed for the respirator the neurosurgeon is deprived of almost all the usual clinical signs on which he relies to detect an intracranial hematoma, or other complications.

Treatment

Pressure monitoring may be of use in indicating when ICP has reached a level which demands treatment in its own right, as distinct from the underlying lesion. It is, however, difficult to indicate a particular level which demands treatment because there seem to be two different groups of patients with high pressure – those with *diffuse lesions*, who have a high baseline pressure on which waves of higher pressure may be superimposed; and those with *focal lesions*, whose baseline is not unduly high but on which there are prolonged plateau waves which reach serious levels. But what is a serious level? This meeting has indicated that no one level can be defined as dangerous – it depends (inter alia) on what is causing the pressure, where the patient is on the pressure-volume curve, and what is the auto-regulatory state.

It is of value to be able to check on the efficacy of treatment for ICP because clinical improvement is a poor guide. Lack of improvement may indicate either that the pressure has not been effectively lowered, or that there has already been irreversible damage. The ineffectiveness of repeated intravenous mannitol has been described elsewhere in this symposium by our team [8]. In other cases not even the first dose may be effective whereas alternative methods may be very effective, e. g. aspiration of small amounts of ventricular CSF through the recording catheter. Monitoring has also indicated that the beneficial effect of steroids bears little relation to the effect of these drugs on ICP.

Prognosis

LUNDBERG and TROUPP [3] and more recently VAPALAHTI and TROUPP [6] have emphasised the close relation between the level of ventricular fluid pressure after injury and mortality. Our own studies confirm that high pressure has serious significance but they do not support the corollary – that normal pressure is usually favourable. Indeed we would regard the discovery of normal pressure in a patient with bilateral extensor rigidity soon after injury, together with other signs of brain stem dysfunction, as indicating severe primary white matter damage of the kind which, although it may be survived for a time, is likely to give rise to a persistent vegetative state [9]. The ability to predict such an outcome soon after injury is of considerable importance in allocating resources to patients with a more favourable outlook [10].

Many inconsistencies remain unexplained, and the results obtained in any case must therefore be interpreted by someone familiar with this difficult area of dynamic pathophysiology – and it would be premature to consider ICP monitoring as an essential tool in every neurosurgical unit. However, today's research is tomorrow's routine – and by the time we next meet I should be surprised if we had still to argue for the value of this as a useful addition to the investigative armamentarium of the neurosurgeon.

Key Words : Intracranial pressure, patient monitoring, diagnosis, treatment, prognosis.

References

1. Guillaume, J., Janny, P.: Manometrie intra-cranienne. Intérêt physiopathologique et clinique de la methode. Presse méd. **59**, 953–955 (1951).
2. Lundberg, N.: Continuous recording and control of ventricular fluid pressure in neurosurgical practice. Acta psychiat. scand. (Suppl. 149) **36** (1960).
3. Lundberg, N., Troupp, H., Lorin, H.: Continuous recording of the ventricular-fluid pressure in patients with severe acute traumatic brain injury J. Neurosurg. **22**, 581–590 (1965).
4. Johnston, I. H., Johnston, J. A., Jennett, B.: Intracranial-pressure changes following head injury. Lancet **II**, 433–436 (1970).
5. Richardson, A., Hide, T. A. H., Eversden, I. D.: Long term continuous intracranial pressure monitoring by means of a modified subdural pressure transducer. Lancet **II**, 687–690 (1970).
6. Vapalahti, M., Troupp, H.: Prognosis for patients with severe brain injuries. Brit. med. J. **3**, 404–407 (1971).
7. Miller, J. D., Garibi, J.: Intracranial volume/pressure relationships during continuous monitoring of ventricular fluid pressure. In: Brock, M., Dietz, H. (Eds.): Intracranial Pressure. Experimental and Clinical Aspects. pp. 270–274. Berlin-Heidelberg-New York: Springer 1972.
8. Johnston, I. H., Paterson, A., Harper, A. M., Jennett, B.: Effect of mannitol in intracranial pressure and cerebral blood flow; Clinical and experimental observations. In: Brock, M., Dietz, H. (Eds.): Intracranial Pressure. Experimental and Clinical Aspects. pp. 176–180. Berlin-Heidelberg-New York: Springer 1972.
9. Jennett, B., Plum, F.: Persistent vegetative state after brain damage. A syndrome in search of a name. Lancet **I**, 734–737 (1972).
10. Jennett, B.: Prognosis after severe head injury. In: Clinical Neurosurgery, **19**, p. 331. Baltimore: Williams and Wilkins 1972 (in press).

Comments to Session 10

B. Jennett and N. Zwetnow

Introducing this session, the Chairman expressed gratification that such a high percentage of participants had remained for this, the last session. Its variety precluded any introductory or summarizing remarks, and comment is restricted to reporting discussion.

Concerning the paper by West et al., Langfitt asked whether there might not be increased production of acid monoamine metabolites as well as reduced absorption, but West thought not.

Brocklehurst sought to question William's assumption that herniation through the foramen magnum was necessarily the cause of the associated spinal syrinx. Symon asked for an explanation of why the syringomyeliac cavity does not usually extend above C_2 whereas the tonsils seldom come this low. Brock questioned the assumption that there was a valve; all that had been shown was that there were different pressures in different compartments during coughing, which might be ascribed to variations in mechanical properties in different sites. In reply, Williams agreed that different interpretations might be placed on the various observations he had reported. There was no doubt about the pressure differences being real, and it seemed reasonable to assume a valve.

A number of discussants questioned the validity and significance of local measurements made by Rivano et al. in retracted brain, in an 'open-head' situation, but Langfitt confirmed that autoregulation of surface vessels on the cortex could readily be impaired in animal experiments (e. g. by a gentle jet of nitrogen gas).

Commenting on the paper by Sundbärg et al., Troupp reported 9 cases of meningitis in 323 VFP recordings, but 5 had other surgical interventions also. Beks asked if there had been any deaths ascribed to monitoring, and the reply was that no deaths and no sequelae had occurred. Beks then asked what action was taken when infection did develop. Lundberg replied it had been usual to discontinue monitoring immediately, but that now the ventricular cannula might be kept in a route for the administration of antibiotics. Price suggested that it might be appropriate to use a prophylactic (topical) antibiotic in the fluid column in the catheter. Nornes showed a new transducer in which the part coming into contact with the patient's CSF was disposable.

As a comment to the paper by Jennett and Johnston, Langfitt added that this group had noted that changes in ICP (e. g. after mannitol) did not produce consistent changes in CBF, and this might go some way to explaining the failure of the ICP level to correlate with clinical state on occasions. Hekmatpanah protested that with the window technique very consistent correlations were observed between the micro-circulation and the ICP. Van Crevel asked whether the paper was really meant to suggest that clinical physical signs were entirely superseded by monitoring systems as indicators of ICP. Jennett replied that whilst certain traditional signs had indeed been shown to be unreliable, one result of continuous monitoring had been to refocus attention on cardio-respiratory changes associated with variations in ICP, about which there had been a number of papers – notably those of Heck and Tindall. It seemed likely that as understanding of these relationships improved there would be more to be gained from clinical observations, which would be more firmly based than previously.

Concluding Remarks

Pathophysiology of Increased ICP

T. W. LANGFITT

1. Mechanics of Increased ICP and Volume-Pressure Relationships

The intracranial space is bounded by thick bone that is essentially non-distensible, and it is filled to capacity with essentially non-compressible contents. These can be divided into three fluid compartments, brain tissue water, intravascular blood, and CSF. The intracranial space is vented from the supratentorial compartment to the posterior fossa through the tentorial incisura and through the foramen magnum to the spinal canal. In addition, intravascular blood and CSF can be expressed into the extracranial vascular system. Thus, the intracranial space contains displaceable fluid in the form of CSF and blood. CSF volume is approximately 10% of the intracranial volume; values for intracranial blood volume have varied from 2–11%.

As a mass (or the brain) expands, fluid is expressed from the intracranial space in order to accommodate the mass, and as long as the volume displaced equals the volume added ICP does not change. If the mass continues to expand, however, ICP begins to rise, because the volume of displaceable fluid is finite. Furthermore, each additional and equal increment in the volume of the mass produces a larger increase in ICP such that when nearly all displaceable fluid has been eliminated a slight further increase in volume produces a very large rise in ICP. By the same token when ICP is greatly elevated a slight reduction in the volume of any one of the intracranial compartments produces a marked fall in ICP. The shape of the volume-pressure graph also depends on the rate of expansion of the mass. A rapid addition of a small volume (e.g. epidural hematoma) causes a larger rise in ICP and brain dysfunction than a much larger mass that expands slowly (e.g. chronic subdural hematoma). On the vertical portion of the volume-pressure graph a relatively slight increase in intravascular blood volume produces a marked rise in ICP. This is the reason why ICP is so sensitive to hypoxia and hypercarbia when a mass lesion or brain swelling is present.

2. Pressure Waves

Pressure waves are fluctuations in ICP that may be spontaneous in origin or due to changes in system blood gases. In discussions that took place during the symposium, it was agreed that the original terminology for pressure waves introduced by Lundberg should be retained except that the term plateau wave should be substituted entirely for the term A wave. Plateau waves are recurring increases in ICP to values of 50–100 mmHg lasting 5–20 min and generally arise from an elevated base of ICP. B waves occur more frequently ($^1/_2$–2/min) and are of less amplitude and of little clinical significance. During a series of plateau waves both amplitude and duration may increase, and a "terminal" wave may follow in which ICP rises to the level of SAP and CBF ceases. There is good evidence that the plateau waves are due to changes in cerebral blood volume. Thus, one can visualize a series of plateau waves followed by a fatal wave as follows: The resistance vessels of the brain alternately constrict and dilate producing a rhythmic change in cerebral blood volume and ICP. As the plateau waves become larger, cerebral ischemia occurs at the peaks producing some damage to the resting vasoconstrictor tone of the resistance vessels. Finally, the resistance vessels fail to constrict at the peak of a plateau wave, and cerebral blood volume and ICP remain elevated. The persistent dilatation of the resistance vessels is termed vasomotor paralysis (or paresis). If the tone of the resistance vessels (the origin of which is unknown) is not permanently damaged, if the vessels are still responsive to changes in CO_2, hyperventilation (or agents such as mannitol) may reduce ICP and save the patient. If the ischemia persists for any length of time, however, blood pressure and ICP become equal and inseparable, and CBF ceases permanently.

3. Transmission of Increased ICP

The term ICP is meaningful only if pressure is freely transmitted throughout the intracranial space. Otherwise, it is necessary to speak of "intracranial pressures", and the problem becomes enormous in attempting to correlate ICP with CBF and brain function. During expansion of an intracranial mass obstruction may occur at the tentorial incisura or foramen magnum preventing communication of pressure among compartments. Obstruction appears to be the rule with very large masses. Contrariwise, as long as there is a fluid connection among compartments ICP appears to be equally and nearly instantaneously transmitted throughout the compartments, obeying Pascal's law. The major issue that has not been resolved is transmission of pressure or force within the brain substance. The brain is a visco-elastic substance, but this says little because of the marked heterogeneity of brain architecture. The blood vessels appear to provide the major elastic component, and it is the elastic component that would be responsible for failure of transmission of force from one part of the system to another, if this is found to be the case. There is evidence from intracerebral and bilateral extradural pressure measurements in experimental animals that a pressure gradient does develop across the brain when a mass expands rapidly, but this gradient may be dissipated by movement (plastic creep) of the brain. Observation of cortical and pial vessels through a transparent water tight calvarium during expansion of an extracerebral balloon also suggests pressure or force gradients in that vessels adjacent to the balloon are collapsed at a time more remote cortical vessels are normal. Further resolution of the problem has been hampered by lack of the instrumentation to accurately measure forces within the brain substance.

4. ICP and CBF

Blood flow through the brain is a function of the inflow and outflow pressures, the diameter of the cerebrovascular bed, and blood viscosity. Normally the perfusion pressure across the brain is considered to be the internal carotid artery pressure minus jugular vein pressure. As ICP rises, however, cerebral venous pressure increases, and there is good evidence that the two pressures are nearly identical at all levels of increased ICP until the veins collapse. Thus, ICP is often considered to be the outflow pressure when it is elevated. At its simplest:

$$CBF = \frac{\text{mean SAP} - \text{mean ICP}}{CVR}$$

when ICP is elevated. The reduction in CBF that occurs when ICP is elevated is due to a reduction in perfusion pressure, according to this concept, and CBF ceases when ICP and SAP are equal. An alternative approach is to use the equation:

$$CBF = \frac{SAP - JVP}{CVR}$$

in which circumstance the outflow pressure changes little, because it is known that jugular vein pressure does not change very much with variations in ICP. Here the emphasis is on CVR, and when ICP equals SAP, CBF ceases not because of abolition of perfusion pressure, which in fact changes very little, but because of vascular compression and collapse resulting in an infinite increase in resistance. There is recent evidence that the entire intracranial vascular bed including the large arteries collapses when ICP equals SAP.

CBF autoregulates to increased ICP in much the same fashion as it autoregulates to decreased SAP. Thus, when autoregulation is intact and ICP is diffusely elevated CBF does not fall until CPP is in the 40–50 mmHg range. When autoregulation is defective CBF follows CPP passively whether the latter is reduced by elevating ICP or decreasing SAP.

In unconscious patients there is not a predictible relationship between ICP and CBF whether autoregulation is intact or defective except at extremely high levels of ICP. Part of the reason is the cause of the increased ICP. Cerebrovascular dilatation increasing cerebral blood volume will increase ICP, and under this circumstance both CBF and ICP are elevated. In contrast, there is evidence that edema may compress the cerebral microcirculation reducing

CBF at a time when ICP is minimally elevated. Thus, the cause of increased ICP appears to be as important or more important than the height of ICP in determining its relationship to CBF.

5. Systemic Responses

Brain compression and increased ICP can cause arterial hypertension, bradycardia, and respiratory irregularities, the well known Cushing triad. There is evidence that compression or interference otherwise with a small region in the medulla is critical for the production of arterial hypertension. However, it is clear that compression of the isolated spinal cord also produces an arterial pressor response. If intracranial hypertension is diffuse, if there are no pressure gradients along the craniospinal axis, the pressor response does not occur until ICP equals or exceeds the diastolic blood pressure. In contrast, a mass lesion that causes compression or distortion of the brain stem may produce a pressor response at relatively low levels of ICP. The increase in blood pressure is due to peripheral vasoconstriction from increased sympathetic activity and to increased cardiac output.

The pulmonary complications of increased ICP are difficult to separate from those caused by a brain injury per se. The most common pulmonary complication in unconscious patients with increased ICP is alveolar obstruction. This results in ventilation/perfusion abnormalities wherein non-ventilated portions of the lung continue to be perfused by venous blood. Venous admixture occurs in the pulmonary veins and left heart causing systemic hypoxemia. Increased ICP and brain compression can also cause acute pulmonary edema both clinically and in experimental animals. The mechanism is not well understood but could be due to pulmonary vein constriction or left heart failure. Acute pulmonary edema appears to be uncommon. Finally, venous admixture and systemic hypoxemia might be produced by neurogenically mediated opening up of pulmonary A–V shunts that bypass the alveoli.

Techniques for Measuring Intracranial Pressure

B. Jennett

It is difficult to dissociate methodology entirely from theoretical concepts or from clinical constraints. Because of the avalanche of data about intracranial pressure (ICP) in recent years, both from the bedside and the laboratory bench, basic ideas about ICP are now changing rapidly – in particular the degree to which pressure is transmitted between different parts of the intracranial cavity and across the dura. As a result there is uncertainty about what it would be desirable to measure, even if it were possible, whilst at the same time technical developments are frequently altering what is possible. This chapter should therefore be read in conjunction with the discussion and summary of Session 1 (p. 37) and Session 2 (p. 70) on methodology.

Although there have been attempts to record changes in ICP by non-invasive methods, such as echo-encephalography and impedance plethysmography, all techniques which give useful measurements involve the implanting of a device within the cranial cavity. Where the methods chiefly differ is how much of the detecting system is implanted and whereabouts in the intracranial cavity the sensor is placed.

Detecting System

This consists of a sensor and a transducer. The sensor may consist of a fluid column in a cannula, a moveable diaphragm or balloon, or a solid state probe. The problem with the first is maintaining a free communication, as there is always the chance of partial or complete blockage by debris by collapse of the surface being recorded from, with either damping (and altered frequency response) or loss of the pressure recording. The problem with diaphragms is their stability once implanted in tissues, and also the possibility of anomalous recording due to sensitivity to forces applied in certain directions rather than to uniformly distributed pressure. The problems with solid state probes are at the technical level, and if these can be solved this might prove to be the ideal sensor.

For practical purposes it seems reasonable to regard all present methods as fluid conducting systems – even the wick method, claiming to measure tissue pressure, is in fact recording from the small fluid cavity around the end. It is not clear how important it is in practical terms to take account of the fact that the brain is not an incompressible fluid, but a visco-elastic substance; certainly under many circumstances it is forces rather than pressures that are being measured, but the area of reference is always unknown – and it is therefore difficult to apply this concept practically: moreover certain devices (e.g. extradural sensors, even if coplanar) record differently under the changing circumstances of rising pressure, eventually measuring stress force rather than fluid (i.e. central cavity/ventricle) pressure; moreover the time at which this change occurs cannot be determined. A problem with fluid filled systems is partial blockage, with its unknown effect on the frequency response of the system.

The transducer may be implanted with the sensor, and the problems then are those of the feasibility of recalibration in situ to correct for drift. Without the capacity for zeroing, such devices can record only changes in pressure, not absolute pressure. It seems to be generally agreed that unless absolute pressures could be measured there is little benefit to be derived from monitoring at all. Drift derives partly from the effect of body fluids on the device, but rendering it impermeable by coating in latex reduces sensitivity. Most transducers so far manufactured show an unexplainable and unforeseeable tendency to work less well in vivo than in vitro – of a batch of similarly produced devices, all working equally well on the bench, only some prove reliable on implantation. It seems likely that there is a commercial problem impasse here in terms of technical development, in that many small laboratories or firms are trying to perfect similar but not identical devices – yet there appears to be insufficient financial incentive for a large and well-equipped organisation to bend its mind and its money to the problem, which clearly must be soluble.

There is no shortage of reliable and relatively inexpensive transducers available for use at the side of the bed rather than in the head, and the problem is the connections between the detector and recorder ends of the system. Telemetry has been successfully used, but the implanted device must then include a power source which increases its size. Wires carry no risk of blockage and very little of infection and, apart from certain experimental situations, there seems no particular advantage in a telemetric system.

The size and nature of the implanted device has practical implications which are crucial to the general acceptability of any method. It is one thing to devise a technique which works well when used by its inventor in his own clinic on his own patients, quite another to establish ICP monitoring as an investigation which is as available and feasible, as say, angiography. Before that happens, not only must the electronics be reliable and relatively cheap, and the risks reduced to acceptable limits, but the procedures involved in placing and removing the implanted device be simple. A catheter or a solid state probe can be placed through a twist drill hole after a tenotome stab, which does not even require an operating theatre; such a method would clearly be widely applicable. On the other hand if not only a burr-hole but special self-threading screws are needed for placement, and a further visit to the operating theatre to remove the device, then there will be fewer patients (and indeed fewer clinics) in which the method will be used.

Data Processing and Display

No one now requires to be convinced of the importance of continuous recording over many hours (and often days). Only in this way will intermittent events, such as pressure waves, be detected; and also progressive changes, such as might indicate complications such as hematomas or brain edema. Great lengths of paper recording, the majority of which may be featureless and of little interest, present a problem not only in practical terms but in how best to analyse and describe the findings.

Two different kinds of solution are possible. One is to record pressure on magnetic tape, and to arrange for this to be erased after certain quanta of elapsed time provided that certain predetermined limits of 'normality' or of 'change' have not been exceeded. This could be elaborated further both to produce a paper record and to set off an alarm whenever these limits were passed. This deals only with the practical problem of clinical detection of abnormality – it does nothing about the analysis of data, which, indeed, it largely destroys as being insignificant.

Mathematical data analysis depends on serial sampling of the recording, and using a computer to construct histograms of average pressures over set periods, and also to record the degree of variation. This kind of system could also be used to activate an alarm system such as is used in coronary care units.

Unfortunately each of these methods is apt to be more elaborate and expensive than the system used to measure pressure – and if more than one patient is being monitored at one time this problem is magnified. In this context there is some merit in the simplest system of all – very slow chart recorders (which may even operate intermittently, for so many seconds in each minute.)

Site of Sensor

Various investigators reported differences between intradural and extradural pressures, simultaneously recorded both in animals and in man; and some had observed differences between extradural pressures on the two sides of the head during the development of a unilateral expanding lesion, and between different compartments of the intradural space. There seemed to be agreement that there was always a difference between extradural and intradural pressures (the extradural being higher), but that if the device was not coplanar then there was a positive intercept and the pressures could not be compared. But even with a strictly coplanar device there are unexplained deviations at higher pressures, presumably as contact increases and it becomes a stress/force rather than a fluid-filled system. It is clearly of importance to calibrate any system over an adequate range of possible pressures.

In regard to pressure differences between separate compartments of the intracranial cavity (loosely termed "gradients" by many authors), it seems important to distinguish between relatively steady-state conditions and rapidly changing situations – such as immediately after an injection of fluid, or even during a slow infusion. Clearly transient pressure differences must have existed to allow the development of the various internal brain shifts and herniae which are the pathological hall-marks of increased ICP. That brain tissue pressure is higher than the pressure in CSF pathways (ventricle or subarachnoid space) is obvious from the way in which brain immediately escapes when the pia or ependyma is breached at operation. It is difficult to know which of the intracranial pressures is the most relevant, but it should not be assumed that central cavity pressure is necessarily the most valid because it happens to be the most readily recorded.

It is clear that there is no one method which is ideal in all circumstances – nor in the nature of the parameter being measured is there ever likely to be. Even in the animal laboratory, where ethical considerations and risk factors do not obtain, the method chosen will depend on the experiment. In the clinic much will depend on the demands of the particular situation; for example, initial screening for high pressure might be carried out by some simple method and more elaborate and accurate techniques used only if raised pressure is demonstrated. Again, what is suitable for a few hours of measuring may not be appropriate for monitoring over several days.

Rather than competing for the 'best' method, it would be more helpful if all investigators recorded faithfully their various methods, their calibration technique and the specifications of their instrumentation; and if every opportunity was taken to run simultaneous recordings by different methods, or in different sites, in order to broaden our understanding of this complex field.

Clinical Indications for Measurement of ICP

N. LUNDBERG

To be of use, quantitative assessments of ICP must be founded on continuous and intracranial measurements. This means opening the cranial cavity, a surgical procedure which will always be accompanied by a certain risk of complications. It is a truism to state that indications for intracranial measurements must always take into account that this risk must be gauged in proportion to the benefit for the patient.

Intraventricular Measurement

In the Neurosurgical Department in Lund we have practised continuous recording of ICP with an indwelling ventricular catheter in 976 patients over the last 15 years. A survey of the complications has been presented to this symposium [4]. As expected, the main risk was infection of the CSF spaces and this risk has been a constant challenge. It was concluded that the present technique has been shown to be sufficiently safe to permit extensive use in patients in whom knowledge of the VFP can be expected to be of considerable importance for diagnosis and treatment.

The indications are of course influenced by the fact that the method facilitates drainage of fluid under pressure control. In acute pressure situations the combination of immediate diagnosis and immediate treatment may be lifesaving and in many patients continuous drainage of ventricular fluid under pressure control has shown to be a valuable aid for prolonged treatment of intracranial hypertension. In addition, the indwelling catheter facilitates ventriculography, sampling of CSF and intraventricular administration of drugs.

Recording of the VFP by an indwelling catheter may be more or less useful in different kinds of patients and in different situations. The following description of our routine may give an idea of our indications: In cases selected for monitoring of ICP, recording is started one or two days before a planned operation. Urgency sometimes makes immediate drainage of fluid necessary; otherwise, to obtain *information on the intracranial dynamics*, the pressure is recorded for at least two hours before the recording is disturbed by e. g. pneumography. In some patients, it may be necessary to maintain the pressure at a low level, usually between 10–20 mmHg, for some days before operation in order to relieve the brain stem or optic nerves from stress.

Pneumography is performed under pressure control. In most cases the procedure is started by lumbar insufflation of gas. If filling of the ventricles is insufficient, gas is insufflated and fluid withdrawn through the ventricular catheter. The risk of deterioration after pneumography due to acute elevations of the ICP is conventionally an argument for immediate operation after pneumography. This routine may be discarded if the VFP is continuously controlled after the examination. Unless operation is urgent for other reasons it will usually be delayed for one or two days after pneumography.

Recording of the VFP during *operation under general anesthesia* has proved very valuable. Among other things it has taught us and our anesthesiologist that induction of, and subsequent disturbances during general anesthesia may provoke dangerous acute elevations of the VFP in patients with intracranial hypertension. (Drainage of fluid or administration of hypertonic solutions should be started before the induction of anesthesia in these patients). Recording of the VFP also helps to detect disturbances of the ventilation, inappropriate positioning of the patient and other things that might jeopardize optimal operative conditions. Furthermore, during the operation the indwelling ventricular catheter facilitates adequate drainage of fluid without additional injury to the brain.

After the operation it is our policy to record the VFP without drainage for the *early detection of a hematoma*, the failure of a shunt or any other cause of postoperative intracranial hypertension. Apart from urgent situations, fluid should not be drained unless the surgeon has decided either to reopen the wound or to resort to non-surgical treatment. Usually the ventricular catheter is removed 3–5 days after the operation.

In patients with *acute brain insults* such as e.g. traumatic brain injury, subarachnoid hemorrhage, stroke, encephalitis, recording of the VFP may serve as a guide to treatment and prognosis; measures against intracranial hypertension such as drainage of fluid, controlled hyperventilation, hypertonic solutions, hypothermia, corticosteroids or surgical decompression become more rational if the indications are based on, and the results controlled by, monitoring of the ICP. Even in such cases drainage of ventricular fluid under pressure control is often the most reliable method of controlling intracranial hypertension.

In patients with e.g. *papilledema of unknown origin* or "*low pressure hydrocephalus*" it may be important to decide whether ICP is normal or increased. In such cases continuous recording of VFP under standardized conditions (position of patient, environment, time, zero level etc.) is the best means of getting reliable information. The monitoring should preferably be done over a 24-hour period; it should at least include the nocturnal variations.

In cases of *hydrocephalus*, recording of the VFP may be used for preoperative assessment and to check the effect of a shunt operation. However, we do not use it in hydrocephalic infants before or after ventriculo-atrial shunting because of the risk of bacterial colonization in the shunt.

Extraventricular Measurements

In recent years a number of methods for recording ICP without ventricular puncture (extradural, subdural, intracerebral) have been introduced into clinical work. Easy application and lower risk of complications have been reasons for preferring such methods to VFP recordings. Reports from several investigators suggest that extraventricular measurements can be used for prolonged monitoring and give valuable information on the ICP. However, available data do not yet permit the different techniques to be evaluated and compared with regard to qualities of basic importance. Provided that reasonable requirements for such qualities [1, 3] are fulfilled, extraventricular recordings should be preferred if overriding reasons for access to the ventricular fluid space are not at hand. Also, extraventricular techniques should be used if ventricular puncture and/or maintenance of free communication is difficult or impossible.

With regard to different facilities and different policies in the neurosurgical departments and the swift technical development, it would not be meaningful to establish in detail indications for monitoring the ICP. As a general guide it may suffice to repeat that this aid should be used when and only when the information provided can be expected to be of potential importance for the treatment of the individual patient. I should also like to refer the reader to the article by JENNETT and JOHNSTON [2] in this volume.

References

1. JENNET, B.: Techniques for measuring intracranial pressure. In: BROCK, M., DIETZ, H., (Eds.): Intracranial Pressure. Experimental and Clinical Aspects, p. 365–368. Berlin-Heidelberg-New York: Springer 1972.
2. JENNETT, B., JOHNSTON, I. H.: The uses of intracranial pressure monitoring in clinical management. In: BROCK, M., DIETZ, H., (Eds.): Intracranial Pressure. Experimental and Clinical Aspects, p. 353–356. Berlin-Heidelberg-New York: Springer 1972.
3. LUNDBERG, N.: Continuous recording and control of ventricular fluid pressure in neurosurgical practice. Acta psychiat. scand. (Suppl. 149) 36 (1960).
4. SUNDBÄRG, G., KJÄLLQUIST, Å., LUNDBERG, N., PONTÉN, U.: Complications due to prolonged ventricular fluid pressure recording in clinical practive In: BROCK, M., DIETZ, H., (Eds.): Intracranial Pressure. Experimental and Clinical Aspects, p. 348–352. Berlin-Heidelberg-New York: Springer 1972.

Glossary of Definitions, Standards and Abbreviations

M. BROCK and C. HARTUNG

Autoregulation (of Blood Flow) : Change in steady state resistance across an organ in response to changing perfusion pressure (JOHNSTON, 1964). The efficiency of autoregulation can be measured by the change in blood flow in response to changing perfusion pressure. The effect of autoregulation in the brain is to maintain an appropriate (not constant) blood flow within a certain range of perfusion pressure.

Blood Pressure : Pressure of the blood in a given segment of the circulatory system. Reference should be made to systolic, diastolic or mean, and to the vessel in which pressure is measured. Units are mmHg.

Brain Tissue Pressure : corresponds to the interstitial or extravascular pressure. The real interstitial pressure of the brain can not be measured with the methods available, and the term "brain tissue pressure" defines, in fact, the pressure within a (very small) cavity in the brain parenchyma surrounding the measuring device.

Cerebral Blood Flow : Volume of blood passing through the brain or part of the brain in unit time. For the brain as a whole it can be expressed in ml/min but regional flow (rCBF) is expressed in units of weight of brain tissue in unit time. This assumes brain tissue density as 1, whereas it is actually 1.030 (MUSCHENBROEK).

Cerebrovascular Resistance : Resistance offered by the vascular bed of the brain to the flow of blood through it. In analogy to Ohm's law, CVR is calculated as the ratio of CPP to CBF (CVR = CPP/CBF). This is valid only for total CVR because calculation of regional CVR requires information on regional CBF and regional perfusion pressure, the latter of which is usually not available. Units are (mmHg · sec)/ml.

Compressibility : Property by which a mss of material decreases in volume when subjected to pressure from all sides (hydrostatic pressure). Biological liquids and solids may be considered essentially incompressible.

Compression of the Brain : Compression is a change in mass caused by pressure from all sides. In the brain, unlike the classical model, compression involves loss of mass, as tissue fluid, intravascular blood and CSF are squeezed out of the tissue. This term is loosely used for deformation and indentation such as occurs with focal masses (natural tumors or hematomas, or experimental balloons).

Conductance of a vessel or vascular bed is the reciprocal of *Resistance* to flow. Units are ml/(mmHg · sec).

Constriction : Active reduction in diameter of a hollow body (vessel or cavity). This term is usually employed as the opposite of dilatation. Passive reduction in diameter of a vessel or cavity should be termed (total or partial) closure, occlusion, stenosis or compression.

Cisternal Pressure : usually employed to mean the CSF pressure in the cisterna magna.

Deformation (of the Brain) : Physically, deformation is a change in geometry caused by a force (compression, traction, torsion, shearing etc.). In the brain, deformation is defined as an alteration of the normal anatomical configuration.

Dilatation : This is usually taken to mean the active increase in diameter of vessels, as distinct from their passive distension.

Elasticity : (see also *Viscoelasticity*): Property by which a material resumes its original state once the deforming forces have ceased to act; the mechanical energy expended to cause its deformation is recovered when the deforming forces cease to act.

Elasto-Viscosity – see *Visco-Elasticity.*

Flow (F) : Biologically, flow is used to mean *Volume Flow* (Q) which is the total volume of fluid (V) passing with a given velocity (v) a section (area) (A) of a vessel per unit of time (Q = v · A). Its unit is m³/sec but for biological purposes ml/sec or ml/min are used. (see also *Cerebral Blood Flow*)

Force : is defined as product of mass (m) by acceleration (a) (F = m · a). It has the properties of a vector and is able to accelerate a body and to deform it.

Herniation (of structures of the CNS): Type of deformation in which the increase in contents of one compartment of the cranial cavity displaces part of its original contents into neighbouring compartments. Herniation is associated with distortion of the involved structures.

Hysteresis : Failure of a system to follow identical paths of response upon application of, and withdrawal of, a forcing agent. The result of this failure to retrace the same path on withdrawal as on application is a hysteresis loop. The area within this loop is proportional to the energy mechanically dissipated during application and withdrawal of the forcing agent. A perfectly elastic material has no hysteresis loop.

Intracranial pressure (ICP) : Generic term to designate any pressure measured within the cranial cavity. There are several intracranial pressures. The term "intracranial" should be substituted by the designation of the compartment where pressure is measured. The term "cerebrospinal fluid pressure" (CSFP), usually employed to mean lumbar fluid pressure, is vague, and representative only if CSF pathways communicate freely. All above mentioned pressures should be measured in mmHg. The location of the transducer and its position as compared to the right atrium should be specified.

Laminar Flow : A flow is called laminar when its streaming lines are not disturbed by any mixing motions. It contrasts with *Turbulent Flow*.

Mean Blood Pressure : This is calculated as the diastolic pressure plus one third of the pulse pressure, a calculation which allows for the shape of the pulse wave and is therefore more accurate than the arithmetic mean of systolic and diastolic pressures. The same applies to *Mean Intracranial Pressure*.

Nutrient Blood Flow : Fraction of the total blood flow of an organ which contributes to, or participates in, the metabolism of said organ. Its opposite is shunt blood flow.

Osmotic Pressure : corresponds to the pressure difference across a semipermeable membrane separating two compartments containing solutions of a given substance with different concentrations. Osmotic pressure of plasma at 38° C is 7.39 atm = 5616 mmHg. *Oncotic Pressure*, more properly called *Colloidosmotic Pressure* refers to the osmotic pressure exerted by colloid solutions.

Perfusion Pressure for a tube or system of tubes is the difference between the pressure presented by the perfusing fluid when it enters and that when it leaves said tube or system. When the expression *perfusion pressure* is used for the brain, the sites of pressure measurements should be specified. For further information the reader is referred to the paper by T. W. Langfitt (p. 361).

Plasticity : Property by which a material remains in its deformed state after the deforming forces have ceased to act. In other words, plasticity is a property of a given material by which the mechanical energy expended to cause its deformation fully dissipates.

Pressure : Special case of normal *Stress*, where the force per unit area is normally directed towards this area. Pressure is measured in Torr, mmHg atm etc. Intracranial pressures should be measured in mmHg. (See also *Intracranial Pressure*.)

Pressure Gradient : This term is often erroneously used for what is in fact a defined difference in pressure between two different sites. A gradient is a vector and has the direction of the higher pressure values. Its absolute value is given by the resultant of infinitesimally neighbouring isobars.

Pressure-Volume Relationship : Relation which defines the pressure change within a given system caused by a change of the volume contained in it or vice-versa, e.g. changes in intracranial pressures caused by changes in intracranial contents. In pressure-volume diagrams pressure is conventionally displayed in the y-axis (ordinate) and volume on the x-axis (abscissa).

Pulse Pressure : Amplitude of pressure oscillation during the cardiac cycle.

Regional Cerebral Blood Flow (rCBF) – see *Cerebral Blood Flow*.

Resistance (see *Cerebrovascular Resistance*).

Shunt Blood Flow : Fraction of the total blood flow of an organ which passes its vascular network without contributing to its metabolism.

Stiffness : From the physical standpoint, stiffness is the ratio of increment in force to increment in length. Applied to the brain, it means the amount of resistance offered by the brain to deformation. In the brain it is evaluated by the pressure necessary to cause a given indentation.

Strain : Relative deformation produced by the application of stress. Strains can be subdivided into:

1) dilational strains, the sum of which represents the relative change in volume of a substance, and

2) distortional or shearing strains, which represent the change of shape at a constant volume.

Stress : Force per unit area. Depending on the type of force, whether it acts tangentially or normally to the area, stresses are called normal or tangential (shearing) stresses.

Tissue Perfusion Pressure (TPP): Perfusion pressure within the parenchyma of an organ. Theoretically it corresponds to the difference in blood pressure between the arterial and venous ends of a brain capillary. Cerebral TPP has also been employed to designate the difference between mean *arteriolar* blood pressure and ICP.

Tissue Pressure (see *Brain Tissue Pressure*).

Transmural Pressure : net resultant between the pressures acting on the inside and on the outside of a vessel.

Turbulent Flow : A flow is called turbulent when a more or less irregular mixing motion disturbs the main laminar flow.

Vascular Resistance (see *Cerebrovascular Resistance*).

Vasopressor Response (VPR) *to Raised ICP :* Increase in arterial blood pressure consequent to an increase in "intracranial pressure" (often known as "Cushing response").

Vasopressor Threshold : Term usually employed to designate the "intracranial pressure" level at which a vasopressor response takes place.

Visco-Elasticity, Elasto-Viscosity : Rheological combinations of the properties of elastic solids and viscous fluids. The term "visco-elasticity" is used for materials made up mainly of viscous fluid, whereas "elasto-viscosity" is used for materials the behaviour of which resembles more an elastic solid.

Viscosity : Physical property of a fluid which causes it to resist a shear force. It is due largely to the intermolecular forces within a fluid which cause one layer to adhere to and resist the slipping movement of the layer of molecules next to it.

Subject Index

Running for Fitness

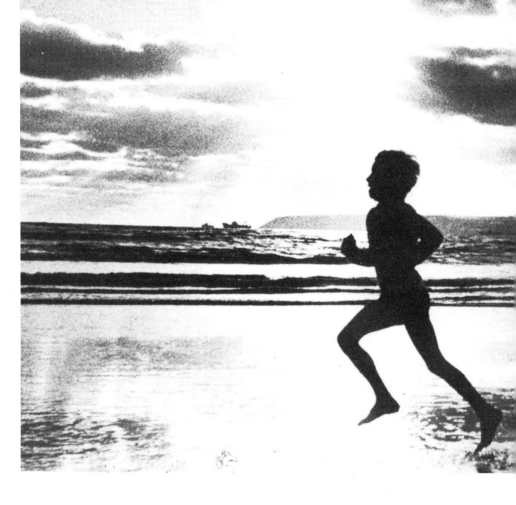
RUNNING FOR

Sebastian and Peter Coe

FITNESS

ROBINSON'S
10
Barley Water

HALLAMSHIRE HARRIERS

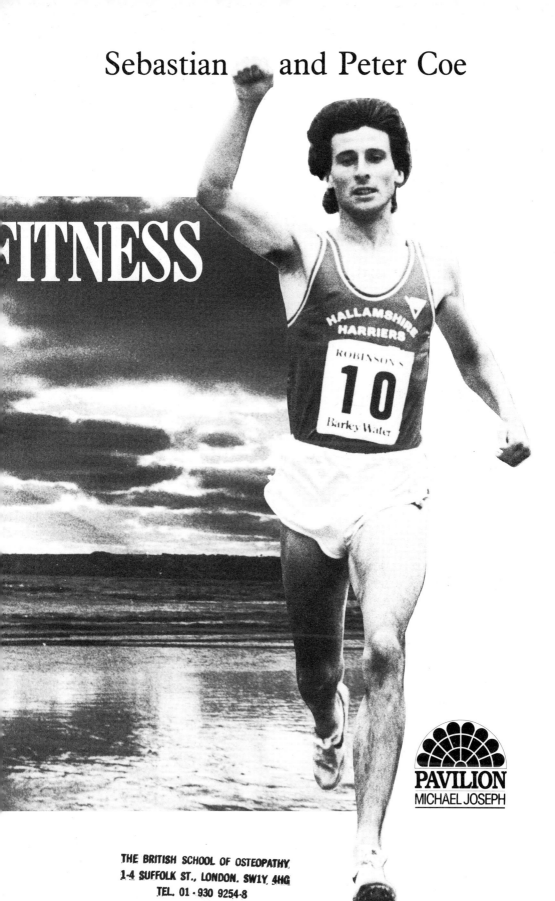

PAVILION
MICHAEL JOSEPH

First published in Great Britain in 1983
By Pavilion Books Limited
196 Shaftesbury Avenue, London WC2H 8JL
in association with Michael Joseph Limited
44 Bedford Square, London WC1B 3DU
September 1983
Second Impression November 1983

Designed by Lawrence Edwards

Editorial Consultant: Nick Mason

Photoset by Rowland Phototypesetting Ltd, Suffolk

Printed and bound in Great Britain by
Butler & Tanner Ltd, Frome

British Library Cataloguing in Publication Data
Coe, Sebastian
   Running for fitness
   1. Running   2. Physical fitness
   I. Title   II. Coe, Peter, 1942–
   613.7′1   GV1061

   ISBN 0-907516-21-1

CON

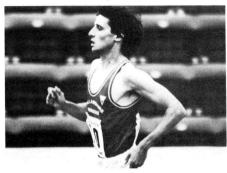
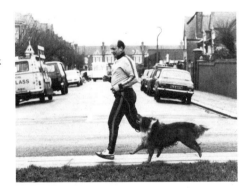
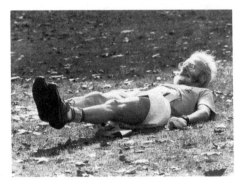

TENTS

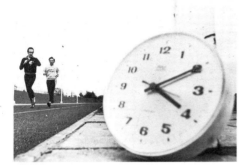

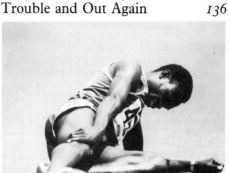

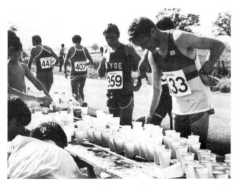

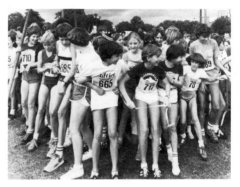

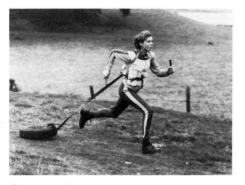

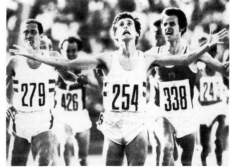

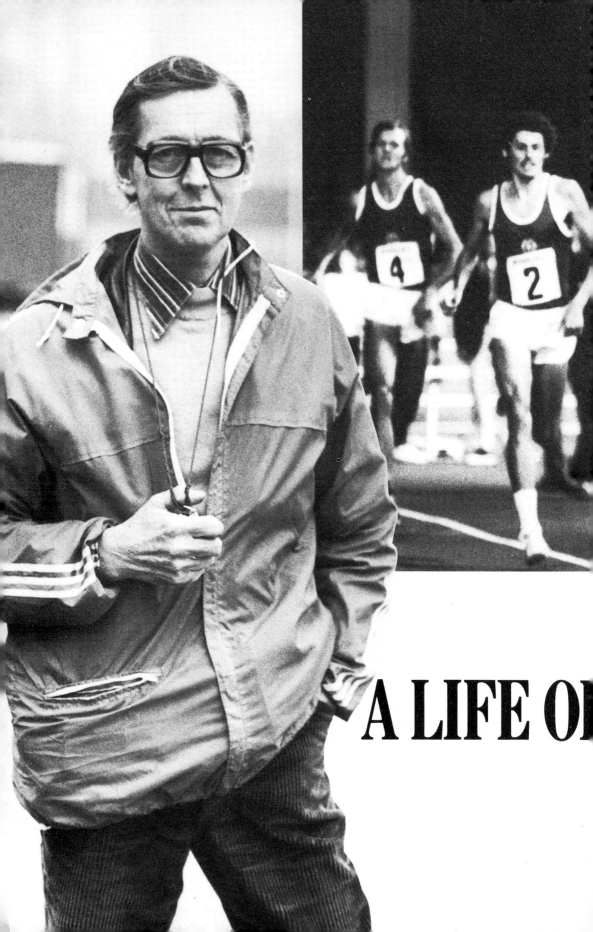

A LIFE OI

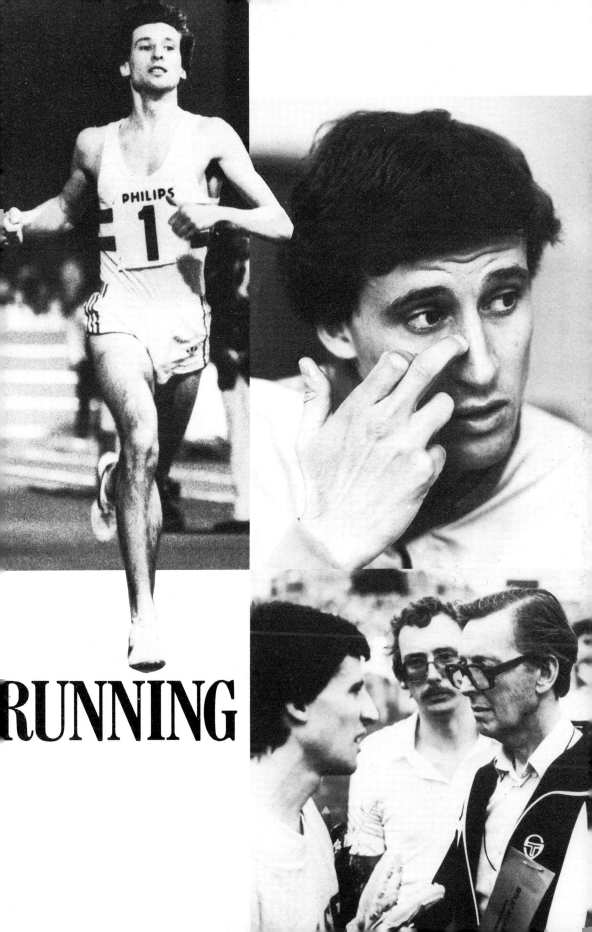

RUNNING

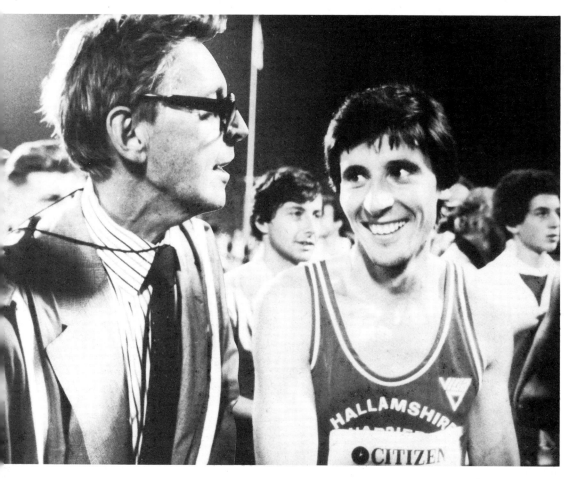

When running has enriched the lives of two people as much as it has ours, and when it has done this in so many ways, the wish to share the pleasure is a very strong one.

We are well aware that while the super-enthusiast is happy in his own world, he is in danger of becoming a bore when he tries to convert others to his own beliefs. Why then should we presume to add to all the other books on running and fitness?

We enjoy the involvement in running at the very highest level. It is not a privilege that can be bought or conferred, it has to be won. It can be achieved only by starting at the bottom and then, with dedication, and resolution and hard work, climbing slowly to the top. As so often in life, the effort is at least as rewarding as the prize – for who can put a value on what has been learned on the journey?

The coach and the athlete not only become aware of the problems that face beginners, they also learn that superstars are not immune to the same problems, in some degree or other. And in facing difficulties that cannot be avoided on the way up they learn how to overcome them. This book is based upon what we have learned on that climb.

Running is a natural thing to do, and as every child runs, or wants to run, it might seem that there is not all that much to it, and not a lot that can be said about it. The first assumption is true, the second is not. There is a lot that can be said and written about running, and the problem is not what to put in but what to leave out.

Of necessity much of this book must contain plain facts and figures. Muscles have Latin names, different shoes have specific functions. But we are writing about more than this; we are writing about running: the whole is so much greater than the sum of its parts. Anyone who runs, at whatever level, will find that he is at the same time finding out about himself and, even through his running, making a personal statement. For many of the men and women now caught up in marathon running, this is especially true.

Running is running. Yet to many it is more than that, it is a way of life. In some parts of Britain for example, cross-country running is King. Its disciples would be adamant – world records and gold medals notwithstanding – that no runner has arrived until he has won the 'National'. You smile? Until you have seen a truly hard-fought National (and every one is hard-fought) with its giant field and its cavalry charge start, you cannot begin to appreciate the enormous pull of the National Cross-Country Championship to competitor and spectator alike. In the not too distant past, for many good track men, miling was something to do to fill in the summer until the real running began once more, and the road running scene which overlaps the seasons and has its own intense excitement, especially with the great distance relays, claims its own fanatical adherents.

The spectrum of the sport is astonishingly wide; from jogging at one end to attempting world records at the other. Between them there are such variations as orienteering, with its combination of navigation and stamina, which offers a unique challenge to those who would like to 'rally' without charging deep into our countryside in cars; or that most formidable challenge to nature at its most raw, the hard companionship of fell-running. Or, if all that sounds too competitive, remember that every kind of running, with perhaps the exception of track athletics, can be enjoyed at your level and in your way without competing against anyone but yourself. You can set out at any time you choose to run the country lanes or highways – you may set off down a hill or along a mountain ridge at your own pace. You are not compelled to race anybody. You can run solo with only a map, or a list of clues by which to navigate. At the end of the day the occasional well earned 'half' will be doubly welcome, but as you rise to your own challenge and reflect, justifiably, on your own modest attainments, achieved alone or in the company of other like-minded souls, you will know that these efforts have their own rewards.

For some, as we have said, running is a way of life. For others, regrettably, it can become more than that. It assumes the proportions of a religion or, worse still, becomes an addiction and an obsession, as its victims become unbalanced

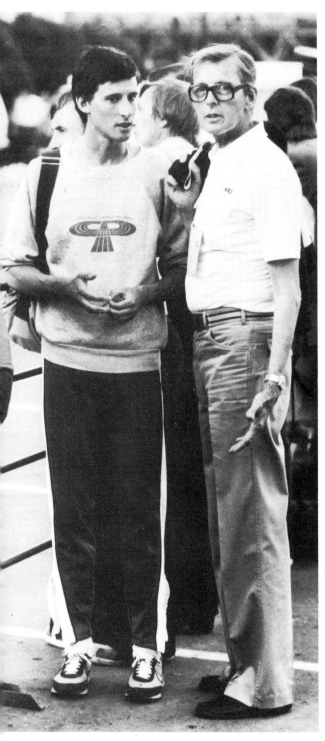

and hooked on mileage mania. From there running can all too easily become a substitute for living and a retreat from the real world – a sad aberration that is being reported with increasing frequency from the United States. Far from achieving the fitness and the sense of well-being that it should bring, it is more likely to end in a frustrating crop of over-use injuries and a lowered level of health from the constant over-stress.

Fitness must be sought after with care. In all the enthusiasm and perseverance we should not forget that in running the real achilles heel is excess. We must always keep the main objective in mind: to run for fitness, but to run for pleasure as well. It is ridiculous to confuse the need to maintain a running programme and its concomitant dedication with an obsessive drive to complete a schedule regardless of the consequences. The total commitment of an Olympic athlete to run in the once-in-a-lifetime final and to hell with the possible consequences is understandable – if not wholly wise – but for anyone else it is quite inexcusable. It was that great hurdler David Hemery who rightly said that a serious test of an athlete's quality is how he behaves when he is injured.

To urge competitiveness and to urge caution in quick succession is not a contradiction. The longer you keep running well the longer you will stay well. And if you are running for fitness, anything that curtails your running will also curtail your fitness. The basis for overall physical fitness is achieved by improving your respiration and your circulation, and to this end the most effective activity is running. Once this base is obtained it has to be maintained, and again it is running, though not necessarily in larger doses, that will do it effectively. Furthermore, running's one great advantage is that it is not an expensive pursuit, and your sessions can be timed to suit yourself. In the unhappy event of your being unable to run for any length of time, the alternative methods of maintaining fitness – cycling, perhaps, or swimming, gymnasium training or even physiotherapy – tend to be less effective, more time-consuming and usually more expensive. In every way it is better to stay unhurt and fit.

This caution is as important in a coach as it is in a runner. Assisting and guiding an athlete to the pinnacle of his or her running success requires a hard and demanding taskmaster. But lasting success has never been achieved without understanding the need for moderation. In preparing training schedules for the build-up, the pre-race and the race periods, the correct restraint is at the very heart of the matter. When applying increasing doses of stress – for that is what a large part of race training is – giving the correct opportunities for recovery requires careful thought. And if the top performers can practise restraint in their training build-up, then so can fitness runners, for certainly the same pressures are not on them.

As runner and coach we have been involved in serious competitive running for fourteen years. Before that, as boy and father, we shared the child's joy of uninhibited running. Since we started serious competition we have also shared the ever-increasing discipline and pressure that continued success imposes. We have shared, too, in a different way, the pride of world records and the ecstasy and agony of victory and defeat in the Olympic Games. But in the end the true experience, and the self-knowledge that goes with it, belongs to the runner and to him or her alone.

This book is written in the hope that it will give encouragement and guidance to those who want to share in the unique experience that running can give. If it were to start some unknown on a personal quest to 'Go for Gold' it would be a delightful bonus. But it will bring equal satisfaction if someone starting out later in life, seeking no more than enjoyment, health and well-being, finds here the same encouragement.

AUTHOR'S NOTE
The greater part of the book represents the joint thoughts and opinions of both of us. In a few places where we have felt it more useful to include expert opinion or personal reminiscence particular to one or other of us, the change is clearly flagged and the first-person section set in different typeface.

Sebastian Coe
Peter Coe
Sheffield, England
Spring 1983

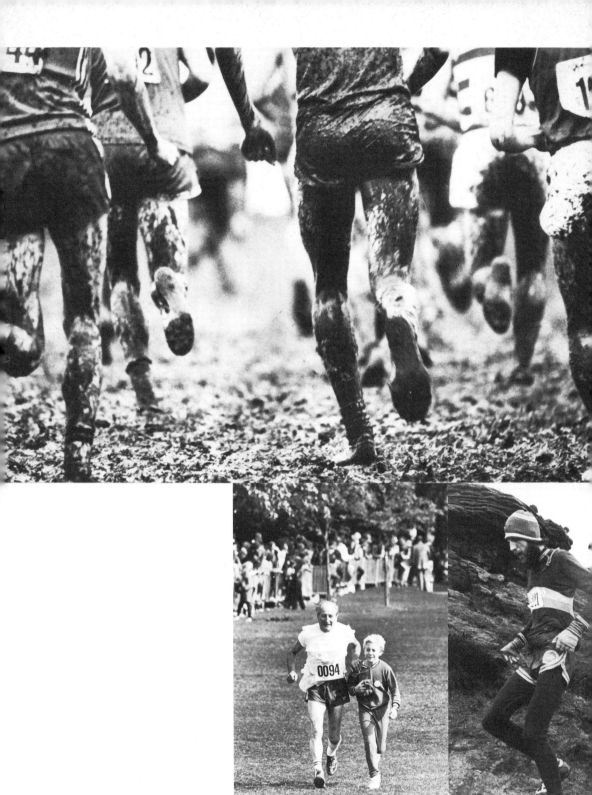

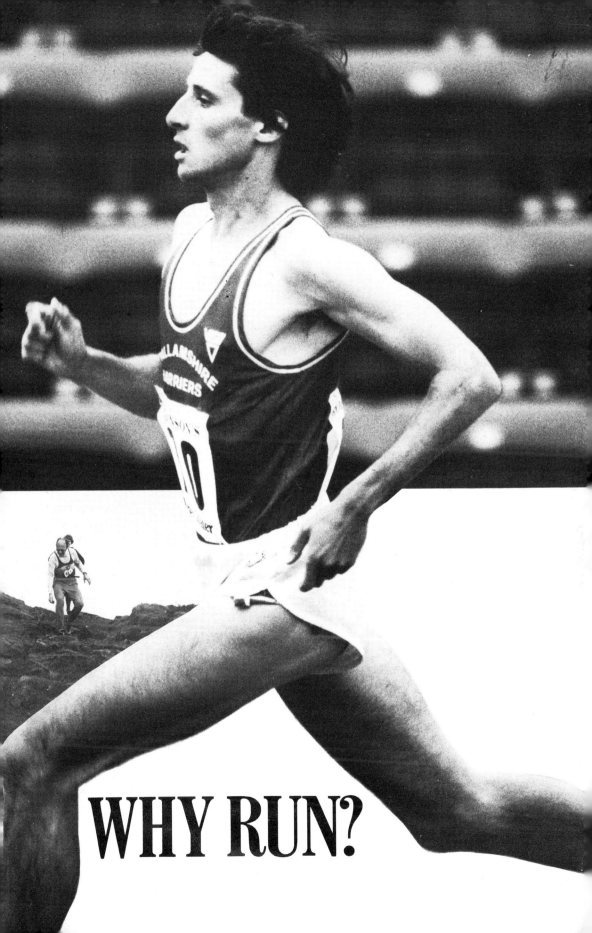

WHY RUN?

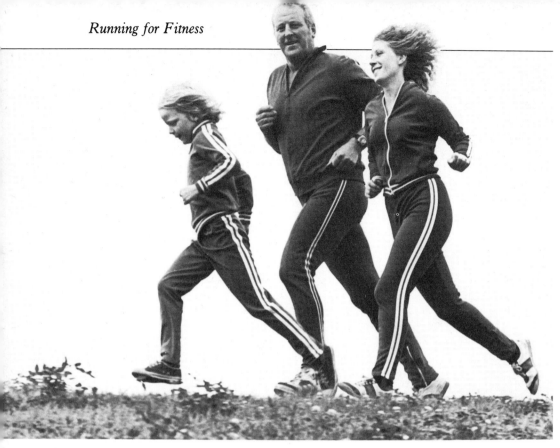

There have been very few, if any, societies in history which have not shown competitiveness in some way. It is hardly within the scope of this book to analyse social behaviour, but it is sufficient to say that sports and games have been with man for a very long time, and that in one form or another, running or jumping have always had their place.

For the majority of people in Western society the physical demands are minimal, and for many the mental demands are also decreasing. Today there are more and more people with more and more leisure – some of it earned, some of it enforced – who are bound to be faced with the problem of time on their hands. There is no real virtue in hard, gruelling work for its own sake, and one of the proper uses of technology has been to liberate mankind from drudgery. But in the Western world modern technology also offers the ordinary man a better diet than he has ever known, notwithstanding many of the junk foods that are on the market.

Thus we face the contradiction that we have enhanced nutrition that is not matched by an enhanced work load. Worse still, the modern man and woman have the additional problems of coping with the foodstuffs industry, from which a large amount of advertising is aimed at persuading people to eat for pleasure – a very different proposition from taking a normal, healthy pleasure in what they eat.

Modern society also tends to regard all problems as having technological solutions. Every doctor knows that many of his patients no longer regard sound advice as therapy, and without recourse to drugs or even surgery they do not believe they are getting good treatment. There are innumerable jars, bottles, tubes, capsules and syringes containing alleged cures and reliefs for ills that arise solely from the way we live. Consider how much orthopaedic trouble has arisen from fashion shoes alone. Think how many people insist on medicine and treatment rather than stop smoking. We owe it to ourselves, as well as to society, to try to live in a more natural and healthy way. There may not be much we can do about our employment, but there is a lot we can do with our diet and our leisure.

A carefully worked out running schedule, coupled with a good diet, will not only help us to achieve fitness, but it will also be one of the best pieces of preventive medicine that we ever undertake. That exercise is 'good for you' has long been believed, but the duration of a belief is not a proof. It has only been with careful long-term studies that solid evidence has become available.

There may indeed be a built-in human need for exercise. Living as we do in a Western industrial society, we tend to forget that there are still parts of the world where people live by hunting and foraging and even follow a nomadic existence, and that our own days as hunters and foragers are only in the very recent past. Before the intervention of modern science and technology, survival went only to the fit.

Both hunting and early agriculture involved hard work, which is exercise after all, and since survival then depended on strength, skill and mobility, it might very well follow that we are genetically programmed for physical work or exercise.

If the play of young animals such as puppies, kittens and cubs can be seen as part of their development, then the games children play might also be showing us the way we were intended to be.

We ensure that our pets are adequately exercised without drawing the proper conclusions from it. Animals confined in conditions that do not allow them adequate exercise become unhealthy and mean-tempered; it's a simple step to draw a parallel to humans. We strongly believe that the best base for mental health is physical fitness. It is worth reminding ourselves just what is the body's most important function. It is to feed and protect the brain, which houses the mind. Without the brain functioning properly we will lack not only an understanding of what we are doing, but also the necessary willpower to meet the demands of successful training. Furthermore, once fitness is achieved, it will need maintaining. *Mens sana in corpore sano* – 'a healthy mind in a healthy body' – is a much quoted proposition, as old as it is corny. But is no lesser an ideal for that, and it remains a neat and realistic conception of health: mental fitness linked to bodily fitness.

When finally listing reasons for running, which range from a biological need to avoiding the excesses of living, it is easy to appear puritanical without meaning to be so. This would be a great pity, because one of the attributes of running is the sheer pleasure of it. Running when undertaken sensibly is a fun thing. Even when some of the fun is driven out by the sheer intensity of the sessions that the most dedicated performers must undergo, the pleasure flows back with the feeling of achievement and the company of others in search of the same goals.

There are any number of valid reasons for wanting to run. Most of these will be totally personal, and could include emulation, mental escape, physical freedom, perhaps even friendship. But whether or not fitness is among your reasons, fitness you will certainly achieve.

As man is a gregarious animal it might well be that an athletic club could offer both the companionship and the advice and support that you feel you need when starting to run – and could be true even if you want to run for fitness rather than to compete. No jogger should feel that he is out of place in a running club: in our own club, the Hallamshire Harriers, there is a place for everybody, including the parents of young members. Indeed, there have been many cases of parents following in their children's footsteps and subsequently becoming active runners themselves.

Athletic clubs vary in size and quality, and the choice is yours. Being comprised of people, they are bound to have the odd crank among the membership, but they are just as likely to have a member or two who have made a study of some aspects of fitness, and who would be glad to help you. Our own club newsletter, which we happened to refer to when we were preparing this book, is compiled by an active veteran runner who finds time to compete, officiate and edit.

For coach and athlete at the highest level running is – and must remain – a very serious matter, and we cannot afford to be flippant when giving advice to others. But that doesn't mean that we have forgotten how much fun running can provide. For every race that fades from the memory into mere statistics, there is another of which the mere mention can start us laughing – if only in the safety of hindsight. Like the appalling mid-winter mudbath of a cross-country race in Derbyshire which started and finished in a bleak wooden hut as a changing room, to which the runners returned, half-frozen, to clean up under one common cold-water tap and with one enamel bowl. Or the potential misery of another bleak evening in the Dales when one of the cars broke down on the return journey to Sheffield. It was the wild, impromptu football match that whiled away the time until the car was repaired which remains in the memory, a match that served up more professional fouls in a deserted Derbyshire school-playground than can have been seen in the whole World Cup!

It wasn't all disaster, either. We shall never forget the international road race at Loughrea in Ireland, when the race was preceded by entertainment and dancing, and followed by a riotous evening in Galway of eating, dancing and incomparable Irish hospitality. Nor the complete contrast to that single cold Derbyshire tap – the day of the Batley road relays when the local swimming pool, complete with warm water, was thrown open to all the runners.

All over the country, every weekend, there are teams on the move taking their own fun and laughter to the competition. For us, bound tightly by our employment and by the work and detailed preparation required for top level international competition, there is far less time nowadays for such fun-and-games outings. But the wit and the laughter of those coach journeys has stayed with us longer than the events they accompanied, and if the glory still goes to the superstars, the most fun in running remains with the majority.

We all know the old saying – everything you enjoy is either illegal, immoral or fattening. Well, running certainly isn't any of these.

One Man's Return . . .

This is the tale of a friend of ours who proved to himself the hard way that being overweight and unfit can subject tendons and muscles to sudden loads that might be reasonable for the fit, but not for the sedentary. The belated preventive therapy that his case illustrates could hold good for anyone looking for a reason to run.

John Edwards is his name. He was our next door neighbour, and he had seen Sebastian as a thirteen-year-old set off on his daily training runs either on the road or round an all-weather football pitch. One day he said rather wistfully, 'I used to do a bit of running myself.'

John's profession was and still is demanding, but only mentally so. Lecturing in a university on control engineering taxes the head, not the body. In addition, and he will not mind us saying it, John has a gourmet's taste with a gourmand's delight for food. In short, he was well overweight. It was the classic situation when 'somewhere, somehow, something's gotta give'. It did – it was his knee.

It was a game of squash that was the turning point; in the middle of a rally he badly tore the tendons in his knee – a simple overload.

His stay in hospital gave him time to reflect upon his younger days and his sport when in the fourth, fifth and sixth years at school he ran cross-country. At university, too, he had run at least twice a week for three years, and while he never made the top, neither did he reach the thirteen stones that helped to finish his knee.

Emerging from his enforced rest lighter and wiser, John's interest in running was further heightened by seeing Eric Miller's fine film of the famous Three Peaks fell race.

He saw clearly that here was a chance to combine his love of nature and the outdoors with the need for enhanced fitness in a positive way. For him it became running for fitness and fell running for the challenge, with road-racing as a back-up sport.

His training is largely done solo. He enjoys running with groups as often as he can, and he would prefer to be with other runners, but the solo running, though harder, provides the solitude that gives him time to think over problems or ideas free from other distractions.

The roads and moors of Derbyshire and Yorkshire over which he trains, while magnificent, make very hard and demanding courses. Although used somewhat differently, it is the same area that stimulates Sebastian so much and provides the hard background mileage on which his training is based.

John commenced slowly, and he steadily built up his strength and stamina through a period of jogging before starting continuous running as part of his training. He now uses road-running and six-mile road races for sharpening his speed but when we asked him why, despite his respect for road speed, he loved fell running we got an interesting reply: 'I feel the macho image and the toughness of the challenge to be the extra ingredients that compensate for the lack of sheer speed.'

Even when involved with extra work, either setting or marking examination papers or other additional university demands, he maintains his training. Depending upon the terrain over which he is running, or on the state of his preparation for a race, his mileage can vary between thirty and fifty miles per week; over the year he maintains his forty-mile-a-week average. From being a regular tail-ender in racing and training, he is now moving up through the field. As he gets older his times keep improving, and he has not suffered any set-back from injury.

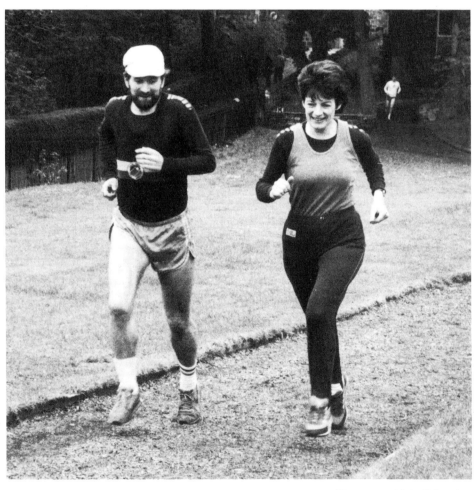

**Margaret and John Edwards:
from perseverance to pleasure**

. . . and One Woman's Arrival

Family reaction to all this has been encouragingly positive. John's wife Margaret's earlier mild humour at John's truly desperate perseverence in the early days slowly gave way to an understanding and admiration, not just for him but for everyone who runs.

Her interest in running, like John's, had first been aroused by seeing the *Three Peaks* film and following the fortunes of their young neighbour, Sebastian. But initially she only dabbled (and this phase lasted for about three years), partly because she suffers from both migraine and asthma, and partly because of her family responsibilities.

Nevertheless, the day came when Margaret decided that brief insights into the advantages of feeling fit warranted going the whole hog and getting thoroughly fit, and running was to be the principal means of reaching this goal.

This time she was to adopt a more thorough approach. On her earlier outings she had found that running on the flat was one thing and that running up hills was quite another. In other words she was proving that if you have a weakness, hill running will find it. Hill running requires a good all-round fitness but also, like sprinting, it requires strength.

Now, because of the previously mentioned difficulties, Margaret looked for a fitness course that she could carry out at times most convenient to herself, and she chose the *Sunday Times Body Maintenance* fitness programme. Ignoring both the sarcasm of her offspring and the advice of the *Sunday Times* to complete the women's programme first, she plunged straight into the men's course and soon adopted a minor running programme on top of it. Very pleased with the result of the *Sunday Times* exercises and, as she puts it herself, 'with all the bits that wobbled under control', she then took to a more serious running programme and to her great joy the hills that had once been insuperable were now quite manageable.

She now runs twice a week at least, and usually manages three outings a week – on Wednesday, Saturday and Sunday. If her work as a teacher allows, she also tries for a run at lunchtimes on Mondays and Tuesdays. A long run is between eight and ten miles, an easy run is four miles. The weekend runs are the ones she can use for distance and any three short runs will total at least fifteen miles.

It is the flexible kind of programme that a working wife and mother must develop.

What does she say now about her new-found fitness? 'Above all, I really do enjoy the extra sense of well-being that I have achieved. And because I was determined to do something about my general condition before I reached a point of no return, the lifting effect on my wounded vanity was reward enough. The good effect on my appearance of the combined fitness exercises and the running is not so much in the reduced inches as in the increased muscle tone and the general firming up that goes with it.

'I have lost only a few pounds, but my shape is so much better. I recall the thrill of this first realisation. I was sitting watching the television. I stirred in my chair and felt firm new thigh muscles for the first time – Oh, the joy!

'Mentally I am better too. I have a lot more confidence in myself, and going for a run seems to get me over that "life has got me down" feeling, even if the run has to be at a time when I really don't want to go. I never regret going for a run, no matter how reluctantly I start out.'

She still has obstacles to overcome. She is still a migraine sufferer, and a headache induced by over-exertion can last all day; and her asthma, though controlled by drugs, is still there. But the children, who thought the running all a bit of a joke, don't laugh any more, and the comments from members of the public have lessened over the last two years, an indication in itself of the social acceptance of running for fitness – 'Anyway, I don't care any more.'

She was pleasantly surprised by the helpfulness of the seasoned and experienced runners who, provided they saw someone really trying, were very supportive, and keen to give help and good tips on running or injuries.

She enjoys running with John because it stretches her, although she is aware that he still has to slow down a bit for her. She is proud that she can run up some of the most testing hills, she has run as much as 15 miles, and she is now contemplating entering a half-marathon. Perhaps the fascination both John and Margaret Edwards feel for fell running can be explained by the size of the challenge.

The 'Big One' is in the Lake District where the standard is 42 peaks in 24 hours. The record is held by Bob Graham who has logged all 42 in 13 hours. Imagine three very hilly marathons including the equivalent of a trip up and down Everest.

In summary it is fair to say that running has changed a thirteen-stone injury-prone man into a very fit eleven-stone injury-free man with a racing weight a few pounds less. For Margaret, the rewards have been less dramatic, but equally satisfying. Could this be you?

These stories of men and women finding rejuvenation through running are not fairy tales made up by the shoe manufacturers. You may not want to fell-run – there's no reason why you should, but there are plenty of opportunities for people with every kind of outlook. Perhaps a good collective noun for fun and fitness beginners might be 'a Bassetts of Runners' – a collection of all-sorts. There will be all manner of shapes and sizes, and all of those who continue with the sport will refine their shapes and achieve a worthy goal.

The Women's Angle

It is easy to forget that the similarities of the sexes are much greater than the differences and in the same way that one can get an odd feeling seeing women's pages in newspapers, and journals labelled magazines for women – as if they inhabited a different world – it seems an odd idea to write a section on women.

As far as running is concerned, women are no different from men. They have become part of the running boom at all distances from fun runs to marathons

Conquest of the mud: the finish of the women's
World Cross-Country Championship at Glasgow, 1978

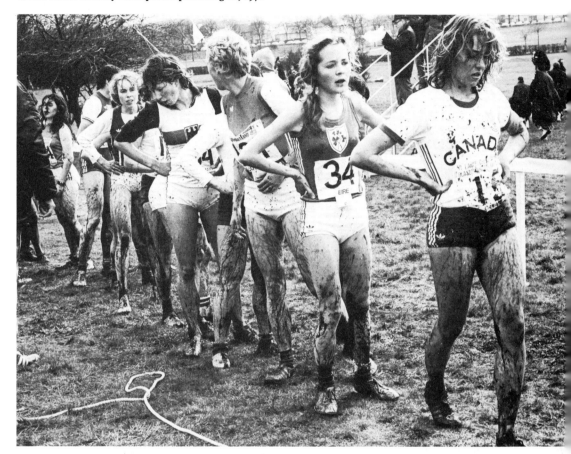

and the fitness that running brings men, it will bring equally well to women. No longer is it difficult for a woman to find running shoes her size, no longer is the sight of a woman training through the streets an occasion for amazement and wolf whistles.

In competition, too, women have rightly begun to play a more important part. In the last fifteen years we have seen a significant increase in the range of official championship distances in women's events. On the track women run all distances up to 3000 metres, and there is soon to be an official 10,000 metre distance for them. On the road they run anything up to a marathon – and some even compete at the 'ultra' distances beyond that.

There are differences, of course. For young women runners pregnancy, and any effect that running might have on the pregnancy and vice versa, is bound to be an important consideration. As one would expect, through the political involvement of the state in sport, there has been more attention paid in the Eastern bloc countries than there has here to the success of women in sport, and also to their reintegration into competition after childbirth. The immensely detailed book *Track and Field*, published in East Germany in 1977 under the auspices of the Leipzig College of Physical Culture, has gone thoroughly into the subject. In summary, their conclusions are that:

Intensive training before pregnancy does not cause difficulty with the first delivery, and the physical condition of the mother after childbirth is better and more stable than before the pregnancy. More than half the pregnant athletes they studied did not suffer loss of form in the first three months of pregnancy and they were allowed to train and compete under medical control.

Pregnant athletes suffering from nausea, sickness, hypertension or anaemia are not allowed to train or compete, but are advised to continue lighter exercise, like gymnastics and swimming.

For the second three months very light training – but not jumps or force exercises with sudden position changes – is encouraged. The light training is designed to keep up the general condition of the cardiovascular system. In the final three months, deep breathing, swimming and extended walks are recommended.

After delivery an immediate commencement of exercise for strengthening the abdominal and pelvic muscles is started and after one month strengthening exercises for the particular event, together with moderate endurance exercises. After three months the athlete can resume real exertion. It is considered that around six months after delivery she should be fit and trained well enough for competition.

The East German study also concludes that training on this pattern does not hinder breast feeding.

There are plenty of reports from America of women who have kept on running or jogging very late into pregnancy, but it should be remembered that the demands on these women will be a lot less than on those in competition, and in any case a woman in late pregnancy should be under medical supervision.

As we write there is further confirmation, this time from Great Britain. In 1978 Jane Colebrook (now Jane Finch) won the European indoor 800 metres championship in Spain. In January 1983, only eight months after her confinement, she convincingly won the WAAA indoor 1500 metre championship at Cosford. This was of particular interest to us, because at the 1983 Congress of the European Athletics Coaches' Association we heard the Russians report that their experience with women showed after the first child their whole organism stabilised and they were capable of enhanced performance, though there was no evidence that subsequent pregnancies continued to further improve athletic ability. All this should help dispel any lingering Victorian ideas that pregnancy is an illness rather than a healthy experience.

The so-called frailty of women is not the only myth to have built up around the comparatively recent entry of women into competitive athletics. Another, quite contradictory absurdity, has recently been gaining ground which, if taken seriously, might be harmful to sport in general and running in particular.

In the past, for various socio-economic reasons, women have failed to achieve their full athletic potential. Now that barriers are at last disappearing the overall performances of women – as one would expect – are improving rapidly, particularly in middle- and long-distance running. These achievements have led to statement like: 'by the year 2000 (or whatever crystal ball date you care to insert) women's records will equal the men's.' Quite simply this is not true.

In *The Physiology of Exercise*, Morehouse and Miller list forty-seven significant differences between men and women and to pick out only some of them is enough to prove the point. Men are stronger than women and, more significantly, their power-to-weight ratio is higher than women's. Their larger lungs and hearts, too, give enhanced vital capacities. Higher aerobic, anaerobic and oxygen-carrying capacities give physical advantages to males that are too big to be ignored.

When the surge due to social changes has finished, and the rate of improvement has levelled off, the very real physiological advantage of males will still be there and then we could be left with the following ridiculous proposition: Ms X achieves a magnificent all-time best performance. However, since she failed to get within so many seconds or minutes of Mr Y's world record, it is hailed not as a great performance, but as a worthy 'failure'.

It is not as silly as it may sound. In one of the finest track races of 1982 David Moorcroft beat Sidney Maree, John Walker, Steve Scott and the rest of a world-class field in a 3000 metre invitation at Crystal Palace, broke the European record for the distance and came within a second of the world best time. At least one national newspaper greeted the superb performance the next day with the headline 'Moorcroft's near miss'. And Sebastian too has won an international race in Europe, only to find his victory announced in England as a 'failure to beat the world record' – a record that he had set himself!

If the 'parity of records' nonsense was allowed to prevail it would prevent many women from going on to reach their full potential: nothing is more disheartening than struggling to achieve impossible and unrealistic targets. Women's times will approach more closely to men's but they will not exceed them. In long-distance events women stars are able to beat many men runners, because the spread of ability in any population group is very wide. But these performances are general, and world records are very specific.

For some time, for reasons both chauvinistic and political, it has been easy to excuse the relative failure of Western athletes compared with those of the Eastern bloc in the race for medals and world records. The reasons given have ranged from drug abuse to state-supported professionalism. State aid, it is true, can be a great help, particularly when there is a state back-up in sports medicine, but it most certainly is not the whole story. Now, with the emergence of brilliant all-round athletes like Daley Thompson, and the grip taken on all the middle-distance records by Coe, Ovett and Moorcroft, all from a small country like England, these excuses are beginning to look decidedly weak, especially as the emergence of younger men like Steve Cram is providing world-class continuity.

So we are now left with another set of female myths. One says: 'You can't succeed at the top and still look like a woman.' (It usually comes clothed in remarks like 'Oh, well – if you want to look like a man.') Another is: 'Do you want to be as big as that?' Or 'They're not really women, are they?' – comments both stupid and wounding.

There will always be people who take steroids illegally, willingly or under some coercion, but this does not account for all the Eastern European success in the women's events – the publicity will always go to the grotesque rather than the normal. But there are world-class female athletes from all countries whose only 'abnormality' is super-fitness and extremely healthy looks. They are attractive and clear-skinned, they do not carry around unwanted fat, and they do not look like men. Exercise, particularly running, does not detract in any way from physical attraction in women, it can only enhance it.

It is not without interest that the very countries which are under attack for doping their way to success (for which there are proven examples and no excuses) also provide excellent advice for women athletes on menstruation and pregnancy, right through to how to resume an athletic career after childbirth, and with a record of improved performances to show for it.

It is one thing to have a firm and valid objection to a political system; it is quite another to shut your eyes and rationalise your failure. All that is required for the women in Britain to join the men of their country at the very top is to show the same will and commitment to succeed. The training knowledge is here, the success should be with it.

The Choice is Yours

For men and women alike, the time is likely to come when plodding around the local streets or the local park is going to lose its fascination, and you will be thinking of branching out into something more specialised. All the following forms of running – whether you are attracted by the competition they can provide or the companionship or the relaxation they offer – will give a whole new dimension to your search for fitness.

Road Running
Almost every section in this book will deal with some aspect of road running – indeed, even the most inexperienced keep-fit runner will have had some experience of, at least, running on pavements – but road-racing is a widely popular sport, and a few words are important for a newcomer.

The spread of distances in competition is enormous, from around three miles to the marathon. And beyond that there are the ultra-distance races and the long place-to-place runs like the London-to-Brighton. Other forms of running are either on closed courses or in open country fairly remote from roads, but road running is on the public highway. It is vital to learn the rules of the sport and to stick to them. In some areas the police are extremely co-operative, but there is already one chief constable who looks upon road runners with as little favour as football crowds.

It is not worth giving ammunition to the prejudiced. Not all motorists see the runner as a healthy competitor doing his own thing on the public highway. They are equally likely to regard you as a mobile obstruction carrying the sole responsibility of avoiding contact with their vehicle. Accidents tend to provoke the simple response from authorities. It is easier to stop people racing on roads than to restrain car drivers.

If you keep to the correct side of the road, do not cut corners or run straight across at intersections without looking about you, and adhere to any signs or instructions from the marshals, all will be well. But if you lose concentration you are the one who gets hurt. One more thing. If you are ever roped in for marshalling *stay alert*. A misdirection, or no directions at all, may not only send a runner off course and lose him a race – it could also send him out of the human race altogether.

Track Running

This is undoubtedly the showpiece of the sport, the branch of athletes from which the heroes and heroines of running are bound to emerge, from which the record books are written, and from which television draws so much of its sports audience.

In all other forms of competitive running, comparisons between races are very difficult to make. No road course is the same as another and cross-country courses are even more dissimilar. You can only get a rough assessment of ability by comparing your position at the finish with those in a number of other races over the same distance. Track racing, though, offers far better opportunities to assess your own improvement.

Track running, too, has graded races. These are events which cater not just for the stars, but for those who have achieved a particular time for their event. For example, if your time for 800 metres is 2min 2sec your race will contain runners whose personal best time is close to this. Finishes are closer and more exciting, and these races provide the best experience in the early days of track competition. They give a better chance of winning, and no runner is going to be embarrassed by being beaten out of sight.

The humble runner who enjoys competition without having a great ability or the opportunities for a lot of training will also be able to run in club and open handicaps – another way of ensuring a more equal competition, and thus a greater chance of succeeding.

Track racing also has the advantage of an almost instantaneous feed-back by way of the observers. While the competitor can have a good feel for the condition of the runners close to him, the observer is in a much better position to read the race as it unfolds. The manner of a run, the degree of commitment, for example, or the changes of pace will often reveal as much about runners' strengths and weaknesses as the actual finishing time for the race.

It is one of the advantages of club life to have keen, supportive friends who

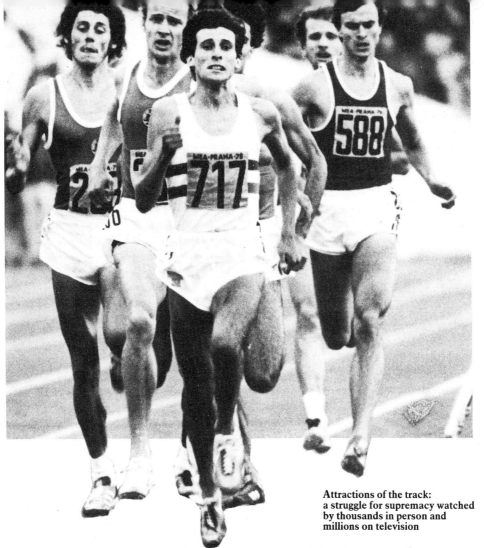

**Attractions of the track:
a struggle for supremacy watched
by thousands in person and
millions on television**

want you to win and who can also give you a fair, unbiased account of your race. Even if you win it is important to know who was finishing quickly, and who may perhaps have been guilty of a tactical error earlier in the race, something worth knowing for the next time you meet. All this information helps you to assess the quality of your own performance, and only on the track is this possible.

In winter, for a privileged few, track racing moves indoors – a season which culminates this side of the Atlantic in the European Indoor Championships in March. The standard track is half the distance of the outdoor one – two hundred metres, slightly banked to allow for high speeds on the tighter bends. Many European and American cities have adequate indoor tracks, but only at Cosford, near Wolverhampton, courtesy of the RAF, can Britain boast an indoor circuit. It follows, inevitably, that for the average fitness runner, winter exercise is almost certain to be taken outdoors.

Cross-country Running
If you are the type who likes a good run for his money, then cross-country running will certainly meet your needs.

Look at the requirements: speed with endurance, strength with stamina, and the ability to change style and pace to suit the conditions. Quite a specification – but before you think of winning the National you will need a bit of experience.

A good tactical sense is essential in all kinds of running, and at 800 metres, as we well know, he who hesitates is lost. But even at 5000 metres, and 10,000 metres, when the leading bunch is on the attack, the complexities of pace-change are not as difficult to cope with as in a cross-country. For a start, conditions on the track are uniform from start to finish, and you can nearly always see the leaders; in cross-country the slopes and hills, the bushes and trees and sharp corners can soon obscure the leaders from the pack. In a road race there may be bends, but the field does not bunch up while it filters one at a time through a narrow gap as it often does in the country.

Up the steep slope, down the slippery bank, through the mud – the course is always changing. If any form of racing needs a good apprenticeship, this does. Experience of the traps and pitfalls and the many combinations of hazards that different courses provide is essential if you are going to do well.

Training for cross-country needs diligence and imagination to find opportunities to experience the sort of conditions you are likely to find in a race.

From the age of twelve, until the time he was eighteen, cross-country provided a grand toughening and testing background for Seb. It helped us to lay the foundation of his strength and stamina over a wide range of distances, and even today the sport provides its share of fitness and fun. And whatever the standard of the field, cross-country makes a grand day out for all, competitor and spectator alike. Regardless of the conditions, a fast, hard-fought race cannot fail to be exciting, and the refreshments after the race and the prize-giving that follows invariably provide warmth, wit and a lot of laughs.

A brief note to parents: give all the support you can to the school races, and the boys' and girls' events in the clubs. Support and encourage, but in your excitement do not push the youngsters too hard. Seb started at twelve, but it took him several attempts to get a good place in an English Schools' Championship at cross-country; if the youngsters are really keen, remind them that it is only as a senior that the wins really start to matter. A disheartened apprentice will never complete his indentures.

And a safety note for all competitors and the parents of young aspirants: make sure you are up to date with your tetanus immunisation. We have only one public track in Sheffield, the centre of which is often used for soccer matches and which frequently serves as the start and finish of our county cross-country championships. Despite the risks of tetanus, the corporation allows it to be used for equestrian events. Remember, don't blame a farmer if you fall or get spiked in or near manure.

Don't let the big mileages or the hard training necessary to shine in big cross-country races put you off. Even if you are only on thirty miles a week you will still be able to finish a four-mile or six-mile run. You won't be one of the first into the finishing funnel, for sure, but after a couple of tries it will be up to you if you want to push on. And however you perform there will always be an excited group of spectators at the finish, and their cheers never fail to lift the runners as they approach the line. Even the weariest of competitors can find the spirit for a final spurt at the end.

Fell Running

All devotees can wax lyrical over the attractions of their own sport, and in some sports the appeal is not always readily seen. But for those who want to add not only extra toughness and some degree of solitude to their sport, but also an extra touch of risk, join John Edwards and have a go at fell running.

Run nigh on full tilt down a loose scree hill, or down a mountainside with all certainty of safe footfall removed; add the vagaries of the weather, the very real possibilities of mist . . . and you will see that this sport demands a certain type of competitor.

No wonder John finds it has a macho appeal. If you are keen to join this hardy breed and flourish with them in their beloved wildernesses, you will find that the basic running gear, as well as the basic observations about training and safety, are the same as for cross-country, though special attention must be given to footwear.

Orienteering

No runner will get very far if he doesn't know where he is going. In cross-country or road running it is easy for competitors to run off-course if the route is

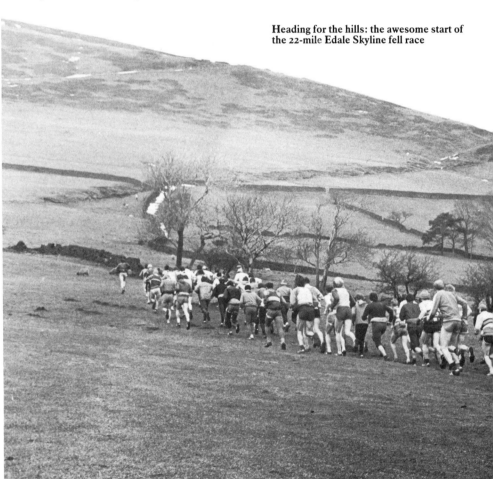

Heading for the hills: the awesome start of the 22-mile Edale Skyline fell race

not well marked, or if there are not 'markers' to call loud and clear directions to the competitors. Well organised races will have reduced this hazard to a minimum, so that even the front runners will be able to follow the course with ease, and can therefore concentrate on their running.

In orienteering, things are quite different. Finding the way is the name of the game, and navigation in woodland and forest is every bit as important as the running. The sport had its origins in military training in the forests of Scandinavia at the turn of the century, and has evolved as an increasingly popular sport in many parts of Europe, particularly in the last twenty-five years.

Orienteering is racing, but runners start at timed intervals, and create their own 'courses' by navigating from point to point by means of map and compass between a fixed start and finish. The points on the map they must visit are listed on a description sheet, and all are indicated on the map the runner carries with him. At each control – distinguished on the ground by a marker flag – he punches his card to prove he has found it, and proceeds to the next control and so on to the finish. It is not – take our word for it – as easy as it sounds.

Though the courses are not particularly long, the terrain can be demanding. It may be that the same degree of physical training is not required for orienteering as for competitive cross-country or road racing but the top exponents will probably be running fifty miles a week in training, and the sport undoubtedly demands more mental sharpness on the day; mental alertness declines as a runner gets tired, and a tired orienteer is many times more likely to lose his way – and with it valuable minutes on the clock – than a relaxed and strong orienteer. We would advise a full programme of distance, fartlek (see page 68) and interval training, and even speed-endurance running if you have any aspiration to top class results.

As with so many facets of running, much of the attraction of the sport comes from the fact that it is open to performers of all abilities. The Southern, the Midland and the Northern Championships, the British Championship itself, and the sport's great four-day Easter Festival, the Jan Kjellstrom Trophy

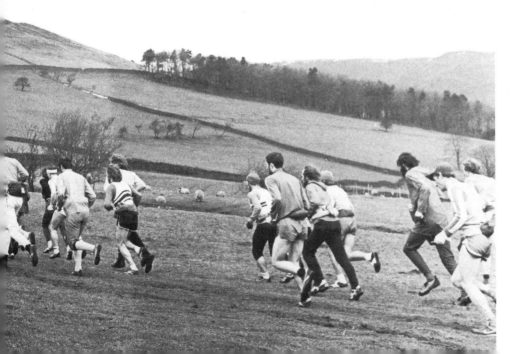

Speed in the forest: map and compass, calm head and sure feet – the essential equipment of the orienteer

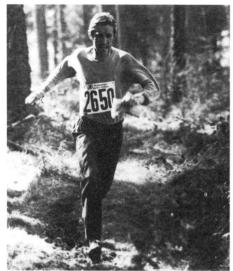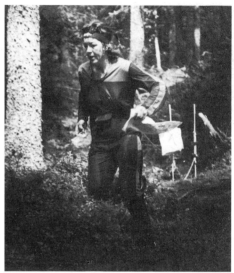

meeting, are all open to all-comers, where the humblest beginner can compete in his or her age group against the best entrants from Britain and Europe – and get lost in the same part of the forest.

The best introduction to the sport is through local clubs, most of which organise Come-And-Try-It events from time to time. Almost any running gear will do to begin with, though it is a rule of the sport that all competitors are covered from neck to toe (primarily to avoid infections being passed on in overgrown, bramble-ridden areas where the same thorns might scratch different skins – it has happened! – but more practically to prevent the unnecessary shredding of skin in rough country). Tough, lightweight tops and trousers are designed for regular competitors, and there are a number of brands of shoe specifically designed for orienteering. Running over rough terrain with one eye on the map and the other searching for landmarks does not give you a lot of time to study your footfall – your feet are going to need the best grip, and the best support, that they can get.

Whether you start running solely for fitness or with the intention of racing, sooner or later this thought will enter your mind: 'How do I compare with others of my kind?' And why not?

There is a real joy at the end of a grand competitive effort, and the losers will have the full respect of the winner. It will not matter that on the way there you may have looked a little less than a golden Olympian, because you will share this truth with most of the others, and as anyone who has tried racing will tell you, the first time you pass another runner a never-to-be-broken spell is cast.

You can both be tired, puffing and wheezing, but the one who can drag himself a few extra inches per minute in front of the other walks tall until the next time.

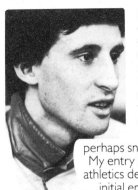

I developed a love of running as a child. I made my entry into the ranks of "serious runners" as early as the age of thirteen – half my life ago. I have been hooked, or perhaps snared, ever since. My entry into international athletics developed from that initial enjoyment I found from simply putting one foot in front of the other at anything faster than walking pace. Then, as now, the faster I ran the more exhilarating it became.

My immediate aim now is further success at the highest levels of the sport, but in my life as a runner, this will be only a temporary phase; I am sure the pleasure of running will not stop with my retirement.

I know that the same things that first attracted me to running – before the competitive side of the sport took over with all the glorious unpredictability that has gone with those select few years – will still be there, and I will once again be able to get back to the simple pleasure of going for a run. The enjoyment of the scenery will still be there, and so will the knowledge that I am keeping up – even at a somewhat lower level – the kind of all-round fitness that enhances everyday life.

It seems to have become fashionable in the last few years to package the joys of taking to the road in the manner of the wild-west salesman, extolling the virtues of their all-curing potions. America, particularly, has been subjected to a barrage of the all-curing claims of running: everything from constipation to cancer can be overcome by putting one foot in front of the other.

I am not making these claims, but it is true that at times of mental stress, whether academic or personal, taking to the trails has always been refreshing and helpful to me. I feel healthier and generally more resilient when in training, and the habit of the daily run will be with me for ever.

The rewards of a carefully planned and tempered fitness routine may not be felt immediately – indeed, you might even feel worse before you feel better. A level of fitness that will last will not be produced overnight, and the efforts that you make towards that goal are unlikely to progress without occasional periods of physical and mental strain.

But if you do feel discomfort please take heart. Every seasoned athlete at any level of sport will have gone into, and passed through, this phase. I always get this feeling when I make the transition between my winter work and the first few faster sessions on the track during springtime. But once I have climbed from this plateau of fitness on to the next, and I have equipped myself for the rigours of international competition, there is no denying the benefits. In just the same way, you will feel the satisfaction of knowing that you have left the land of the tired and breathless and have, by your own endeavours, joined the ranks of the fit.'

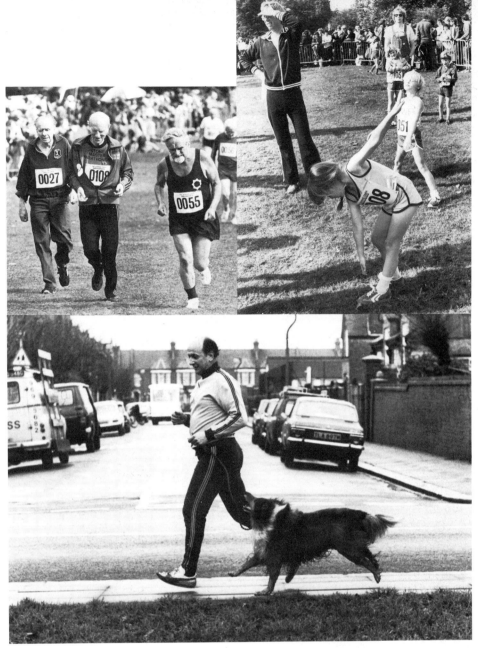

STARTING UP

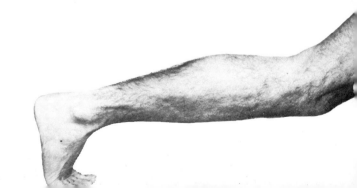

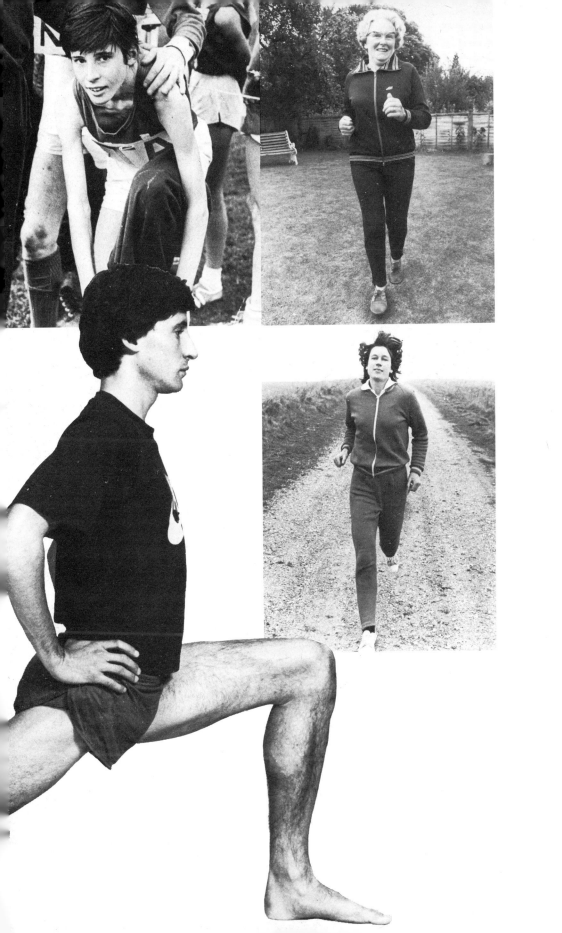

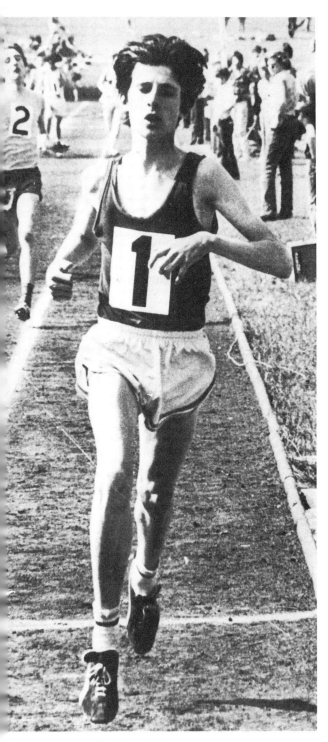

**Early days: Seb at 14,
Sheffield Schools 1500-metre champion**

Once the helter-skelter running of childhood ceases, a general slowing up of the body begins. For some this process is delayed by organised sport and games in schools but, alas, for many, late adolescence sees the end of regular exercise. This has never been more true than today, with large sections of the population slumping into a television sloth at earlier and earlier ages. So now is the time to begin.

In the sense that it is always easier to maintain fitness than to achieve it, age *is* important for anyone thinking about running. It is a good example of the sooner the better, because if you do leave it too long, it could become too late. The best advice is to form good habits at a time when it is easiest to form them, but that said, there are several cases of men starting to run in their fifties and sixties and going on to run in marathons.

Age also offers a loose guide to the level at which you should start running, and the rate at which you should progress. We say 'loose' because any age group will be made up of individuals with widely different fitness levels. When you are thinking about fitness running you would be wise to start considering at the same time whether or not other aspects of your life are conducive to the fitness you are seeking. Running will take effort and time, and it does not make sense to waste either of them in a busy life. Attention to diet is important, and sleep is necessary – the more exercise you do, the more recovery you are going to need. However, slothful dozing in armchairs at every opportunity is neither wise nor necessary – it is probably best described as interval training for death.

'Do I need a health check?'

Before they start running some people will understandably be anxious about their health. Running may be good for my health, they will think, but is my health up to running? The answer to this is in two parts. First, those at risk from making a sensible and careful start to jogging and running are few (it is worth noting that, under medical advice, diabetic and epileptic runners for example, compete successfully at a high level). Secondly, running programmes have been used very successfully for the rehabilitation of patients, including those who have had heart trouble.

'Risk', for runners, is generally meant to be the degree of expectation of coronary illness. Most other ailments are so limiting that pain or decreased mobility would prevent running as an exercise until cured. Diseases of the lungs, for which you should certainly be receiving medical attention anyway, would preclude running for fitness until a doctor gave you the go-ahead.

Who would be in the categories at risk? Anyone who could not pass a stress electro-cardiogram test (known widely as a stress ECG). Other clinical tests would give strong contra-indications, including an ECG taken at rest, but a stress ECG would be the most conclusive. Unfortunately, the average person in Britain would neither know where to obtain, or want to bother himself with, this test. So apart from a routine check with your GP who, if he was sufficiently sports minded and had doubts about you, might recommend a stress ECG, the following list gives an indication of factors that you should consider if you are an inactive person or one not taking regular exercise:

Family history: do you have relatives who have had heart troubles?

Personality: are you a hyped-up go-getter? Is your working day a long one in a stressful environment?

Obesity: are you overweight? The condition places an unwelcome and unnecessary strain on the heart.

Smoking: the habit is often indulged in by those under real, or imaginary, stress. Heart attacks are more often fatal with smokers than with non-smokers, and among those who die from heart attacks the life span is dramatically shorter for those who are heavy smokers.

Blood Pressure: high blood pressure increases the risk of rupturing arteries.

Generally: anyone who feels at all distressed by increased efforts of a normal kind – stairs, gardening or hurrying for the bus – should seek medical advice before starting to run.

In short, prevention is always better than cure. If you have any doubts see a doctor first.

In a free world, we all have a choice in most things, and to whom you go for your medical advice is one such choice. It is important that you choose your physician carefully. Try to find one who will give you all-round advice, fairly presented. Our own orthopaedic specialist is candid in both diagnosis and prognosis, and he spells out the choices and what you may expect from them. He freely acknowledges that his own love of winter sports will eventually result in a permanently fixed ankle. He thinks the cost is acceptable to him.

If you need medical advice, then seek it comprehensively, but while you need this knowledge, remember that it *is* advice, and that the decision must be yours. A good doctor will *want* to help you.

We shall have more to say later about the effects of smoking, but to anyone who argues for ignoring the warnings about smoking and health on the basis that there is no direct proof – only statistical evidence – we offer the following observation: insurance companies and betting organisations live by statistics, and very well too, it would seem. Why be a punter with your own life?

Getting Moving

It would be possible to break down the population into groups representing various categories of age, sex and initial fitness and to prepare running schedules for all these people, but that would require a book of its own. We propose to tackle three groups of men and women, all of whom we presume to be in normal health.

The first group is all those who are aged thirty and under, the second those between thirty and forty, and the last group all those over forty. Any divisions you care to make will be riddled with exceptions. Clearly a forty-four-year-old living outside London who leaves his or her cycle at the station each morning having ridden the four miles from home, and who plays the occasional game of squash after work, will be a lot fitter than a twenty-nine-year-old who does little or nothing beyond walking the dog to the pub.

However, the under-thirties should be able to start a modest jogging programme immediately, and the next group should be able to ease themselves into jogging with a little extra care and preparation.

The over-forties probably represent the group with the widest range of fitness, and therefore need the greatest care in starting up. Provided that there is nothing sufficiently wrong to exclude them from trying, the approach we recommend should enable anyone to get started on the road to fitness running. But for these men and women we do propose a very simple and careful beginning. If you are young enough or fit enough you can start more ambitiously, but remember, exercise was never spoiled by caution.

The Warm-up

Serious athletes will always warm up before an event, and part of their warm-up procedure will include stretching and suppling. Even brisk walking, if you are not accustomed to it, will cause the legs to tighten up a bit and some suppling exercise will help you to avoid, or at least alleviate, the effect of stiffening up after exercise.

There are reflex actions built into our nervous system which are designed to protect our joints and muscles from damage due to over-stretching. This reaction is triggered off to work before harm is done. However, if stretching is done jerkily, particularly with muscles cold or not well exercised, this protective reflex can itself be the cause of injury. So when muscles are being stretched so that the limbs can have an increased range of movement, it is much safer if this is done by static stretching – that is, slowly and comfortably getting to the limit of stretching, and then holding the position for ten to fifteen seconds. In this way you will not invoke the stretch reflex, and the increase in the range of movement will be safely achieved without muscle damage. If flexibility exercises are part of your warm-up routine, do not do them first. Gently jog around until you feel warmer, *then* do the exercises, after which you can continue your warm-up.

When you start exercising seriously, either for the first time or after a long lay-off, there are specific areas that will need extra attention.

For those approaching jogging via walking, it is advisable to include a number of exercises specifically for walkers – which partly overlap with those more suitable for middle- and long-distance runners. Walkers need to concentrate particularly on shoulders, spine, hips and ankles, whereas runners are more likely to be concerned with the hips, ankles and knees as the key areas. But since modern living hardly encourages us to use our bodies through their full range of movement, a full range of flexibility exercises is best for everyone.

First steps

There is an old proverb which says that it is better to learn how to walk before you try to run. This is good advice for older beginners, or for people who have dieted enough to feel ready to run.

First, let at least two hours elapse from your last meal. Blood is diverted to the stomach, away from the muscles, after eating; if you begin exercising too soon, the blood will be diverted away from the stomach to the muscles before it has finished its work, which can give rise to extreme discomfort in the stomach. Wear the shoes you are going to wear for running. Now you are ready to start.

Sedentary people have pulse rates of something between seventy and eighty beats a minute, and to sustain double this rate without discomfort is a good indicator of your condition and your progress. Begin by taking a fixed distance of one mile on a smooth, level path or pavement and walk this distance as briskly as you can without undue discomfort. Drawing deep breaths for a change is all right, panting and wheezing is not. As a guide a brisk pace would be four miles (6.5 kilometres) per hour, or one mile in fifteen minutes.

Immediately you reach the end of your walk check your pulse rate. Count for fifteen seconds and multiply by four, to give you the number of beats per minute. On successive walks, still maintaining an even pace throughout, increase the pace until you achieve a pulse rate of 140–150 per minute. From this point you can go on to extend the length of your walk to a mile and a half, and then two miles – always at an even pace. It is worth checking your pulse at one-mile, or even half-mile intervals, just to make sure you are maintaining this pulse rate throughout the walk.

It is worth making one further safety check. After you have finished your fast walk, allow five or six minutes for recovery, preferably still moving, but quite slowly. If as a beginner your pulse rate has not fallen to 120 beats per minute, then (if your finishing pulse rate was taken accurately) your effort was probably too hard.

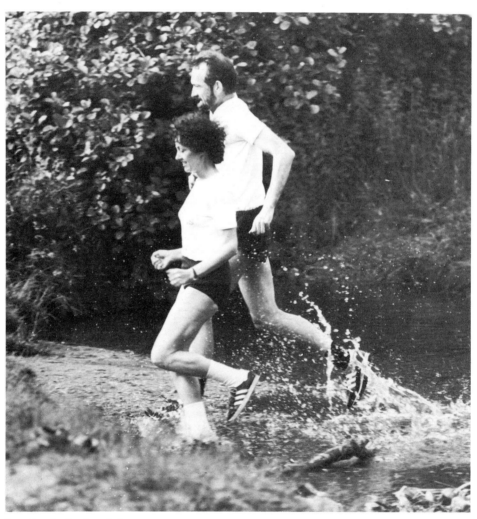

**Easy does it: the shared pleasure
of a run in the country**

Once you have found that you can walk for thirty minutes at a pulse rate of 140–150 per minute, you can extend this in easy stages until you can keep going steadily for one hour. You are now covering about four miles, and as you progress you will find that your pulse rate is falling, that is, you are covering the same distances in the same times with a decreasing pulse rate. You are now showing increased fitness and you are ready to try jogging. You will have certainly become used to your running shoes by now.

If at any time you suffer a chest pain, or giddiness or nausea – stop. You are either training too hard or these are symptoms of illness. If a chest pain should occur again on the next occasion you train, see a doctor as soon as possible. This is an obvious precaution, but you would have to be pretty far gone already to be injured by careful exercise.

'How much should I train, and how often should I train?' These are the questions that everybody asks sooner or later. Walking is not as stressful as running and it is a different action, so if you are starting by going through the walking phase, train every day if it is comfortable, or perhaps two days on and one off if you find you need some recovery time when you first begin.

Housewives, or people working short hours or part time, may find it possible to work out twice a day. A good walk or jog morning and evening is fine once you have become accustomed to exercise.

Provided that these simple checks on your condition are maintained as you progress, this should constitute a safe and simple introduction to aerobic exercise. As your programme increases so will your health, but always keep an honest eye on yourself – not the neurotic vigilance of the hypochondriac, but the sensible check on over-enthusiasm.

Now you are ready to jog. You have found that walking at an increased pace for an hour is no longer taxing (maybe you were one of the fitter ones anyway) and you want to push on. Right, get changed, warm up and go out. Start walking briskly and then increase the pace until you feel it would be easier to break into a slow run, which is what jogging is. Continue at this pace until the fatigue is moderately uncomfortable. At that point start walking again. Repeat alternate walking and jogging when you have recovered sufficiently.

There will then come a moment when you feel it becomes too uncomfortable to start jogging again. This time walk all the way back home. Next time you go out and on each successive outing, extend the jogs and the total distance.

This is the old boy scout way of alternate running and walking by which you increase your daily distance in your own way at your own rate of progress.

This jog-walk method offers you the broadest approach to continuous running with the choice of three immediate goals – duration, distance and continuous running. For example, if your goal is half-an-hour of continuous movement you walk-jog until this time is achieved after which you progressively shorten the walking periods until you achieve the full thirty minutes of continuous jogging, or you can set up a target distance, say three or four miles; then you shorten the walking recovery periods until you complete three or four miles of non-stop running.

We feel that the first aim – duration – will provide the best basis for distance running. This, after all, is what we are aiming at and in aerobic training, once a pulse rate around 140–150 is achieved, duration is the aim. Although our genetic inheritance is the ultimate decider of our running ability, endurance is somewhat easier to foster than speed, and in any case endurance is the better base on which to build.

Building Up Distance

For those who want to go on to compete, building up running distance must be the aim. Ultimately, what constitutes fitness will be decided by you, and for us to say you should reach this goal or that would be quite arbitrary. It would over-extend some and perhaps place a false limit on others. But for anyone who has the time and inclination to measure their progress carefully, and who likes testing themselves and securing points against a table, they could well use a graduated (and cautious) training programme, like the one suggested by Kenneth Cooper in his excellent book *The Aerobics Way*.

However, for that non-existent average man, middle-aged, middle-active and middle-weight, a weekly mileage of around twenty-five miles would be enough to help him keep a lot healthier than those who do not run.

Fitting in twenty-five miles of running into your weekly routine should be no great problem. If you take two days off running each week, you are left with five miles each, or five times thirty-five to forty-five minutes. Allowing for changing and freshening up, all you need is to set aside one hour a day at the most, five times a week.

Those who have adequate lockers and facilities at their place of work are the luckiest, because being able to run to or from work is a great advantage. It is healthier and cheaper at the same time. Alternatively if your commuting distance is too long, fitting in some lunchtime training may be possible. The weekends generally offer more opportunities for running, and a six-mile run on both Saturday and Sunday would leave only three more runs of four miles each during the week, say thirty minutes per run.

When broken down like this the total doesn't appear so formidable, and remember, all over the country there are runners logging up totals from forty to eighty miles per week and living normal lives.

A Place to Run

Where should I run? What surface should I run on? These are almost the same question. It is easy to list the desirable qualities of where to run, but in modern urban living it would be rare to find the perfect combination of the ideal and the practical.

Beginners should start running on smooth surfaces which are as true as you can find. This is the time when ankles and feet, which are unaccustomed to running and have not had time to strengthen, are at their most vulnerable. Until you have become used to running on uneven surfaces, try to keep to good paths or on grass that you can trust. Having to look carefully at every footfall while running is boring, and it could get you set into a bad style. By all means scan the ground ahead of you, but keep your head up – if your surroundings are pleasant, enjoy them. While good smooth grass is the best surface on which to run it does mean that you have to live near large open parkland. The paths in most urban parks are well maintained, and they offer the next best choice.

If as an inner city dweller you are forced to be a road runner there are some important do's and don'ts you should observe.

The first requirement is to stay away from main road traffic as much as possible. The concentration required to avoid being run over, particularly when going round parked cars, makes it difficult to slip into the kind of running detachment which makes for pleasure in running. A runner can get into a complete mental and physical rhythm – running on auto-pilot – that allows you

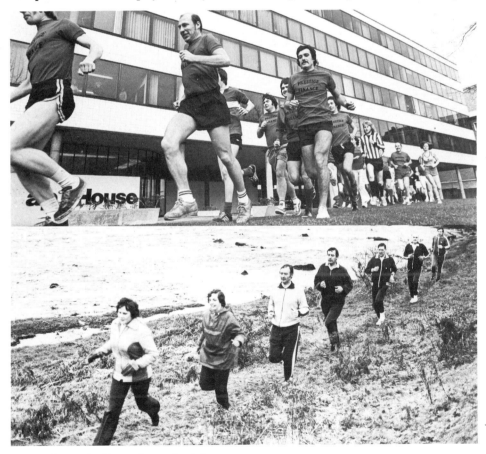

Town and around: office workers at lunchtime,
families at the weekend –
two faces of the jogging club

to complete a run leaving your body healthily worked and your mind refreshed. This is neither easy nor safe on busy roads, and busy pavements are by definition impossible places for safe and satisfying running.

Wherever and whenever main road running is necessary, if at all possible avoid them at peak traffic hours. Running to and from your place of work is fine, but a heavy concentration of cars and lorries means a heavy concentration of exhaust gases; carbon monoxide is poisonous, and so is the lead in petrol fumes. Find the quietest roads you can, and if they are free enough the pavements are the best to run on. You may have to step off when you cross junctions but the pavement will be flatter than the road, which will have a camber.

If you are near to rural or semi-rural roads, then of course you will run in the road. The classic golden rule of running in the road is: face the oncoming traffic except when this would mean running on the inside of a tight bend, when you cannot be seen and cannot see what is coming.

Unfortunately what is good for road safety is bad for your legs. Continual running on a sloping surface is very likely to set up imbalance injuries – stress fractures are not unknown and knee pains are common, and there is a marked tendency to a sideways tilt of the pelvis and the lumbar region of the spine.

Running on the crown of the road reduces this risk, but substitutes that of being hit in the back by a lorry. The next best thing you can do is to alternate between sides, say every half mile, and look carefully when you switch over.

In summer, with longer hours of daylight, your choice of courses or routes is wider. Winter running restricts this choice to adequately lit roads. Determined runners, who believe they have good night vision and who wear bright reflecting clothing or over-vests, do go night running. Their precautions may even extend to a small bulb at their back, powered by a battery attached to a belt. Night running on unlit roads with its attendant risks is a personal decision, but what might drive a top competitor to train regardless is not so necessary to a fitness runner.

Crisp dry snow that is not too deep is good to run on. The higher knee lift required is strengthening and good for your running action, and the additional effort can be as hard as you want to make it. The general atmosphere is cheerful and refreshing, particularly when you are out with a group. But it does have a few hazards of its own. Don't run on unfamiliar ground. Don't run unless you have a good idea of what is under the snow. If there is only a thin layer of powdery snow on the grass or tarmac this is fine, but an apparently smooth layer of snow merely covering hard and rutted ice can be dangerous. You may not actually fall over or slide into an obstacle, but there are other ways of getting athletic injuries. In these conditions a runner instinctively tries to curl his toes into the ground to scratch for traction. This can give rise to shin splints, soreness in the fibula or a very 'bruised' feeling in the feet. All these injuries are common from running on uneven, hard-packed snow. Groin strain from trying to stop legs from slipping away sideways is another danger and in our experience these ill effects last a long time, sometimes as much as six to eight weeks. The more obvious risks are low park railings, sometimes only inches off the ground, or lightly covered pot-holes. If you are likely to be running in snow in winter, it is worth studying the ground in the autumn.

In extreme snow and ice, in order to run at all, you may have to wait until traffic has lessened and use a restricted course on roads that are well cleared and gritted.

This kind of restriction necessarily cuts down your choice of route. Varying your runs between flat and hilly courses not only adds variety but should be an essential part of the correct application of the running load. Top athletes know the advantages of phasing hard and easy sessions, and the beginner should not make every run the same length or tackle it with the same intensity.

The degree to which you need and seek variety in your routes depends entirely upon yourself. You must explore your own areas thoroughly and with imagination. When training in Sheffield finding hills is never a problem; in Loughborough this is quite another matter. You know your own area best.

If you decide to do your running on the local track, please respect it. Unless you are a sprinter and need to practise bend running or relay handovers in marked-out zones, or you need accurately measured distances for comparative times in sets of repetitions, there is very little need for training on tracks. But if you must use the track for winter lighting, freedom from traffic or whatever, please keep out of the two inner lanes. These are habitually churned up by people plodding round, getting in the way of those who are using the facility properly. On cinder tracks this is a nuisance; on synthetic tracks the cost of relaying the principal lanes, particularly the inside lane, is considerable. If you feel you must know exactly how long one lap is when running in any of the outer lanes, just measure the distance from the inside edge of the track to the centre of the lane you have chosen, subtract 30cm (one foot) and multiply by 6.286. Add 400 metres and this is the length of your lap.

The change of scene so important in avoiding boredom is rather easier at weekends, and more so in the summer. If you have a car, drive out into the country, and use an ordnance survey map to look for suitable rights of way or large estates open to the public – which could provide pleasant running surroundings. Indeed, for any runner looking for fresh routes the ordnance survey maps are worth an hour's study; and booklets describing country walks often include stretches that would make suitable running routes – sometimes fields, sometimes roads, sometimes both.

Such spaces as Chatsworth in Derbyshire, Clumber Park in Nottinghamshire, Wimbledon Common and Richmond Park in Surrey, and the Downs in Sussex are all attractive and explorable. Coupled with a picnic such places could provide a pleasant compromise between a family weekend outing and an agreeable new running experience.

It might also give a husband and wife the chance to run together – something that varying work patterns often make difficult at other times. But even during a busy week it might make a pleasant change to run together – and might solve the potential problems for women running unescorted on the darker winter evenings.

Stretching Exercises

We all of us, athlete and non-athlete, share with the animals a common experience of stretching, particularly after sleep – it is the natural way of easing ourselves into activity.

We do it because after a period of rest, and especially when the rest follows spells of activity, the fascia of each muscle tends to contract. This tension – which can be severe after muscle spasms caused by cold or by bad posture – puts pressure on nerve fibres which can cause irritation or even pain – so the fascia has to be restretched to allow the muscle to relax fully.

Repeated use of any muscle through the sort of limited, unvarying range that a runner submits it to will make it increasingly hard and tense; the bigger the muscle becomes through training, the more it and its associated tendon come under tension. So a more elaborate programme of gentle stretching, to release this muscle tension, is advisable for all runners. If done properly it will produce many of the benefits of a relaxing massage – the soothed and smoothed-out feeling of relaxation.

The exercises should be done in the warm – they are best not attempted if the conditions are cold and you are unable to warm up thoroughly before you start. Too many runners have been injured by attempting incautious exercises before they have properly warmed up.

If you have a sedentary job it is worth cultivating the habit of stretching (simply, not the whole programme) after an hour or two of sitting. Students should stretch between classes and those who have to adopt rather fixed positions at work should stretch during lunch and tea breaks.

As we grow older, our natural suppleness is gradually reduced, and a good programme of stretching can do much to keep us supple, relaxed and comparatively free from tension.

The trouble with stretching exercises is that they really are rather boring. I know that they have to be done, but I got so fed up years ago with doing them in sequence in a long session that I have now got into the habit of spreading them out through the day.

I may be sitting chatting to someone when for no apparent reason I'll get up and start trying to push the wall over – all I'm doing is exercising a calf muscle; or I'll find myself sitting watching television with my leg folded under me doing hurdling type exercises. It's far more practical, stretching like that, than by setting aside half an hour to go through the whole routine. And I find I can fit as much in during the day as I used to in a formal session. I think this is the reason those workout books and tapes have become so popular lately: people know they want to get fit and supple, but they *are* looking for a bit of flavour to keep the work interesting.

There are times, though, when these exercises have to be done in a concentrated sequence. Obviously before a race or before a fast training session I can't leave anything to chance – I've got to stretch all the muscles I might have to call on in a hurry. And in winter, too, I tend to do a lot of stretching before I leave the warmth of the house. Cold muscles are more at risk anyway, but there are added hazards in winter.

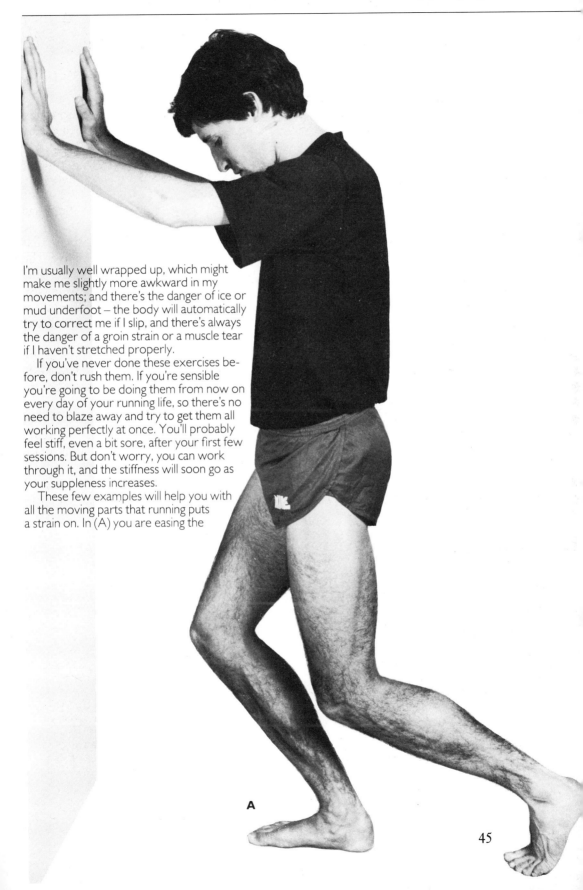

I'm usually well wrapped up, which might make me slightly more awkward in my movements; and there's the danger of ice or mud underfoot – the body will automatically try to correct me if I slip, and there's always the danger of a groin strain or a muscle tear if I haven't stretched properly.

If you've never done these exercises before, don't rush them. If you're sensible you're going to be doing them from now on every day of your running life, so there's no need to blaze away and try to get them all working perfectly at once. You'll probably feel stiff, even a bit sore, after your first few sessions. But don't worry, you can work through it, and the stiffness will soon go as your suppleness increases.

These few examples will help you with all the moving parts that running puts a strain on. In (A) you are easing the

A

45

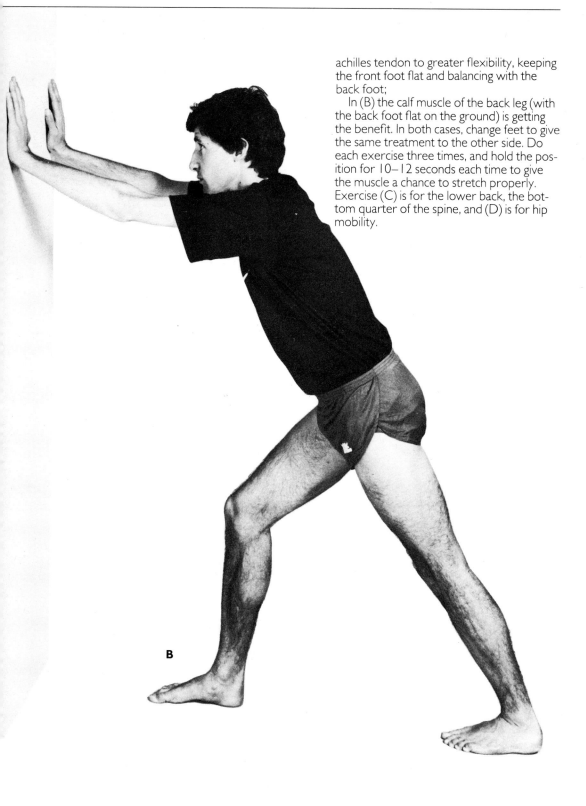

achilles tendon to greater flexibility, keeping the front foot flat and balancing with the back foot;

In (B) the calf muscle of the back leg (with the back foot flat on the ground) is getting the benefit. In both cases, change feet to give the same treatment to the other side. Do each exercise three times, and hold the position for 10–12 seconds each time to give the muscle a chance to stretch properly. Exercise (C) is for the lower back, the bottom quarter of the spine, and (D) is for hip mobility.

B

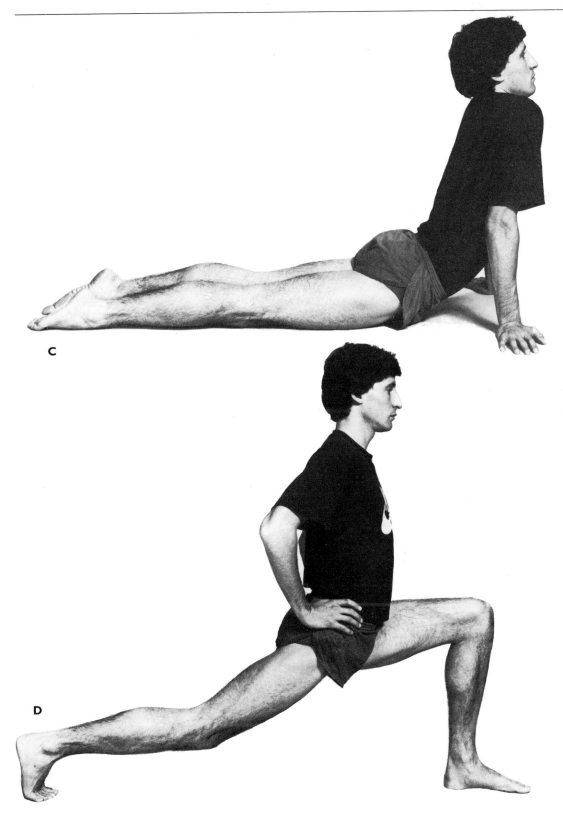

C

D

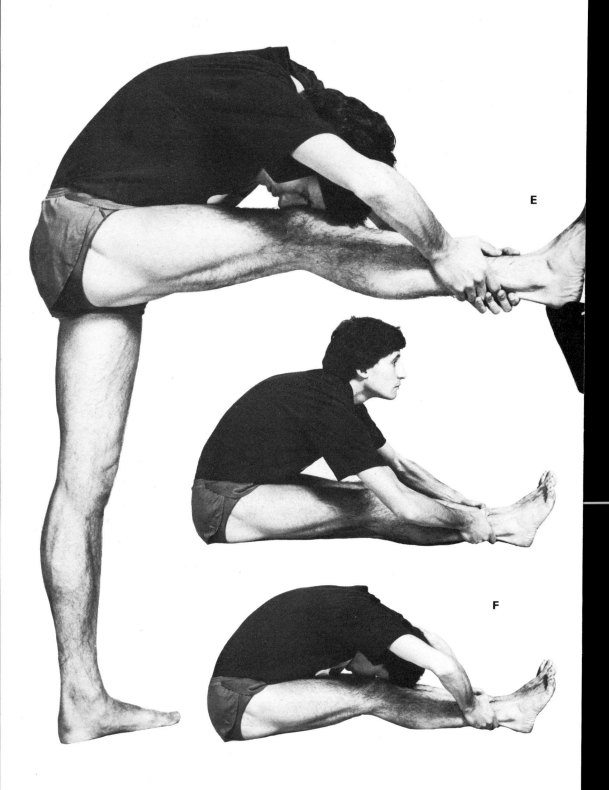

E

F

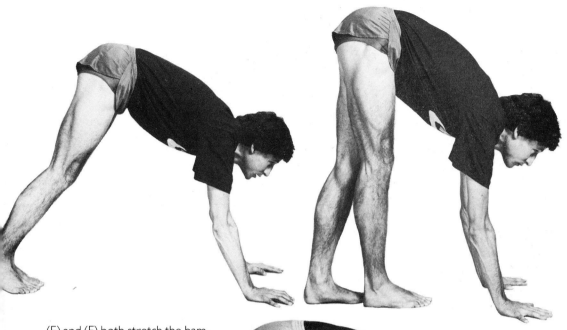

(E) and (F) both stretch the hamstrings (the former, of course, to be done with both legs outstretched in turn), and (F) also gives even greater flexibility to the lower back.

Finally (G) is a really good all-round stretching and flexing movement. A lot of you will hardly be able to move forward at all to begin with, but in time you should be able to walk right up to your hands, even with palms and heels flat on the floor.

None of these is a jerky exercise. You should apply the pressure gradually in every case, hold each position for about 10 seconds, and gradually take the pressure off. Remember, you are *easing* your muscles into greater flexibility, not snapping them into shape.

G

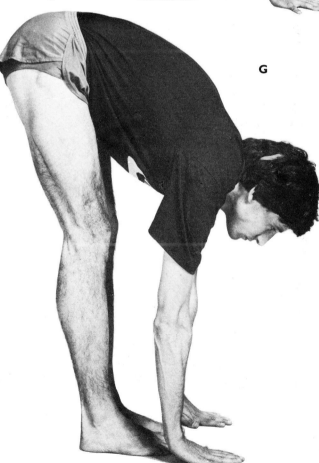

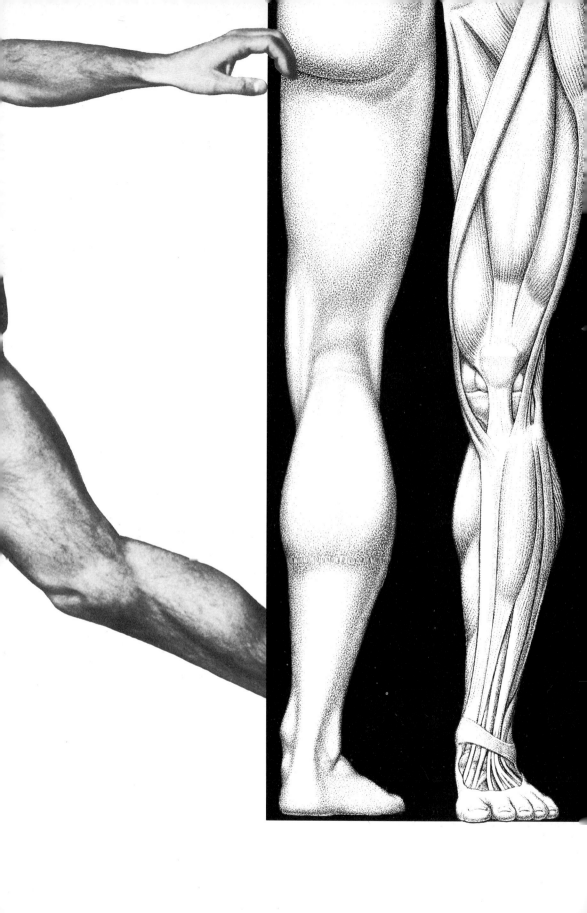

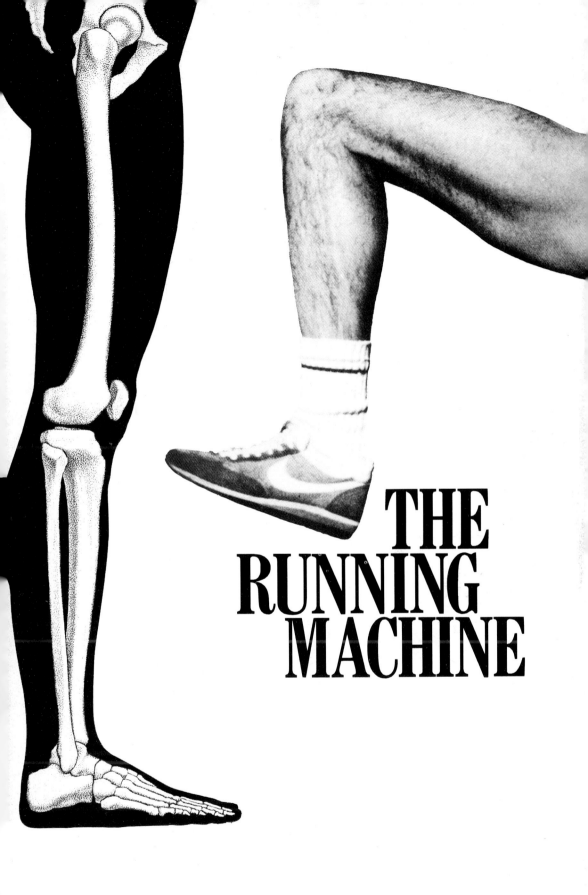

THE RUNNING MACHINE

'Stiffen the sinews, summon up the blood . . .':
priming the finely-tuned machine

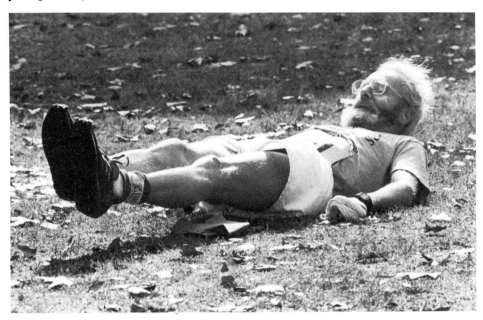

Now that you have decided that your goal is fitness, and that you are going to employ running as a means to that goal, it might be worth looking at just what is meant by 'physical fitness'.

Fred Wilt's *Run Run Run* gives a definition that we rather like. He defines fitness as 'the development of a body to a state or condition which permits the performance of a given amount of work, when desired, with minimum physical effort. The efficiency of physical effort depends upon the mutual development of the muscular, respiratory and circulatory systems.' This is a particularly useful description, because it introduces the idea of changing the state of the body.

If you are going to achieve physical fitness by running, you are going to have to run with sufficient intensity to produce significant physiological changes in your cardiovascular system (your heart, lungs and bloodstream) as well as in certain muscle groups; improved efficiency of the cardiovascular system is a basic requirement for all-round fitness. The effect of running on the muscle groups is rather more specific to running.

You are running to become and to remain fit, not to earn a Ph.D., and in attempting to explain the physical effect of running we do not propose to give a potted degree course in anatomy. Sports medicine and physiology are sciences, and a runner needs only to know enough to use them as a useful tool. It is more important for you to know where to go for information and advice than to try to turn yourself into an encyclopaedia of sports medicine, but it is as well if the runner can learn to cope with the occasional physical problems that might arise, and he will certainly have a better understanding of the complexities of the human body.

Training and the Body

Running for fitness will have a number of specific effects on the body; all will help you to run better and also, to a large extent, all will be beneficial to the efficiency and well-being of the body in general.

First, training brings about the enlargement of muscle fibres (not their number – that is determined at birth), giving them the power to work harder and more effectively, given an adequate supply of fuel.

Training will increase the number of the minute energy sources in the muscles – the *mitochondria* – which use the oxygen extracted from the blood to provide the energy needed for muscle contraction. More mitochondria will mean easier and faster fuelling of the muscles, which in turn means more efficient muscles.

This increased production of fuel will call for an increased supply of oxygen from the blood. To this end, a trained body will have an increased number of capillaries – the tiny vessels carrying the oxygenated blood to the muscles (tests have shown some 40 per cent more capillaries serving the thigh muscles of trained athletes than in the thighs of untrained subjects).

Finally, to meet this increased demand for oxygen, the heart-lung system will have to work harder and more efficiently. The heart, and the muscles which help the lungs to breathe deeply, will themselves grow extra capillaries and will work more efficiently, and your cardiac output will increase – the heart will need to beat less often to pump the same amount of blood around the body.

That, at its simplest, is what the walking, the jogging and finally the running will eventually do for you. The effect of running for fitness will be to produce a more efficient fuelling of the muscle mechanism for its task of moving the bones.

The Working Parts

It is quite possible to drive a car for your entire adult life without the faintest idea of what is going on under the bonnet. If, however, you take up motor racing, and need to get the best out of your car, you will quickly become obsessive about torque and gear ratios and anything which will contribute to the conversion of fuel into speed.

In just the same way a human, who is quite content in his pre-exercise existence as long as his body gets him adequately from place to place, tends to become fascinated by the working of this body once he is asking it to perform more efficiently. At top levels of competition this fascination, and what it reveals, becomes crucial to performance, but we felt that anyone determined to take the trouble to alter his or her body by running would welcome a more detailed summary of how a running body works, and why it works better as we get fitter.

The body is a machine, albeit a very complex and elegant one, and the Oxford

Dictionary defines a machine as 'an apparatus in which the action of several parts is combined for the application of force to a purpose'. When we think of applying force, we usually think first of levers, and human levers are part of the skeleton.

The Bones

Our skeleton has two main functions. It provides a framework to protect the organs contained within it, and it provides points to which muscles can be attached, thus converting it to a machine for exerting force.

Our long bones in the limbs form the levers for lifting and locomotion, and our joints are the hinges and pivots of the machine; the levers themselves are held in place by the muscles and ligaments, and the whole frame is built on and around the spinal column.

Bones are beautifully constructed to give the best strength-to-weight ratio to suit their function. The short bones and some of the irregular bones are made to take compression but the long bones – the long levers of our arms and legs – are *hollow*, with a thicker wall in the middle, and they cope with a lot of bending and torsional stress as well as compression. They all contain bone marrow, which is the source of the blood cells.

Bones are strong, but stress is seldom applied to them simply. They are frequently subject to a combination of different forces – bending, twisting and compression at the same time – and they can quite easily be broken without any apparent impact. It only takes prolonged overuse, coupled with an imbalance of some sort, to effect a stress fracture.

An examination of the microstructure of bones reveals the special alignment of the bone substances to meet the forces imposed on them. Exercise maintains and improves this microstructure; inactivity reduces the strength and density of the bones. What we can do, by maintaining muscle tone and by the sensible choice of running shoes, is to protect them from unnecessary stress.

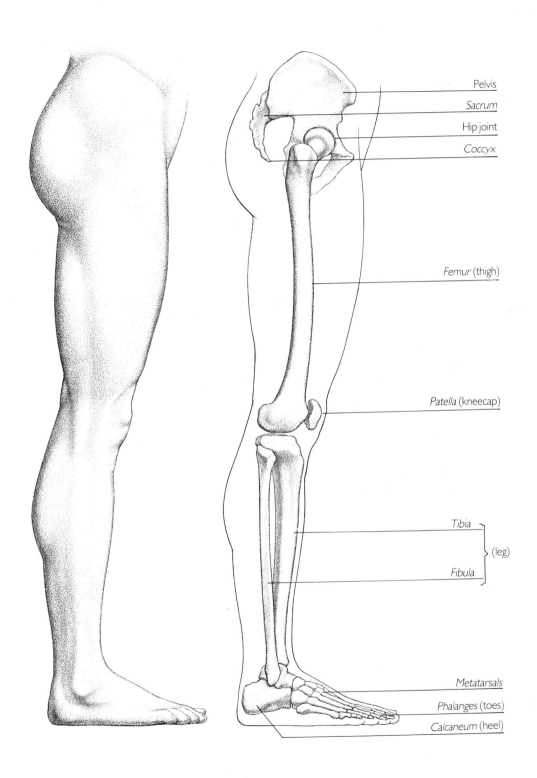

Pelvis

Sacrum

Hip joint

Coccyx

Femur (thigh)

Patella (kneecap)

Tibia

(leg)

Fibula

Metatarsals

Phalanges (toes)

Calcaneum (heel)

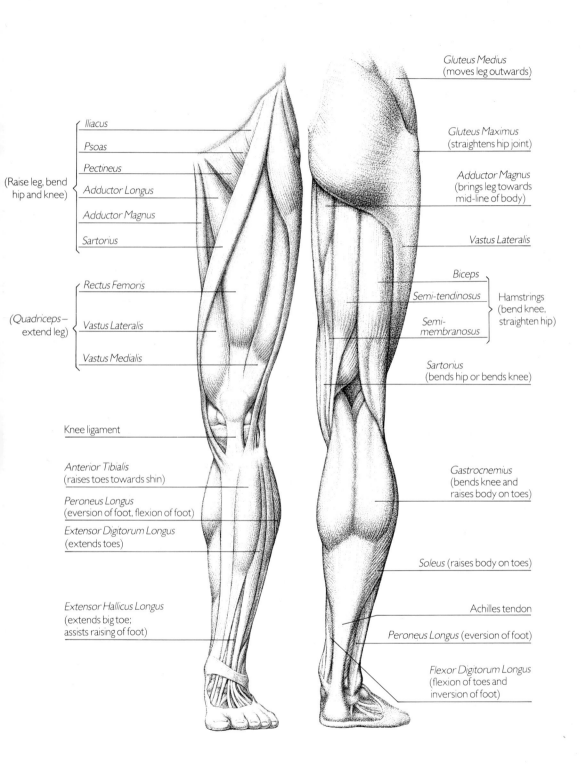

Gluteus Medius
(moves leg outwards)

Iliacus

Gluteus Maximus
(straightens hip joint)

Psoas

Pectineus

(Raise leg, bend
hip and knee)

Adductor Magnus
(brings leg towards
mid-line of body)

Adductor Longus

Adductor Magnus

Sartorius

Vastus Lateralis

Rectus Femoris

Biceps

Semi-tendinosus

Hamstrings
(bend knee,
straighten hip)

(Quadriceps –
extend leg)

Vastus Lateralis

Semi-
membranosus

Vastus Medialis

Sartorius
(bends hip or bends knee)

Knee ligament

Anterior Tibialis
(raises toes towards shin)

Gastrocnemius
(bends knee and
raises body on toes)

Peroneus Longus
(eversion of foot, flexion of foot)

Extensor Digitorum Longus
(extends toes)

Soleus (raises body on toes)

Extensor Hallicus Longus
(extends big toe;
assists raising of foot)

Achilles tendon

Peroneus Longus (eversion of foot)

Flexor Digitorum Longus
(flexion of toes and
inversion of foot)

The Muscles

Muscles are agents for moving things, and the skeletal muscles – the ones which move the long levers of our bones, are the ones that most concern the runner.

Skeletal muscle in the limbs is generally spindle-shaped – thickest in the middle and tapering at either end where it becomes tendon. Muscles are encased in tough, non-elastic membranes called *fasciae*, which not only surround them but also form part of their attachment to the bone. Muscles stretch and contract like elastic bands; tendons, which are tough, fibrous strands of varying thickness and form the cables linking muscles to the bone, stretch very little.

All skeletal muscles link two or more bones; they are anchored to the fibrous covering (*periosteum*) of these bones, generally with one tendon at the fixed end (known as the *origin*) and the other at the moving end (the *insertion*). Under certain conditions or injuries these endings can become detached.

Muscles cross the joint which they move – some cross more than one joint, and therefore produce movement in more than one place (the biceps, for example, which cross elbow and shoulder and cause flexion of both joints).

Mobility, then, is simply achieved by muscles contracting or relaxing, and so allowing the bones to move in the required direction. But not quite as simply as that. For the muscles achieve something every bit as vital as that – they *control* movement: depending on the signal they receive from the brain, the voluntary muscles – the ones that move when we want them to – can react either strongly or weakly.

As an example, bend your arm. The movement itself is pronounced, but the effort is minimal, and there is only the very slightest sensation of effort – even if the movement is done quite quickly. Now bend your arm again, but at the same time resist that bending by trying to keep it straight. You can still bend the arm at varying speeds, but also with as great an effort as you want to apply. Quite simply, the triceps, the muscle down the back of the arm, has been trying to restrain the biceps, the muscle in front, from doing its job. One muscle has been monitoring the action of the other, as it were by a paying out process.

This is the secret of any animal's ability to make the most subtle and refined movements: muscles involved in driving the body tend to work in pairs or in combinations, grouped round joints each having opposing actions. These muscles are known according to the movement they produce; every flexor muscle (for bending a joint) is opposed by an extensor (for straightening it); a supinator (turning upwards) by a pronator (turning downwards); an internal rotator by an external rotator, and so on.

Almost any physical action needs the combined movement of many pairs of muscles, and this action is known as muscle co-ordination. Even the act of standing still involves the use of muscles controlling the ankle, knee, hip, vertebral column, and head – a co-ordination that is very difficult, and takes a long time to master, but once learnt can be performed at will with ease and without thinking.

Muscles have other functions besides movement. With ligaments they hold the body together by helping to keep the joints in place. For example, the strength and condition of the knee joint depends very much upon the strength and tone of the quadriceps, the front thigh muscles. When a muscle is at rest it is still very slightly in tension. This tension and any slight movement generates heat, so that a good muscle condition – or muscle tone, as it is called – is important in both protecting the joints and in maintaining the body temperature. The effect of good muscle tone is particularly obvious in winter.

There are three kinds of muscle each with its own function and structure. We naturally tend to be most concerned about our *voluntary muscles* – those which remain under our conscious control. To these muscles the brain sends out signals via the central nervous system, and the muscles contract to order.

The *involuntary muscles* are not under our conscious control, but take their instructions from the autonomic nervous system. This system is concerned with regulating the automatic functions of the body, among them the heartbeat and the dilation and constriction of blood vessels; the automatic adjustment of their functions is very important, no more so than when we start running. When a conscious decision is taken to run, the autonomic system also becomes involved, automatically issuing special instructions to those parts of the system not under conscious control.

The *heart muscle* is a bit of an exception. While it is an involuntary muscle, it does have a somewhat similar micro-structure to the voluntary muscle, but it cannot sustain prolonged contraction.

The Vital Question

We are now going to get technical. In order to understand how running can help fitness, or why our diet might need changing, and why our cardiovascular system might need improving, we need to have a reasonably detailed answer to one simple question. How does a complex bundle of fibres try to pull its ends together and so move the working parts of our body?

Without going into photo-micrographs and a detailed study of electro-chemical reactions and the nature of enzymes and a description of the whole nervous system, this is roughly what happens.

Skeletal muscles, as we have seen, are wrapped in a sheath (fascia) and tapered at each end. Inside the outer sheath are bundles containing muscle fibres, each surrounded by a membrane (the *sarcolemma*). Each individual fibre is a round elongated single cell. Inside this cell are even thinner elements called myofibrils; these are the cell's contracting elements.

The myofibrils consist of two even smaller elements of protein – the larger is myosin, the smaller actin; and all these tiny filaments move in a fluid containing protein, glycogen and phosphates; this fluid reaches the muscle fibre through the sarcolemma and, in a two-way exchange system, waste products are carried away into the blood stream once the fuel in the fluid has been broken down.

It is believed that the muscle contracts when, on command from the brain, a temporary affinity of the myosin for the actin filaments causes each thin actin filament to slide over the thick myosin filament by means of a minute ratchet system. This action needs energy, and the energy demands fuel. In this case the fuel is adenosine triphosphate (ATP).

The continued replacement of this substance is absolutely necessary if we are to keep moving, and yet there is only a minimal amount of ATP present in the muscle at any given moment – enough to sustain contraction for just half a second before it needs to be replenished. When this is used up, a further five seconds' worth of fuel is found by breaking down another compound, CP (creatin phosphate) to produce more ATP. Then, when this is finished, some of the glycogen stored in the muscle is converted to ATP by a process called *anaerobic glycolysis*; this will keep us going at an intense level of activity for a full three-quarters of a minute.

Now that all the resources stored in the muscle have been used, the body has to think again – and call on a different system.

The Oxygen Process

Those first three steps in the muscle's use of its energy supply can all take place anaerobically – meaning 'without oxygen'. In these anaerobic processes, when chemical bonds are being broken down, by-products are created which – if they cannot be recycled or eliminated quickly enough – will build up, clog the system and eventually stop the muscle moving. When glycogen is broken down without the aid of oxygen to form ATP the process forms lactic acid as a byproduct, which so increases the level of acidity that the muscle cells cannot work. This is why neither you nor the best runners in the world can sprint flat out for, say, 400 metres before seizing up.

Any runner, trained or untrained, will breathe faster and deeper if he begins to run very quickly. He soon exhausts all the energy stored in his muscles, and his body is demanding an increased supply of the one substance that can now be used to enable the muscle to carry on continuous work – oxygen. You can carry stores of fuel, but the body cannot store oxygen.

The level at which you can maintain sustained work depends upon the amount of air you can get into and out of your lungs and the amount of oxygen you can extract from the air that you are breathing in. In fact one of the simplest guides to your progress towards fitness is how much longer it takes you to get out of breath when running at the same pace. It re-emphasises that the basis for all-round fitness is the improvement of the respiratory and cardiovascular systems.

The oxygen is carried round the body by the haemoglobin in the blood. In the muscle a substance is waiting called myoglobin, which has an even greater affinity for oxygen than has the haemoglobin; the haemoglobin readily yields up its oxygen to the myoglobin, picks up in turn the carbon dioxide which is the useless byproduct of the energy-making process, and takes it back to the lungs where it is breathed out.

Meanwhile, in the muscle, the process that allows long-distance runners to run long distances is taking place. It is called *aerobic glycolysis*, and involves the conversion of the muscle's glycogen, by means of the oxygen, into the ATP so necessary to sustain movement. This process takes place inside the mitochondria – tiny units (anything up to five thousand of them in a single cell) which produce the requisite enzymes, break down the proteins and the oxygen, and manufacture the necessary fuel for the muscle.

And, conveniently for all of us who want to see improvement in performance when we start running, mitochondria will grow in number when the muscles in the body begin regularly to demand more fuel.

The Blood Supply

This increased supply of fuel to the muscles, though, can be maintained only as long as the blood supply is increased. But the minute, fern-like capillaries at the end of the blood-line cannot cope – if they have been used to the comparatively leisurely blood flow of a sedentary individual – with a sudden increase in the demand for oxygen-rich blood.

They, too, will increase in number in a body in training, ensuring an easier flow of oxygen to the muscle cells; and at the same time, by the body's system of non-return valves and with some help from the contractions of the muscle itself, carry away the waste product, and CO_2 can be returned to the lungs more quickly and efficiently via the increased number of capillaries serving the veins.

This increased blood supply throughout the body is achieved in part, of course, by the heart simply beating faster, and in the early stages of fitness running this will be the only way that the heart meets the extra demand.

But in time your body will undergo the most important physiological change of all. Your heart will pump out more blood per beat than it did before – so your body will be getting the same blood with a heart beating slower . . . the machine will be, once again, operating more efficiently, and your pulse taken at rest will chart the improvement.

The heart, considered purely as a pump, generally has a low mechanical efficiency (estimated at only 10 per cent when at rest) so even the most modest increase in this efficiency can be seen as a large improvement.

For example, take an untrained person with a heart-rate at rest of 72 beats per minute. If, under a work load (say running) his rate increases to 180 beats per minute, this would theoretically increase his cardiac output two-and-a-half times. After proper training, though, his resting heart-rate would be as low as 40 beats per minute. So when he runs hard enough to increase his heart-rate to 180 beats per minute he is increasing his cardiac output four-and-a-half times – a dramatic 80 per cent improvement.

Not all this increased efficiency is felt by the skeletal muscles. The heart itself is a muscle and a non-stop muscle at that. It too will need extra capillaries to serve its own extra demand. And so too will the muscles which the lungs depend on. Extra blood coming round the body is no use unless it carries the vital oxygen with it, and the demand for extra oxygen means extra work for the lungs.

To fill our lungs with the air we need we increase the size of the thoracic cavity, the space inside our chest. While we are at rest, the diaphragm does most of this work, simply by raising and lowering itself and varying the available space; the movement is quite small – perhaps half an inch or so up and

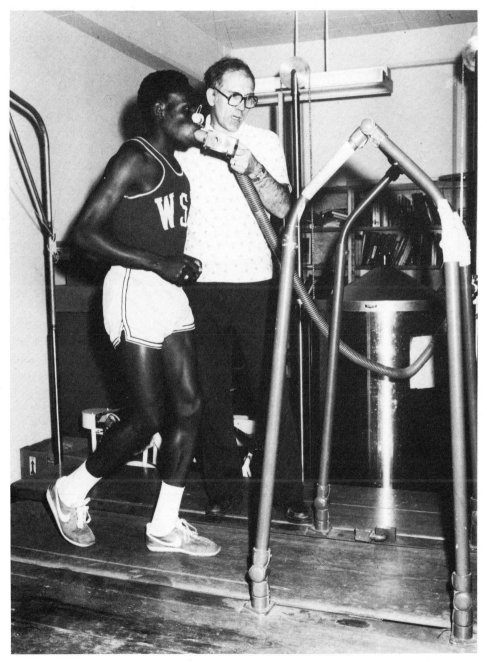

**Looking under the bonnet: a test-bed
examination of the high-performance Henry Rono**

down – but deep breathing can increase its movement to three or four inches.

During hard exercise we are demanding even more air. Now the intercostal muscles will raise and lower the rib cage, thus further increasing the space in our chest, reducing the pressure inside and allowing the atmospheric pressure outside to force air in and inflate the lungs to their maximum. The very act of breathing itself, as we know, can become hard work, and indeed some 10 per cent of that increased supply of oxygen we are taking in is going to be used to fuel the breathing mechanism alone – most of it to overcome the natural resistance found in our air passages; no wonder, when we start breathing hard, we need to use our mouths as well as our noses.

Once the air is in the trachea, conducting airways divide and subdivide to conduct air to the minute alveoli – some three hundred and fifty million of them in each lung – from which the oxygen diffuses into the blood and through which the returning carbon dioxide is taken from the blood to be breathed out.

The cycle, then, is both ingenious and straightforward: air to the lungs, oxygen to the haemoglobin of the blood, blood pumped round the body by the heart to its farthest capillaries, haemoglobin transferring oxygen to the myoglobin of the muscles, mitochondria using that oxygen to synthesise ATP, muscles using the ATP as fuel and returning the waste carbon dioxide to the blood, capillaries returning carbon dioxide to the veins and back to the lungs, lungs breathing out the unwanted carbon dioxide and starting all over again.

In a body which has achieved any degree of fitness by running, the lungs will accept increased and continuous supplies of air without difficulty; the heart will pump more oxygen-rich blood through the body at every stroke; there will be more capillaries to carry the oxygen to the muscles; there will be more

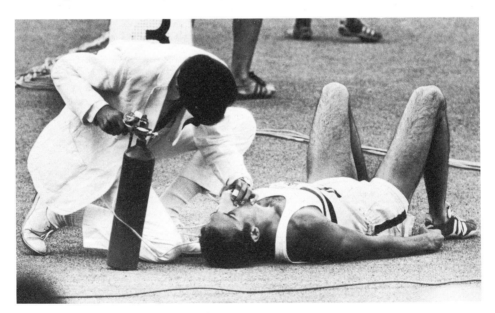

Running out of fuel: a lungful of much-needed oxygen at the high-altitude Mexico Olympics

mitochondria to use the oxygen to fuel the muscle; and the muscle fibres themselves will be thicker and more tightly packed, and will thus contract with greater force.

A word about Smoking – Don't

The whole respiratory tract is an air filter. It starts by removing the largest dust particles in the nose where they are trapped by moisture or hair. In the airways in the lungs some of the surface area is cilliated. This means the surface cells have small hair-like whips which exert a non-stop concerted flailing action, a fast upward movement with a slow return. The whips are covered with a thin sticky mucus which holds any particle which falls on them; the mucus, and the rubbish it holds, moves steadily up the airways to the throat where it is either swallowed or spat out. This process can tolerate a lot, but cigarette smoke will slow it down, if not stop it altogether. In other words, smoking prevents our breathing machine from operating its own self-cleansing mechanism.

Furthermore, at the very end of the airways, inside the alveoli, another process occurs by which small scavengers called macrophages finally clear up and dispose of any unwanted matter at the very point where oxygen is taken into the blood. Again, smoking will impair this important function. So even if you don't believe lung cancer will happen to you, it is clear that smoking is actively working against your maintaining health and achieving the fitness you are running for.

So many people lead such sedentary lives that they will not notice the physiological effects of smoking until any real physical effort is required. Then the limiting effects of smoking are clearly felt. Depending upon the time elapsed between the last cigarette and the start of physical effort, for the same load smokers will have a heart rate which is ten to twenty beats per minute faster than that of non-smokers.

Smoking, too, will increase airway resistance two- or three-fold, thus multiplying the greater part of the effort of breathing. Again, if you are sitting slumped in a chair, with the lungs demanding very little air, this may not seem to matter. But when you are running, trying to meet the body's demand for oxygen, it becomes very important indeed.

The haemoglobin in our blood has an affinity for oxygen, but it has a far higher affinity for carbon monoxide. Smoke contains some 4 per cent carbon monoxide and since haemoglobin is naturally going to pick up the carbon monoxide first, the oxygen-carrying capacity of the blood is immediately reduced. This is the very opposite of the condition we require for enhanced fitness. Furthermore the body does not have any means of making up the deficiency during exercise or hard work. It is also worth considering that a concentration of 0.1 per cent or more of carbon monoxide in the air is highly toxic and would soon kill you.

Smoking tobacco was, is and always will be bad for you.

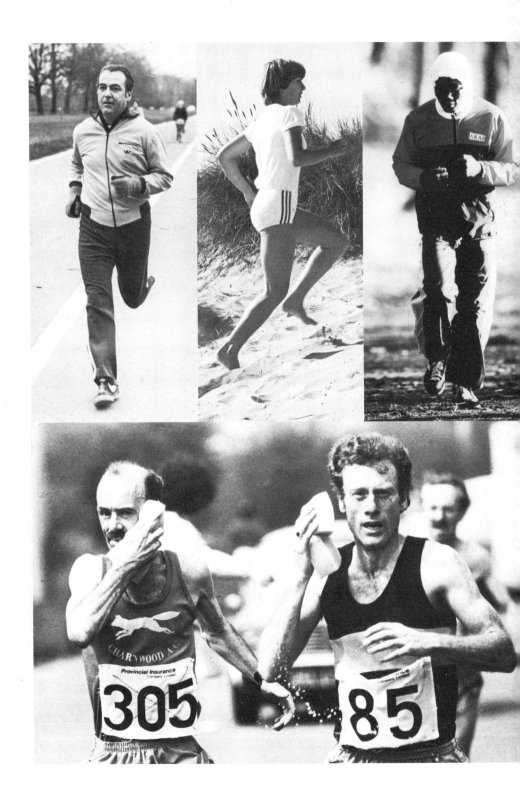

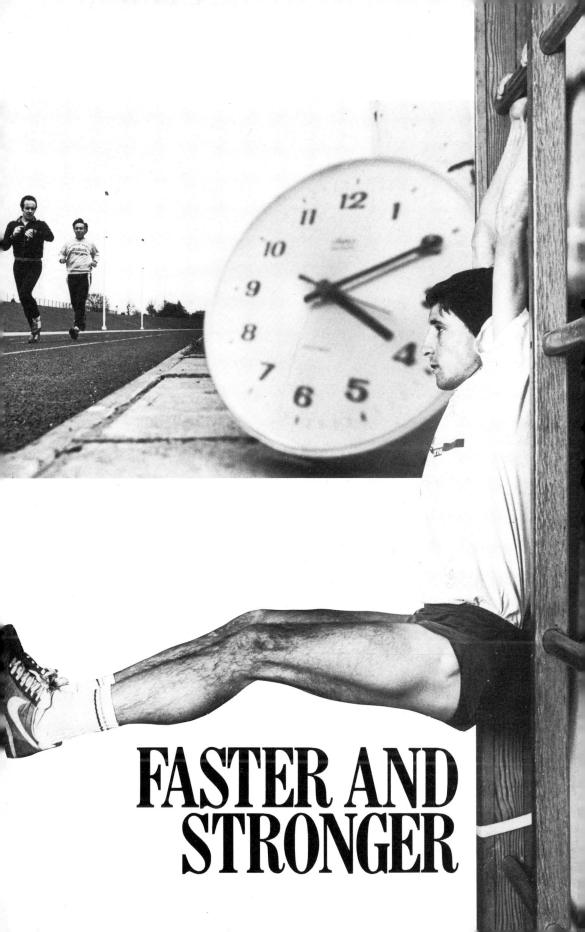

FASTER AND STRONGER

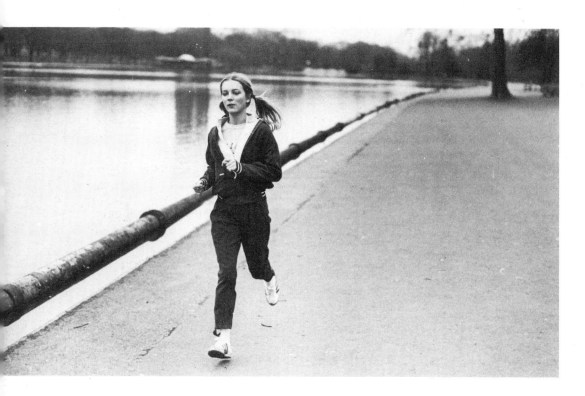

Now that the beginner is on the road, happy with the running he or she has undertaken, and perhaps aware already of some of the changes that it is beginning to bring about in the body, we can think about adding strength and distance and perhaps speed, too. From mere running, we are turning to something more like training.

Training means different things to different people. For many athletes it will be a means to a specific and very clear end – a particular race or an area championship. For others it will be the transition from a relaxed winter to a summer of active competition. To the newcomer, it might mean the eventual achievement of a best distance, or a personal best time on the local track – or just the further satisfaction of measurable progress. In a later chapter we will be looking at the question of training for a specific purpose. Here we can consider training in its most general terms – in increasing strength, in running more economically, in dressing properly, and so on.

The Basic Principles of Training

We have seen that running can produce changes in the body that will enable the body to work better. Training runners is an extension of that same theory – it involves changing their bodies sufficiently to improve their performance significantly.

If you apply a stress to the body, it will respond with an adaptation to that stress, so that it becomes capable of meeting the new demand. By carefully applying work loads, and allowing the proper recovery periods, the trainer will slowly and steadily raise the runner to a plateau of excellence beyond which the loading would become too severe and the runner would break down. This process calls for great care and subtlety on the part of the trainer – to maximise the runner's potential and yet avoid going over the top.

For most runners, operating at lower level and in most cases training themselves, the same principle applies. All runners, once moderately fit, will want to test themselves further; all will recognise the benefits of recovery periods – of hard and less hard training weeks; and all will know of, though few would be silly enough to put themselves at risk from, the dangers of seriously overdoing it – in their case indeed, it is likely that their bodies would rebel before they reached any danger point.

For the runner at the higher level, the trainer is now likely to apply the *principle of specificity*. This says that for the various tasks required from the body, there are exercises specific to that function. Curling with dumb-bells, for example, is specific to the biceps, swinging Indian clubs is not. As far as we are concerned, running is specific to running, soccer, though a perfectly good and enjoyable exercise, is not.

The application of this principle is further refined by applying different types of running training to improve the response of all the body's energy systems to their best advantage. Once again, runners at the top level are likely to use all the types of running described below – particularly those training for middle- and long-distance events.

Steady distance running: aerobic training, as we have seen in the previous chapter, can improve lungs, heart, and muscles for endurance work. The resting heart-rate will drop, the body will take in more air, and will take more oxygen from that air, and the network of blood vessels supplying blood to the muscles will increase.

Faster, interrupted running: known as interval training, this can powerfully stimulate the stroke-volume of the heart. It is not a method that should be used by the very young, or by those without an adequate background of distance work.

High-speed running: these sessions (anaerobic training) will eventually help to cope with these occasions when the byproducts of the muscles are creating conditions in the body which are unfavourable to further exertion.

Training schedules combining all three methods, and based on the general principles we began with, can be applied to any runner on an individual basis by a knowledgeable coach. All, too, in their way, can be of benefit to the fitness runner, though he or she is likely to lean far more on steady distance running, perhaps spiced with some interval training, than on the high-speed work.

There is a fourth type of training discipline whose main virtue is that it is *not* discipline. It can be used equally well by fun runners, club athletes and international stars, and it has the thumbs-up from coaches and runners alike. Peter Coe explains:

Fartlek is a Nordic word loosely translated as "speed play". It is an all-the-year-round component which allows the runner the freedom to choose his own variations.

Staleness is psychological, not physical. If it were physical athletes could not perform so well at the end of a hard season. In 1981 Seb progressed in July from a near world record 1500 metres in one country to breaking his own 1000 metres world record in another four days later. That was physically demanding. To follow this up with two world records in the mile a month later after six big meetings in between would have been the perfect recipe for physical staleness – if such a thing existed. Staleness is a loose word for being mentally jaded, and mental fatigue, whether caused by loss of concentration or through boredom, is at the root of staleness. Seb describes it best himself: "During and after such a season I was able to recharge my mental batteries with the refreshment of fartlek, I can do my own thing in my own way just as easily or as hard as I want to make it. Running round the lakes in Norway, or round the hills and parks of Sheffield, the refreshment of close contact with nature is invaluable."

This break from road and track – which can include a very hard session if you want it – is the great advantage of fartlek, and it is open to anyone at any level.

Fartlek is no more than varying the going in your time in your own way. Jog ten minutes, walk three minutes, run fifteen minutes, walk five minutes, sprint twenty seconds, jog three minutes, sprint fifteen seconds, run eight minutes, walk four minutes, run at a fast pace for three minutes, jog five minutes, run four minutes. That is an hour's training, and you can mix it up to suit yourself. Look at the trees, think your thoughts and come back feeling good: you write the programme as you go along.'

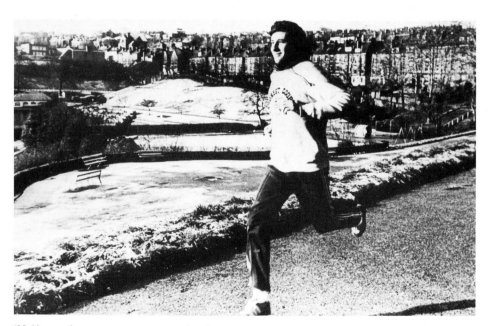

'Making up the programme as you go along'
– a free-and-easy run through the streets of Sheffield

Now that we are running seriously, it is time to think seriously about what we are going to wear.

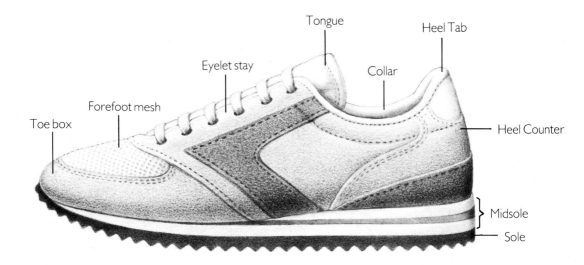

Shoes

Like building a house, a good place is to start from the bottom and where better for a runner to begin than with the feet.

There are no fewer than twenty-six bones in each foot, and these delicate structures have to withstand the considerable forces applied by the human body against the ground.

Running a seven-minute mile can mean 1000 foot strikes, and as each foot-fall has an impact of hundreds of pounds per square inch, 5000 strikes of this intensity in a five-mile run will be giving your feet a problem if they are not properly protected.

A comfortably-paced run lasting an hour is nothing special for most people after a period of training to this level. However, eight or nine thousand foot-strikes are likely to be something for the feet to complain about. Worse still, if the feet are not right to start with, any problems in that area will be reflected throughout a large part of the body, particularly in the knees.

First, before you start running, let's look for a moment at the state of your feet. The chances are that the more you use them the more you abuse them. There are very, very few shoes for everyday use that are not modified in some way because of style and fashion. There will be very, very few readers of this book who are not influenced by these factors. So even if you have chosen sensible shoes for your running, don't blame them for the trouble you may have stored up yourself by wearing shoes for every day that are orthopaedically damaging. Women are often prone to ankle swelling and strain when they start running. They have not done anything traumatic, they are just paying the price for high heels and narrow fittings.

But however badly you've been treating your feet in the past, your aim, now that you are running, must be to give them all the help they need.

If you are to extract the maximum pleasure and benefit from running, which also means avoiding overuse injuries, it is vital that you select the correct type of shoe for your particular needs. And getting the specification correct is not enough if it is followed up by careless fitting. Ideally every running-shoe shop would have trial shoes you could borrow in good condition in all makes, sizes and fittings for a trial. Since this is a non-existant Utopia, the final decision will be yours, and it should be made from the shoe specification and from how it feels on your foot. Here are a few points to remember:

1.   The toes must be free to spread, and the tips of the toes should not rub against the front of the shoe.
2.   When the shoes are laced, the space across the instep between the eyelets should be big enough for you to try more than one method of lacing, but not so wide that it diminishes support.
3.   Friction generates heat. Make sure that the fit that appeals to you does not permit rubbing. Blisters can form quickly.
4.   Wear the same size and type of socks for the fitting as the pair you intend to run in.
5.   If you are not sure into which class your foot-fall belongs, get another runner to observe for you. It requires a different design of shoe if you are a fore-foot or mid-foot striker from the type you need if you are a heel striker.
6.   Obtain guiding literature from the makers, or from the specialist running publications. The best is well written and informative. Buy from an interested sports shoe shop, preferably one run by runners for runners.

It is as well to study the basics of shoe design. If you are a heel striker you will need some 'meat' under the heel – not too spongy, but enough to be shock absorbent. Special inserts can help, but they often spoil the fit with a tendency to lift the heel too high out of the shoe (care must be taken about this, too, if lifting pads are fitted to ease achilles tendon trouble). A fore-foot or mid-foot striker needs the cushioning in the soles. For them heavy heels are no more than a dead weight.

Unless you are involved in serious racing, when you may need four or more different shoes for different surfaces, you will be well able to use one type of shoe for running on roads or grass. Track running, though, is different. At slow speeds most shoes will do, but at faster speeds, on cinders or shale, spikes will be necessary to obtain a safe grip. On synthetic tracks in dry weather a good road-racing flat is a good choice, but in the wet or at fast speeds, spikes again will be needed – not the same as cinder track spikes, but restricted in length – usually to about 5mm – by local track regulations.

These are general points that should set you on the way to a satisfactory pair of running shoes, but anyone preparing to pay the prices asked by shoe retailers today, or to choose between the dozens of models available, might find extra value in considering what the shoe of his choice should provide:

Protection: Since you will hammer the ground with your feet millions of times, you will want to protect them, particularly from the shock which will be transmitted to the rest of the body.

Support: The additional load placed upon the feet by running will strengthen the feet if it is slowly and carefully applied. But support for the intricate structure of the foot and its ligaments will be necessary, particularly when you start running for the first time. An important area of support is the heel counter which must be comfortable but rigid.

Flexibility: It is painful and causes stress to walk in stiff shoes, let alone run in them. The average runner will flex his shoes some thirty degrees, and if the shoe does not bend easily under the ball of the foot it will hurt. The upper shoe should allow for bending without the fold cutting into the foot. A shoe which is insufficiently flexible in the right place will throw painful stress on the calves and the achilles tendons.

Stability: A shoe must support the foot, but the cushioning effect of the shoes must not be so mushy that it throws too much sideways bending force on the ankle. This could be reflected in pain elsewhere in the lower leg.

Arch support: This is important, but its benefit can be negated if the shoe is cut away under the arch. This area of the shoe must be flat on the ground, otherwise it will tend to deflect or even collapse, making the interior build-up useless. No shoe with this defect is a good shoe. Flexibility in the fore-foot area is good but *not* in a distance shoe under the arch.

Wear: Shoes that are badly worn cause foot troubles. Since repairs are both expensive and time-consuming, a runner will be tempted to continue running on mis-shaped soles. He would be wrong to do so.

Midsole and sole formulation: This should be selected by manufacturers to give the characteristics they believe to be the most important. Do not choose shoes on price alone, or you will wind up with a pair of running shoes produced to cost rather than on good design.

Weight: A shoe's weight is quite secondary to the preceding requirements. Within reasonable limits, weight is of little significance except to racers. Leading shoe company research has shown that even in racing lighter is not necessarily faster – quality of the overall design is far more important.

Traction: Your shoe must provide a good grip, whatever surface you are running on. This can be obtained from soles that are ribbed, studded or cupped, or sometimes by a combination of any of these. A sole with a well designed and pronounced raised pattern has an additional advantage. It will not only give a good grip but by limiting the area in contact with road or track it will reduce the risk of overheating on hot surfaces. Fast running on tarmac or synthetic tracks in very warm weather creates a real problem in this respect. Make sure the pattern on the soles is not so widely spaced as to create local pressure points. On the other hand a well spaced raised pattern is worth looking for. Take care if you are running in marathon-type flat shoes in summer. The good are very good – the bad are blister-raisers. The light fast flats may seem attractive, but as with plimsoles and light tennis shoes, the soles may not offer enough protection from stones and small bumps. Bruises on the soles and particularly the heels must be avoided.

Uppers: These are very much a matter of horses for courses. Leather is heavier, and more so when wet, but it lasts longer and is cooler. Nylon is lighter, not so durable, and hotter. Different requirements may be best met by different materials and a wise combination of both is often the solution. A good nylon mesh, incidentally, makes for a better ventilated and cooler shoe.

The Tongue: This must take care of any point or line pressure from laces, it must be soft and cushioning and above all stay in its place and not wander down the foot when you are running.

Lacing: Eyelet arrangements that allow for a wide variety of lacing methods are important not only for snugness and support but also for relief. It is not uncommon to have the odd bump or knob on top of the instep, and to be able to arrange the laces so that this area is free from unwanted pressure is a big plus.

Inside the Shoe: To protect the toes a shoe should have a firm box, but this advantage can be spoiled if hard lines of stitching are left, or if there is too abrupt a change from firmness to flexibility. Always run your hand slowly and carefully around the inside of the shoe to feel for anything that could irritate after you have run a few miles.

Many insoles are now removable. This is a plus point, because frequently the insole is worn through at pressure points – behind the little toe, perhaps, or behind the big toe. These hollows are usually accompanied by some scuffing or wrinkling of the fabric covering of the insole – all potential trouble spots. But be sure that the removable insole stays in place and does not become a hazard by wrinkling or moving around. There is no point in improving hygiene if you are going to raise blisters.

Examine, too, the mid-foot region. Check that whatever method gives additional support to the saddle or arch bandage does not also leave an edge or a rib of stitching to cause discomfort later on.

Think very carefully and take *expert* orthopaedic advice if you are considering buying shoes that have a built-in correction for various foot abnormalities such as excess pronation (foot rolling when making contact with the ground). What might be ideal when exactly right could be very dangerous if wrongly chosen, and prescribing for the abnormal foot is not for amateurs.

A special note for runners who may not have experience of cross-country running but are intending to try their hand. Most runners will be taken up with the problems of studs versus waffles versus ripples, or whether spikes are possible on all sections of the course and how waterproof *are* these shoes? They will be overlooking a major hazard – *mud*. Those shoes that you thought were so snug and comfortable, the ones where you *had* to undo the laces to take them off, can change their nature completely in mud. The shoes may be waterproof, but mud changes many things. A foot in a puddle in some runs can leave your foot almost dry – but not mud.

You run down the slope to cross the stream and suddenly you are in mud. Over the top and down inside the shoes it goes. You now have a very slippery pair of extremities. Does your foot come out of the next mud patch cleanly? No it doesn't – the next thing you know you are groping around in mud looking for a shoe, or shoes, that have been sucked straight off your feet.

In the old days, when there tended to be much more 'plough' around the course and mud was more likely, there were several remedies: special shoes with a strap around the ankle was one; a section of motorcycle inner-tube, slipped over both shoe and foot, sometimes cut to fit round the ankle, was another. Seb's shoes had two eyelets punched into them, one on each side of the heel, and a soft tape threaded through them and tied in front of the ankle.

Beware of gimmicks: shoes over-cushioned around the ankle, for example or the enlarged heel tab claiming protection to the achilles tendon, which can cause unnecessary pressure and irritation.

Two final points on the subject of shoes: when you first buy a pair, especially if you are a beginner, just walk around in them at home for a while, to get their feel, before you set off for a run.

And last but not least, keep them in good condition and in good repair – badly worn shoes can bring on imbalance injuries, and imbalance injuries could stop you running.

Clothing

This is an area of great personal preference. If during the run you kept cool enough or warm enough and were always as comfortable as could be reasonably expected, then what you have been wearing is right for you.

There are some guidelines, though, and fashion is not one of them.

Cold Weather

Wind is the real enemy. A low temperature that is bearable on a calm day or night can become intolerable or even dangerous if the wind picks up. Athletes who run in climates that regularly have very cold winters, part of North America, for example, are well aware of this problem, and the wind-chill factor

**Warm work in the cold:
a crisp winter run in the Brecon Beacons**

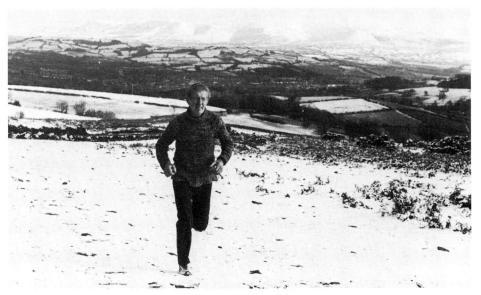

has a real meaning for them. The most important requirement for clothing in very cold conditions is that it should be wind-proof. Genuinely wind-proof outer garments will enable you significantly to reduce the total amount of clothing.

The light-hooded two-piece waterproof over-suits (track wetsuits) are ideal for this duty. The effect is to prevent the circulation of air and so keep in the heat, but remember that while you are keeping in the heat, you are also keeping in the moisture from perspiration. The best types of these waterproofs have well ventilated backs, and the newer materials claim greater permeability – that is they breathe more. While these waterproofs allow you to wear the minimum amount of clothes, what you do wear should be absorbent, and cotton is superior to synthetics for this purpose, though there are some new synthetic materials which are claimed to syphon off the moisture from the skin to the outside of the garment without the material staying damp. Wool is warm and absorbent, but it is easily felted and does not suit all skins.

If this type of waterproof clothing does not suit you, do not go to the other extreme and smother yourself in layer upon layer of gear. Remember, as a child you often ran about to keep warm, so realise that work done means heat released, and if you are overdressed you will soon overheat. Choose clothes that use the idea of small air pockets for insulation – they are warmer and lighter; the old World War Two commando string vests were very effective.

The Face
In intense cold a smear of protective oil or cream on the face is helpful, and in cross-country racing, where large areas of skin on the arms and legs are exposed, a smear of oil all over (even petroleum jelly on the inside of the thighs) is a good

water-repellent. This prevents chapped skin, chafing or soreness from allowing the skin to soften. Although used in Scandinavia and North America, face coverings have not been a great success with most runners in Britain.

The Hands
If you have to run in gloves, then the lighter they are the better. Covered hands warm up quickly, and thick cosy gloves soon become a nuisance. Light wool or cotton gloves can be tucked away in a pocket, heavy ones cannot. Experienced winter runners often find that after a period of almost painful cold, hands warm up again and stay warm.

The Body
Most of your autumn running and even some winter running will need only a running vest and briefs or shorts under a fleece-lined tracksuit with perhaps a light sweater at most. Track suits should be of an easy fit, neither too snug nor too loose. The trousers are best straight or only slightly tapered, with long zips in the sides of the legs to facilitate pulling them on over your running shoes. Do not have elastic stirrups going under the foot. You may feel it is the style you like, but they are inclined to become uncomfortable and a nuisance.

The Head
In dry weather what you wear will depend upon how thick a head of hair you have and to what extent your ears are vulnerable to the cold. Some people develop painful headaches if their forehead gets too cold, but beginners soon become accustomed to the rigours of winter. Some runners are happy in a rainsuit hood, even with drawstrings around the face; others prefer a water-proof cap with a peak that protects from driving rain. Those with thin hair, or who want to limit heat loss from the head, may find a round knitted hat, which can be pulled down round the ears if necessary, the best protection. Balaclavas do seem to irritate around the face after a while.

Socks
Running is only pleasurable if your feet are happy, and the serious considera-tion they deserve does not end with your careful choice of shoes. Running feet are not short on circulation, as your extremities sometimes are at rest, but most people need warm socks when running in winter. Wool is warmest but it does not wear well; it also stretches and thus wrinkles very easily, and long woollen socks are inclined to slip down.

The best sock is a heavy cotton with a Terylene or nylon reinforcement. Those with a towelling type of foot and a cushioned sole are ideal. They keep their shape, they're very absorbent and they wear well.

Try to settle on a choice of socks and stick to them. It is important to know the socks you prefer running in and to have a pair with you when you choose your running shoes. Do remember that socks which are too tight will cause corns and will restrict circulation. Socks that are too loose will be uncomfortable, will wrinkle and will cause blisters.

Finally, unless you are lucky enough to have changing facilities at your place of work or study, your winter runs will be of the circular or out-and-home variety. In windy conditions start off into the wind, so that if you work up a good sweat it will not be so unpleasant on the way home. To get well warmed up – and thus damp – and then turn into a freezing wind is something to avoid.

Cold splash in the heat: a grilling marathon in Taiwan

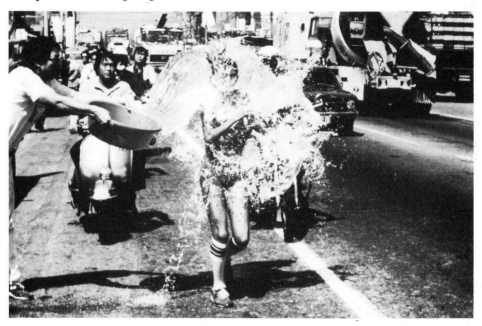

Warm Weather

Choosing clothing for good weather is easy: a singlet or T-shirt and a pair of shorts. Headgear is slightly different; some hair styles require a headband which may also serve to absorb perspiration. In intense heat and glare you may favour a loose-fitting cap with the added protection of a peak. Whatever the type of headgear you choose, good ventilation is always important.

Running vests and shorts should never be too snug a fit, air circulating over the skin as freely as possible is important for adequate cooling. But also avoid the extreme of clothes so loose that they flap. They can cause chafing, particularly from baggy shorts, if you have to run in the rain.

Synthetic materials for summer wear do have advantages. Synthetic shorts do not become as waterlogged as cotton ones do. They are less apt to cling to the skin and they have the advantage of drying quickly.

Look for gear with seams that are as flat and smooth as possible. Even very small irritations not noticed at normal times are magnified a hundredfold when running.

The snug elasticated pants – they are hardly shorts – favoured by some women track athletes are not ideal for distance running, particularly in summer when they reduce cooling by restricting the free circulation of air.

Summer or winter, nearly all shorts and tracksuit bottoms are elasticated today. Be sure that the waistband is only tight enough to stay up; many athletes pull the waistline low on to the hips to avoid constriction when a draw-string support could be much more comfortable.

For those who wish to run in long socks, remember elastic restricts circulation. Soccer players use tapes, not elastic garters, a far better method in that tapes are adjustable to keep the garment in place, and no more. A little more trouble using tapes when dressing can avoid a lot of irritation on a run.

The Woman Runner

In general, advice on running gear is very much the same for women as for men, with the exception of the difficulties some women experience in finding a suitable bra for running, despite the increasing number of companies now producing sports bras.

Our experience in this area is a bit restricted, but it would perhaps be worth a woman asking herself, before she makes a choice, how much tolerance to active movement she builds up naturally at her work and at home. A job where she is continually reaching and pulling, say on a production line, is very different from one which involves sitting reading proofs. The large variety of shapes and sizes of women means that the best design solution could well be unique to each individual, and may, after some trial and error need a bit of high-class do-it-yourself to get the best results, particularly since what may be satisfying for the beginner may not necessarily work when distances increase.

Dry materials behave differently when they get moist from sweat; elastic constricts, fastenings can rub and cause sore spots. Would the increased use of Velcro help? We find it odd that while shoe manufacturers can supply reams of informative literature on product design, sportswear manufacturers are not doing the same for this essential piece of equipment – there must be many design improvements that could benefit serious women joggers and runners.

Looking good

Looking good often means feeling good and in most activities the best are always well turned out. If running gear is well chosen for its functional properties, then it only needs to be kept clean to look right.

Fashion sportswear has become deeply entrenched in sports like tennis and soccer, and it has now arrived in running. There are only two criteria that matter when choosing running gear: Is it suitable for its purpose, and does it fit? Club colours can add a touch of brightness if that is what you want, but the old grey sweatsuits – to which Seb is addicted – are above all functional.

If you find you need a sweatband, use one. If you find a wristband is useful to wipe away sweat, use one, but don't buy them because they look pretty. For all the peripheral gear, the recommendation is try it before you buy it, borrow it if necessary. The last thing a sensible runner needs, whether in competition or running for fitness, is a case of the cycling disease where large sums of money change hands for minutely modified equipment in the belief that it will make you go further and faster.

The ventilation on wet weather running gear is more important than the colour, and zips in the legs, long enough to ensure they slip easily over running shoes, is more important than stripes or coloured panels.

Strength Exercise

Training for running is not solely running. To increase all-round strength as the running becomes more demanding, as well as simply to make a change in the fitness routine, there is considerable benefit in introducing yourself to a series of exercises.

For runners there are two kinds of strengthening exercise. The first group is for the development of explosive strength – for sprinters, jumpers, throwers and the like; these are usually performed using free weights or a multi-gym, and in most cases they are geared towards the development of a specific muscle or muscle group.

The other type is used for developing all-round strength with endurance, and is also a general conditioner – and it is these exercises – used singly or in sequence – that are more likely to concern the fitness runner.

When the various exercises in this group are performed continuously in a series of sets, with prescribed intervals between sets, we have the basis of circuit training. The variables here are the number of different exercises in a circuit, the number of repetitions in each set, and the recovery time between each set. A further variable for the really tough is the number of circuits that can be completed. An additional refinement is placing a time limit on a given number of repetitions and an overall time for a full circuit.

Circuit training is best done in a gymnasium or a sports hall where you can move easily from one exercise to another, each already set up in its own area. But it is quite easy to select exercises which can be done separately, or in pairs or threes, in the home, which is probably the best way for beginners to start. Your local authority will know if any of the schools have gymnasium facilities open on any evening in the week, or whether there are any evening institutes or polytechnics with classes suitable for your strength and circuit training. This aspect of your training can often seem attractive in itself, and it is good practice not only to have a rest day each week, even when you have become well adjusted to running, but to do an evening's strengthening exercise as a complete change from running.

Weight training is a specialised form of exercise, and we would advise you to seek expert advice before you start, and only to use weights under supervision at first. The gymnasium exercises, though, can be performed alone, or by people in pairs, after some preliminary description and explanation.

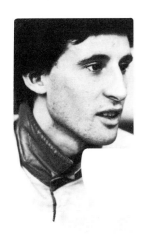

Depth Jumping To develop elastic strength – the strength involving contractile and stretch components in movements done at speed and under load. A useful exercise for developing sprinting speed and fast uphill running. To avoid injury, keep both feet together at all stages. Pause slightly at the top of each box, the first of which should be slightly lower than the others in the sequence.

With all these exercises, begin gradually, and build up the number of repetitions and/or sets of repetitions to meet your own fitness targets. The depth jumping and bounding are called plyometric exercises, and require extra care when attempted for the first time.

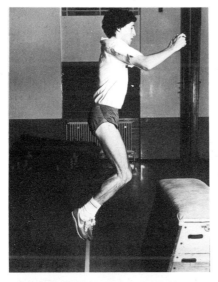
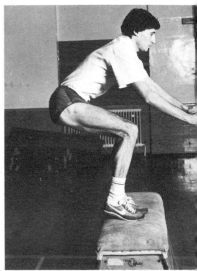
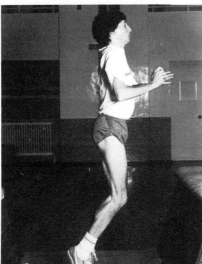
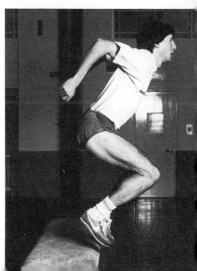

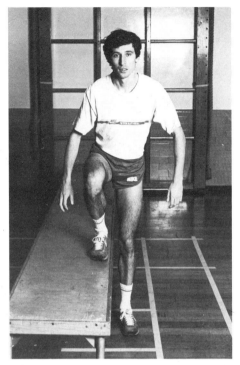
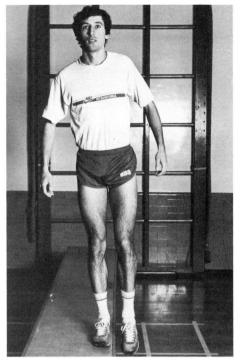
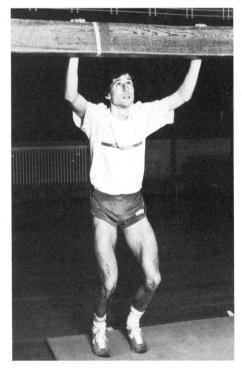
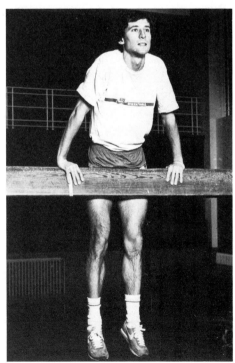

◀ **Bench Step-ups** Select a box or a bench that will raise the thigh to the horizontal. Raise the body, not too slowly but without jerking, by lifting on the bent leg. Do not use the other leg to assist take-off. Alternate with an equal number of repetitions on each leg. A good strength endurance exercise, but the repetitions should be built up cautiously.

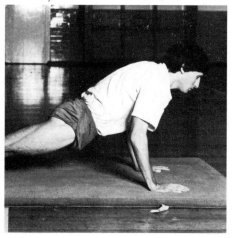
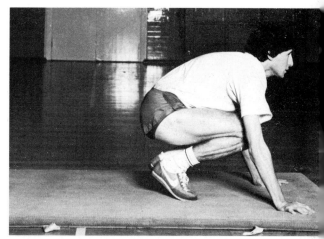

▲ **Burpees** A combination of squat thrusts and vertical jumps to condition the gluteal and quadriceps muscles and to develop dynamic strength. The legs should extend fully backwards, and in the recovery the feet should return close to the hands to obtain a good jumping position. The best results come when the whole exercise is performed as quickly as possible.

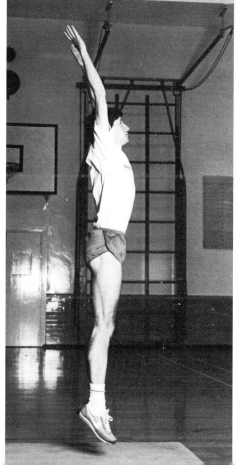

◀ **Beam Jumps** Start with the beam within reach of the arms with the feet on the floor. Later an even more helpful effect is achieved by progressing to a beam height which requires a jump to reach it. Combine the spring and the follow-through in one smooth, continuous movement. A good exercise for co-ordination, dynamic leg strength and upper-body development.

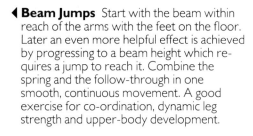

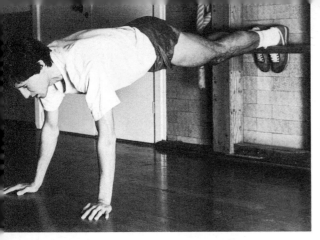

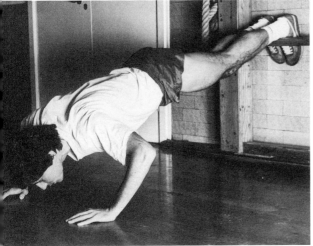

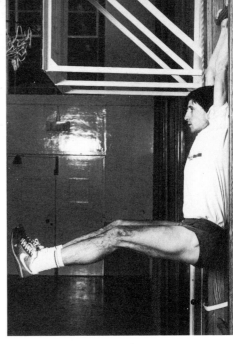

the body). This spin off, by which the exercise is done hanging from the wall bar, is excellent. During this phase the spine is fully stretched, which helps problems of tension and postural defects.

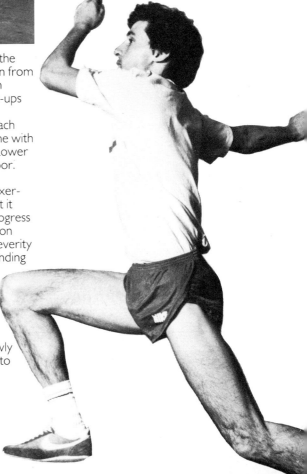

Inclined Press-ups These increase the load on the arms and are a progression from ordinary press-ups. They are tough on triceps and pectoral muscles. All press-ups are a good all-round torso toughener, though older exercisers should approach them with caution. Hold the head in line with the back, and keep the back straight. Lower the face to within two inches of the floor.

Bounding Like depth jumping, this exercise develops dynamic leg strength, but it places a greater load on the ankles. Progress carefully. A useful variation is hopping on one leg, then the other. Increase the severity either by longer repetitions or by bounding uphill. Or try reducing the number of bounds or hops required to cover a fixed distance.

Leg Raisers To strengthen abdominal muscles. In this exercise the legs should be kept straight and raised slowly to at least mid-way (i.e. at right angles to

Total time elapsed (minutes)	Exercise	Duration	Recovery	Repetitions per set	Recovery between sets	Number of sets
	Gymnasium circuits					
	Run to gymnasium, or start with warm-up run	1-2 miles				
10	Extra warm-up and loosening	10 minutes				
30	Static stretching exercises	20 minutes				
55	Leg raising, from wall-bars	20 seconds	20 seconds	5-12	2 min	2-3
59	Depth jumping from boxes [progressing, with more boxes, to ...]	20 seconds [60 sec]	30 seconds [60 sec]	1 [1]	2 min [2 min]	3 [2]
64	Bounding	5 minutes				1
69	More stretching exercises	5 minutes				1
70	Sit-ups	1 minute		30-60		1
75	Rope-climbing	5 minutes				1
77	Beam-jumping and pull-ups			5	1 ½ min	2-3
81	Scissoring (hanging from beam with legs raised – rotating pelvis and crossing legs while keeping legs straight)	10 seconds		1	3 min	2
83	Back strengthening (lying on stomach, arching back)	10 seconds	10 seconds	6		1
84	Press-ups with feet raised			25		1
88	Step-ups on box or beam (with or without weights)	until tired				
	Stretching after each circuit	10 minutes				

The Stronger Runner

With increased confidence from longer running sessions, and perhaps with some extra strength gained from work in the gymnasium too, the runner is going to be looking for other ways of improving both his speed and his endurance. Three types of training we would recommend all tackle the problem in a different way, but all play their part in improving the performance of your body.

Interval Training
This is probably the most common type of running training attempted when the conventional steady long distance running has given all the early benefit that it can offer.

The principle of interval training is that of spaced work. A work load is applied, generally from thirty to forty seconds, which speeds up the heart. This is followed by a recovery period. The subsequent intervals of work and recovery periods are adjusted in duration and number to suit the athlete and the level of training reached.

The duration and intensity of the work should be sufficient to raise the heart rate to a target time, and the recovery period long enough to allow the pulse rate to fall to the threshold rate at which the work interval should recommence. As a rough guide add 20 per cent to your best time for the distance run, and allow a recovery time which is three times longer than the running time.

The aim of this type of training is to increase the volume of blood pumped by each heartbeat. The underlying idea is that when the work load ceases and the muscles are recovering, the powerfully stimulated heart continues to fill and pump at almost the same level as during the working phase. The end effect is to achieve a greater dilation of the heart, and indeed very big increases in stroke volume have been recorded at the end of three or even two months.

Among the experts there is some divergence of opinion on the effectiveness of interval work. The pro-interval coaches claim it is a more effective method than steady distance running to increase cardiac output and oxygen uptake. The pro-steady running camp argues on the other hand, that the effect it achieves is more transient, and that to consolidate the base of your training steady running is best.

We use both methods in our training but regular interval training does not start until March.

There is, incidentally, evidence from French sources that interval training can have an enlarging but *thinning* effect upon the artery walls if performed by young athletes. It is presumably for this reason that in East Germany it is restricted to those over fourteen years of age.

In any case, the application of interval training has to be done very carefully and we would emphasise that the schedules need to be specific to the individual and his current condition.

Its plus point is that an athlete can undertake a lot more fast work in a short period because the lactate levels in blood do not become intolerable. It is also a rapid way to become used to fast work, and even if the development of the heart is not the main aim we find it has a specific role between steady running and speed endurance training.

The recovery period is variously prescribed as a rest or walk/jog recovery. An important factor in the choice is the weather (if it is cold or damp, then jog) and/or the feelings of the athlete. Some runners doing fast work tighten up even in short rest periods, and they would be better off keeping on the move and jogging in the recovery period.

It would be unwise to use this method as the main plank of training for fast middle-distance work because the lactic acid level in the blood does not reach the levels obtained by hard speed endurance training, which would use runs of two minutes or more with short recoveries. The latter is much closer to actual race conditions and to the lactate levels that will be experienced.

But we have found a special use for interval training. If Seb has been out of normal training through injury (*not* illness) and has managed to keep active by way of swimming or cycling or both, then after only a little steady running a few sessions of interval training, say 12 x 200 metres, increasing to 20 x 200 metres, soon brings back some snap and speed into his work. Provided the training base and his condition is sound, it provides us with a rapid return to near form.

We repeat that it is *not* recommended for a fast return to form after illness, because it is all too easy to overstimulate the heart.

Later in this chapter we make some suggestions for newcomers to interval training and speed-endurance running on how to go about planning their training sessions.

Speed-endurance Training
The old adage that speed kills is certainly true. Quite a few people find they can run quickly, and many will find that after some distance training they can keep going quite comfortably for a few miles. But ask any of them to run very quickly for only half a mile, and they will soon be in trouble.

If we think of speed endurance training as having two complementary meanings then we can understand the training better. It is making endurance running faster by learning how to endure speed.

Maintaining speed causes you to use more oxygen than you can extract from the air. You rely on the immediate release of energy in the muscles, which is soon spent. The by-products of this energy-release build up in the body, and the alkaline buffers in the blood cannot take up any more acid. In the end, which comes all too quickly, the whole machine stops through exhaustion.

Here psychological factors are important. Not only does the body have to learn how to delay this process, but the mind has to learn how to force the body to continue functioning while the brain is continually receiving signals to stop. For certainly the body can continue working longer than you think, painful though it may be.

This type of training, more than any other, requires careful assessment of the proper recovery period – not just the rest between runs, but the intensity of the training on the next one or even two days. Speed endurance is the most stress-inducing of all the training methods and can be destructive if over-used. Athletes refer to its misuse as a 'breaking down', as opposed to a 'building up' which is the real aim of training.

Speed endurance training consists principally of repeated extended high speed runs. The distances used are usually 600 metres, 800 metres, 1000 metres and 1200 metres. The best effect is obtained from running with an effort of 95 per cent or better.

Only experience can teach the coach and athlete how best these sessions can be applied but the following simple mistake should not be made. Do not think that the total distance of a set of runs gives the same effect regardless of the length of the run. For instance, if the proper recovery times are observed 8 x 600 metres is not as hard as 6 x 800 metres, and 4 x 1200 metres is harder still. The 4800 metres run is the same distance in each case, the effect is not.

Learning to cope with these runs with a recovery time of twice the running time (when running 1200 metres, recovery is only the same time as the run itself) is very hard, but it is a vital piece of training for all runners for racing between 800 metres and 5000 metres, or even up to 10,000 metres.

Maintaining an even pace is the most economical way of running any race above 400 metres, but in practice there will always be the moment when however, tired you are, you will want to produce a sustained burst. This type of training will help you to meet that requirement.

Resistance Running

This comes in many forms, but only two are relevant here; both involve hill running.

Running up inclines is hard work and is good for style, since the arm action is more vigorous and a higher knee-lift is required. Sessions of running up steep hills, preferably with inclines of one in six or more, is a great conditioner but the first few sessions should be approached with caution.

The most testing form of hill running is up long steep sandhills, which calls for the most pronounced, laboured exaggeration of running movements. Pulling the feet out of the sand, lifting the knees even higher and driving the arms extra hard is exceptionally tiring. Sandhill running is also the most searching. It seeks out any weakness anywhere, and the calf muscles and the achilles tendons get severely worked.

These sessions must be approached with the greatest caution. If you have access to such an area where this work can be carefully incorporated into a regular schedule, well and good, but it is unwise to approach this kind of training on a one-off basis without slow familiarisation. Don't go on holiday, look for long high sand dunes and have a hard workout. The chances are you will limp around miserably for the rest of your stay.

Easing into Session Training

Interval training will be quite new to most runners, and like all first-time training it must start slowly and be progressively increased. We would recommend one session a week for the first month before incorporating any speed endurance into the programme. In any case, two sessions per week of interval training will meet the needs of most runners.

Repetitions of 200 metres is not the only programme used. Runs up to 400 metres are quite common, but 200-metre repetitions are easier to handle when you first start.

Warm up carefully – don't forget your stretching – and start off with a set of ten runs. Keep to sets of ten until any soreness or stiffness which may have resulted from these runs has disappeared. If your first set of ten does not cause any problems, progress to sets of fifteen runs, and so on. For a distance runner we would suggest lengthening the sets of runs up to about thirty runs per set rather than reaching twenty runs per set and then increasing the speed of the run, which is a possible variant. Rather than increase the speed, the distance man could decrease the recovery time.

Once you have managed a few sets of 20 x 200 metres, we would expect you to find it easier to maintain a faster steady pace on the road.

Speed Endurance: again, for the general type of runner, we would recommend lengthening the sessions to 1000 metres or six-tenths of a mile before increasing the speed of the 600-metre or 800-metre runs. Also at this distance it is still better to cut the recovery time rather than to increase the speed of the 1000-metre run.

All the time, remember to check your pace judgment and keep looking at your watch. As with interval training, these sessions will improve your steady running speed.

Putting on the Style

Everybody runs in a different way, and most runners, unless they are reaching for the heights, are unlikely to modify their style very much. Activities depending upon fluent movement, like ballet and gymnastics as well as running, need the faults ironed out very early on, and the correct movements practised as soon as possible. At some stage it becomes too late to start correcting ingrained faults, and for older fitness runners correction becomes so difficult that there is a danger of it becoming counter-productive. But this does not mean that style is not important in running, or that it is not worth examining the running body in detail.

In engineering, particularly on the design side, there is an old saying that goes like this: 'If it looks right, it very likely is. If it looks wrong, it certainly is.' This is equally true of running style. A good style does not guarantee that you are a great runner but a bad style almost certainly guarantees that you are not. There will always be a few exceptions to this rule, but not many.

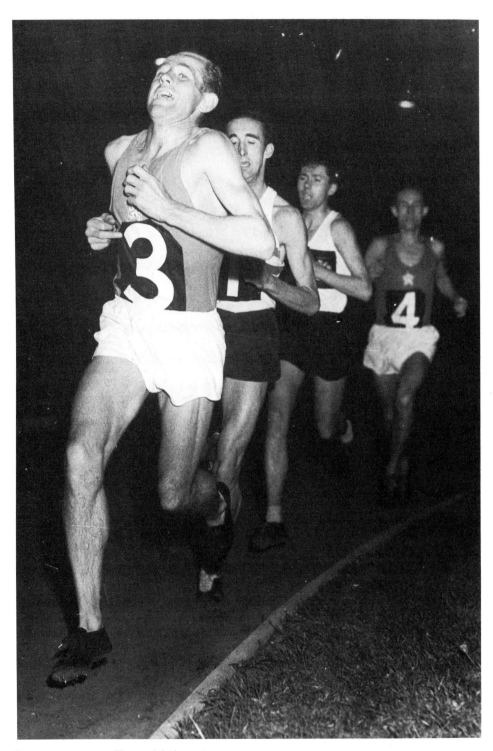

**Supreme runner, appalling model: the grotesque,
agonised, head-rolling style of Emil Zatopek**

Imperfections in some areas, of course, are not as important as others. Anyone who remembers Zatopek might argue that style can not be all that important. The answer to this is that Zatopek would certainly have been an even better runner without the gross waste of energy caused by his tight arm action and the agonised head-wagging. That the whole is greater than the sum of the parts is never more true than of style.

There is a magic about the all-together athlete, a beautifully balanced pouring-out of well concealed effort. Good style and efficient movement are inseparable. Starting at the head and finishing with the feet these are the key factors:

Head
This should be well poised on the shoulders – not too far back, as in exaggerated effort – this restricts breathing and at the same time causes the stride to shorten. Keep it still, the head must not turn. Running head down also restricts breathing, and as the head is a heavy weight, it will alter the line of carriage just to balance the body.

Neck
A well poised head is easier to balance, therefore the muscles have less work to do and neck strain is considerably lessened. Neck strain soon shows with the sterno-mastoid muscles standing out like tight cords. Remember, neck strain does not contribute to forward propulsion.

Shoulders
'To every force there is an equal and opposite reaction.' In high speed running one depends more on the reaction of the arms to offset the drive of the legs, and when you are running with a fast cadence, contra-rotation of the shoulders to any degree is hardly possible. Whenever the fast runner is tiring, though, he starts to labour and roll the shoulders, but at slower speeds some contra-rotation is natural because the arms cannot move with as much vigour. Again, this must not be excessive. Overstriding, which is mechanically inefficient anyway, will tend to distort shoulder movement. While running do not stick out the chest by forcing back the shoulders – it creates tension, which means wasted energy.

Arms
A very essential part of running. Upper-arm development is important to all runners. Sprinters need good muscular development to provide the mass for the reaction to the powerful leg drive required for their event. Middle-distance runners have to attack hills, which requires a good knee-lift and a vigorous arm action. Long-distance runners require endurance-toughened arms that do not drop with fatigue. At any cross-country event, and on hilly sections of long runs, you can hear the old parrot-cry 'use your arms' or 'drive with your arms' often directed at schoolboys and attenuated ectomorphs who have neon-tubes for arms. The under-trained and/or under-equipped can often be seen dropping

their arms from the sheer fatigue of maintaining the arm position and action.

Steady fast running requires a vigorous action with the elbow *unlocked*. The angle between upper and lower arm should be about ninety degrees, but not with the elbow locked. During the backward motion the arm should be slightly extended, and then slightly flexed to something less than ninety degrees on the return.

The carriage of the arm should be low, for two reasons. First, it is less strain on the shoulders if the arms swing close to the body with the upper arm hanging more or less vertically, and the elbows in rather than sticking out spikily. Secondly, arms cannot be lifted into the driving position if they are already there. In the driving position the arms are best moved in a plane parallel to your direction (the sagittal plane) but in distance running, with its far less robust action, the arms will want to swing slightly across the body.

A clenched, high arm action is more tiring and mechanically does not provide the same reaction as the lower arm carriage. The wrists should be loose (though without the hands flapping wildly), fingers should be relaxed, usually with a light curl and with the thumb resting lightly on the index finger. Clenched fists betray unnecessary strain.

Hips

The part played by hips is not readily seen except through the general carriage of the runner, and especially in his stride length. When runners lack flexibility in the hips they often attempt to attain a good stride length by increasing the forward lean of the body. This tends to be self-defeating, because it hinders front knee lift and toe-off comes earlier. While some rotation takes place, the accentuated hip rotation cultivated by the race walker is not desirable in a runner. It often shows as an exaggerated roll as a runner reaches for stride length, especially when tiredness sets in.

Knees

Seen from the front the knees should not describe a circle, but should move in an arc parallel to the sagittal plane. In an all-out drive in flat-out running, or when attacking a hill, the knees should allow the leg to straighten fully in the driving phase. A good knee-lift is an economical way of preserving stride length. It increases the flinging effect of the loose-hanging lower leg so that it flicks forward easily but not too far at the end of the recovery phase. If the leg is fully straightened, at this stage, it throws a stress on the knee joint as the leg snaps out straight, and the runner over-strides. Over-striding places the foot strike too far in front of the centre of gravity of the body. This has a retarding effect, tends to promote a heavy heel-strike and unnecessarily jars the body.

Knees should also allow for a high heel lift of the swinging leg – the faster one runs, the higher the heels. When the heel is tucked up close to the buttock the leg is folded into half its length and this brings the centre of gravity of the leg closer to the pivot point, which is the hip joint. Now the leg is a much shorter lever, and the effort required to swing the leg forward to take up the supporting phase is much reduced. Further, when the heel is dropped it falls freely under gravity and being free to swing is easily flung forward without effort. Remember, good style promotes efficiency.

Ankles

The requirements of the ankle exemplify the basic requirements of all athletic endeavour: strength with flexibility. The ankle is at the receiving end of heavy loads with shock, tension and bending combined. The ankle must be strong to cope with uneven ground, with slipping or with any other accident, but in the context of style our main concern is with flexibility, because of the effect it has on stride length.

When the foot hits the ground the ideal foot-strike is the one that makes contact first with the ball of the foot but allows the heel to lower and kiss the ground immediately after the touchdown, when the leg is then in the supporting phase, slightly bent at the knee. Meanwhile the body is continuing to move forward so that the runner with the greatest range of movement in the ankle will be the one who can leave the foot in *flat* contact with the ground the longest.

This delays toe-off to the very last moment and extends the duration of the driving phase in which the very powerful calf muscles can contract and contribute to forward propulsion rather than pushing the body upwards.

The fault of over-striding has been emphasised. It is in the driving phase where stride length is effectively increased.

Toe-off

By this we mean that as the heel begins to lift it should be driven by the forceful contraction of the calf muscles, rather than just being a foot lifted off the ground. This drive should be continued right through to the toes, which should maintain driving contact until the very last moment. Place the foot flat on the ground and note the position of the ankle bone by placing it in line with the leg of a chair or table. Then still leaving this foot *flat* on the ground take a stride forward. See how far you can stride with the stationary heel still in contact with the ground.

As soon as you feel the tightness in front of the ankle or in the calf you will realise that with more flexibility the stride could be longer. Now slowly raise the heel from the ground and the ankle bone will lift and move forward. Continue this movement until the ball of the foot is off the ground and only the toes are in contact. The distance the ankle bone has moved horizontally from the chair leg is the distance you have added to your stride. Since this also depends upon the range of movement allowed by your ankle it is easy to see the contribution to your stride that ankle flexibility provides.

Feet

When running, feet seldom make contact with the ground in such a way that a line drawn across the ball of the foot makes instant contact along its whole length. The side of the foot is the first point to touch, after which the foot rolls to flat contact with the ground. This is called pronation, and is only safe and allowable over a limited range. There is a considerable risk in distance running from excessive pronation, and here prevention is much better than cure. Orthotics – inserts in the shoes – may be necessary.

The Body as a Whole
Generally, seen front on, a runner should progress in a straight line with the knees moving smoothly in a vertical plane and not seen to move in and out across

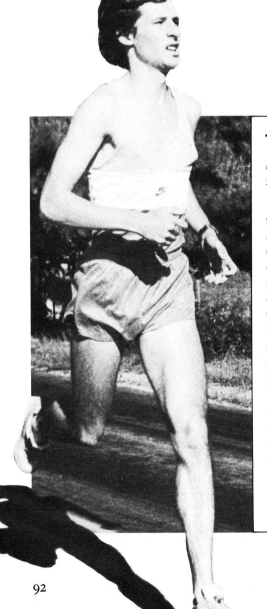

The Critical Eye

Point by point Peter Coe, coach, analyses the style of Seb Coe, runner.

1 & 2 The head well poised avoids the neck straining to carry an off-balance load.
3 Leading shoulder without excessive contra-rotation.
4 Shoulders neither hunched forward with a pinched chest, nor forced back with out-thrust chest which would cause tension in the back.
5 Upper arm hanging naturally, elbows in. The arm moving forward is flexed to 90 degrees.
6 The other arm has 'unlocked' the elbow and is straightening as it moves backwards.
7 In steady pace running the hand may move comfortably slightly across the body.
8 Unclenched fingers, hands and fingers loosely carried, well relaxed.
9 Lead leg nearly straight (*never* lock out.)

the body. The heels, too, should not be seen to move inwards during the toe-off. It is, in fact, often seen in an exaggerated form with some sprinters during the start and early acceleration – and it is wasteful. Style is not merely a matter of aesthetics, it is harmonising a series of separate movements into a single economical effective motion.

Seen from the side, the main features we would look for would be: head well poised, trunk either erect or with just the slightest forward lean, arms held easily, hands and neck relaxed, a clean knee lift, good foot plant, with the knee nicely bent on contact *under* the centre of gravity (or just a few inches in front) and generally a smooth flow. Even the casual and uninformed observer seems to have an immediate appreciation of a smooth, elegant, purposeful and effective style. Remember, once again, 'if it looks right, it very likely is – if it looks wrong, it certainly is.'

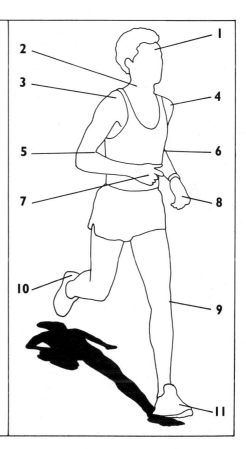

10 Good heel lift – not as much as in sprinting, but enough to produce a forward fling.

11 This is important. The leading foot has slowed and has nearly stopped moving forward relative to the ground. The knee will start bending and the foot will touch the ground without any forward motion and will have dropped so that the strike is on the ball of the foot and the heel contact following on very close to first contact.

Still photographs are deceptive – it would appear from this one that the heel will strike first – but it will not. Some runners *are* heel strikers, though, and the shock on the achilles tendon and the spine is proportional to the degree to which the heel takes the load rather than the forefoot.

N.B. Not a style point, but an important one: note the use of the crown of the road rather than the camber, to avoid the danger of imbalance injury.

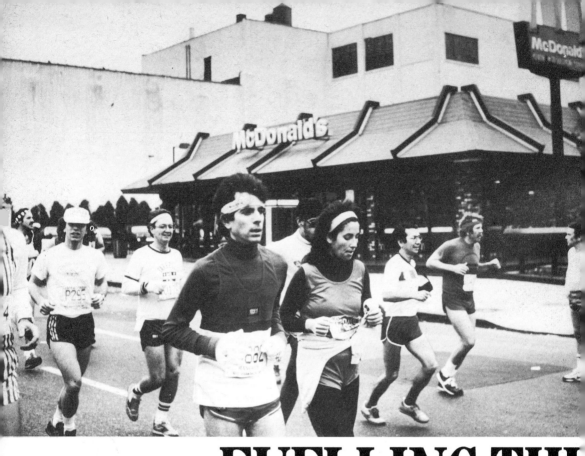

FUELLING TH

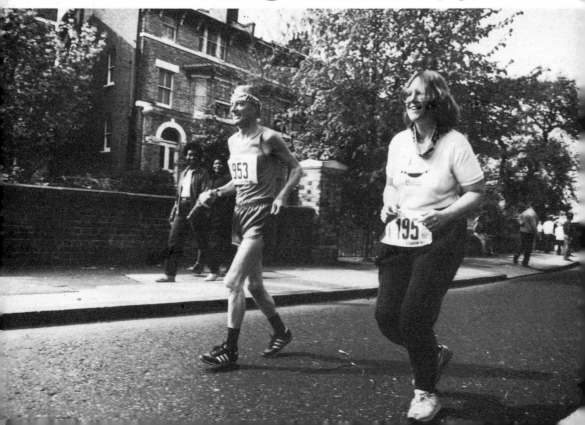

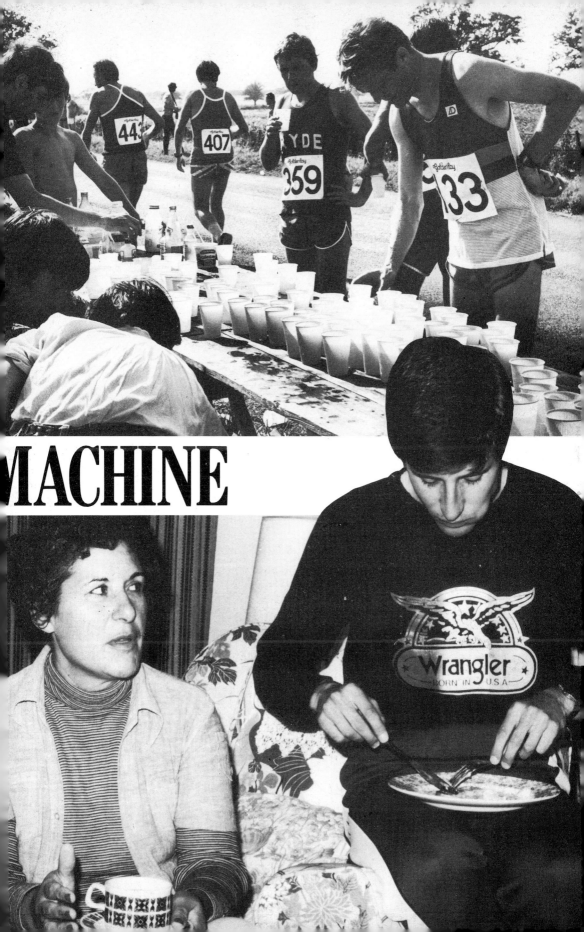

MACHINE

Stocking up on carbohydrate at the Pasta party before the London Marathon

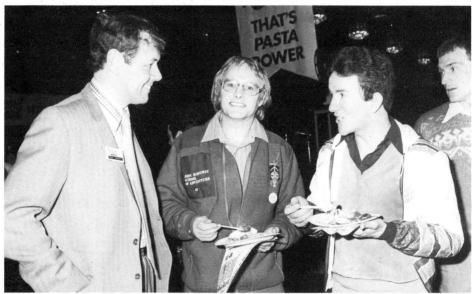

Fitness cannot be achieved solely by exercise. Even if the machine is made more efficient by running, and consequently works better, most of the fuel – all except the oxygen, in fact – is obtained by eating. The condition of your body, however well you train, will be determined to an important degree by how much you eat, and by what you eat. In short, if you want to keep your body in shape, running is not a substitute for dieting. On the other hand, diet, and some knowledge of nutrition, can be of real help to the runner.

Digestion

For our purposes the digestive system is not treated in any great depth because it is not 'trainable' in the sense that other components of fitness are. We are concerned with food only as a source of energy and growth, though the way the digestive system processes certain foods will influence our diet and, on the practical level, the time at which we eat and train.

We need food as fuel to burn for energy, and also, after we have reduced and reassembled it, as the building material for growth and maintenance of the body. In addition, it has to supply those essential ingredients which the body cannot synthesise for itself.

The greater part of the human body is water, about 60 per cent in males and 50 per cent in females (fat contains only a little water, and women normally have a higher percentage of fat than men). Water is composed entirely of hydrogen and oxygen, so 99 per cent of our body consists of hydrogen, oxygen, carbon, calcium and phosphorous. The remaining one per cent is mainly sodium, potassium, iron, magnesium, chlorine and sulphur, plus a few trace elements.

Our principal foods are proteins, carbohydrates and fats – protein mainly for tissue replacement (protein makes up approximately 12 per cent of the human body); carbohydrate as the quick source of energy, in that it is quickly burned as a fuel; fat as the most convenient way energy can be stored and as protection for the body.

Proteins are compounds of nitrogen, carbon, hydrogen and oxygen, together with essential minerals. A molecule of protein is made up of hundreds of molecules of amino acids. Most of the amino acids can be synthesised in the body, but those that cannot, the essential ones, must be contained in the diet, and animal proteins are a better source of these than vegetable proteins. Proteins are also the only source of nitrogen for the body.

Protein which is surplus to the requirements of body maintenance is converted to glucose and burned off as fuel, but if our diet is deficient in energy foods the protein will be consumed for energy; if this condition is prolonged the body will be robbed of replacement material and muscle wastage will occur which, if continued, will ultimately result in death.

With the best balance of essential amino acids as the criterion, the following foods are ranked in order of merit: eggs 100 per cent; fish, meat 70 per cent; soya beans 69 per cent; milk 60 per cent; rice 56 per cent; corn 41 per cent.

Carbohydrates are simpler compounds, containing only carbon, hydrogen and oxygen. They are the quick energy foods in that they can be metabolised faster. Carbohydrates are taken in simple form as sugars or in more complex form as starches; starchy foods such as potatoes, pasta and bread also represent the cheapest of the energy foods.

The speed at which they can be digested must be considered when planning pre-exercise meals; unlike fats they can pass through the stomach quickly.

Carbohydrates, when converted to glycogen, can be stored in the liver and the muscles, but only in a very limited quantity, enough perhaps for one inactive day. Carbohydrate does not supply any of the essentials that the body cannot synthesise, and any surplus is quickly deposited as unwanted fat. Unfortunately carbohydrates are the main ingredients of the sweet and tasty foods and confectionaries.

Fat is generally held to be the villain in the diet war, but even though the average diet contains too much fat it is still necessary for its essential fatty acids and, because some of our necessary vitamins are fat soluble, a fat-free diet would lack these. Fat also yields twice as much energy as protein or carbohydrate, and can therefore save meals from being too bulky.

Nevertheless, more oxygen is required to reduce fat, which is a serious consideration for a runner. And although fat feels more comfortable to eat, and stops you feeling hungry too quickly after a meal, it stays longer in the stomach and so delays the start of serious exercise or heavy exertion.

It is slightly inconvenient that whereas animal protein is the best source of essential amino acids, vegetable fats are the best source for the essential fatty acids, the absence of which might lead to damage of the arteries by allowing excess quantities of cholesterol to accumulate.

The fatty acids themselves come in several forms, which will be familiar, if only in name, to those who have seen cholesterol climb high in the unpopularity ratings in the last few years. A *saturated* fatty acid is one which has taken up all the hydrogen atoms it can; an *unsaturated* fatty acid is one that has not. The former are found as solid animal fats such as butter and lard, the latter are more often liquid vegetable oils. A further division exists in the unsaturated fats between mono- and poly-unsaturated types; it is the latter that is lowest in cholesterol. In this respect margarine is better than butter, but it is still a matter for selection, as some brands of margarines have a far higher content of animal fat and thus more undesirable mono-unsaturated fats than others.

Vitamins are essentials that the body does not have the enzymes to synthesise. An all-round balanced diet will contain all the necessary vitamins for well-being, so that additional vitamin supplements should not be needed. Only the

Vitamin	Source	Symptoms of deficiency
A	Milk, butter, liver, cod liver oil, fresh green vegetables	Lowered resistance to illness; bad skin.
B	Wheat germ, yeast	Lack of appetite; indigestion; wasting.
B_2 complex (B_3, B_6, B_{12}, Choline)	Wheat germ, yeast, nuts fish, meat, milk products	Lack of appetite; indigestion; wasting.
C	Fresh green vegetables, citrus fruits	Scurvy; lowered resistance; poor healing.
D complex	Cod liver oil, eggs, cream	Poor bones (e.g. rickets).
K	Green vegetables, and body bacteria	(One form can be synthesised, so it is hardly an essential).

smallest amounts of the vitamins are required for normal health, and while the excess intake of most vitamins can easily be eliminated by the body, too much vitamin A or D could be harmful, since they are fat-soluble and can therefore build up in the body. A vitamin deficiency could possibly arise from the way the food has been stored or prepared. Overcooking or boiling, or even the wrong storage of fruit or orange juice, could destroy sufficient vitamin C to make the diet an inadequate source, but this would be unlikely in practice. It is rare, certainly in this country, to see obvious symptoms of vitamin deficiency, which goes some way to show that supplementary doses of vitamins are rarely necessary. However, we feel from personal experience that an increased vitamin C intake does help to combat colds and hasten body repairs.

The accompanying table lists the more important vitamins, their sources and their uses.

Minerals are also essentials not synthesised in the body. Some minerals combine with others to carry out their function, and many of these trace elements have functions not as yet understood.

All our cells are bathed in fluid, and the correct balance of this fluid is of vital importance. The first group of minerals are necessary for this. Prolonged efforts like marathon running, particularly in high temperatures, need these minerals to maintain the proper electrolytic balance. The proper function of the electron transport chain, which is how energy gets to our muscles, depends upon the proper balance of *sodium, potassium* and *chlorides*.

The other group has many different functions. *Iron* combines with protein to form the oxygen-carrying haemoglobin. *Calcium* is necessary for bone growth and *magnesium* combines with calcium in this process. Minerals are essential to enzymes, the material-synthesising tools of the body, and for the correct functioning of various body processes.

An iron supplement for an athlete in heavy training is often wise. Runners seem to break up red cells more readily than non-runners, and although the body retains the iron from the haemoglobin when, after the normal lifetime (three to four months), the red blood cells break up, some extra may escape.

Women lose around 30mg of iron per month, and should certainly watch for periodic anaemia if they are considering heavy training or long-distance races, and take a supplement of iron.

Our bodies normally only take up 10 per cent of our iron intake, but will absorb more if the need is there.

Diet and Exercise – the Double Defence

Today there is a lot of talk about diseases of the heart and cardio-vascular system. Arteries become 'clogged with fatty deposits' and cholesterol is made to sound like a death sentence. It may be true that by limiting the amount of fat in the diet, and by selecting poly-unsaturated fats, this risk is reduced, but there are other factors involved. First, a genetic disposition to this kind of body disorder; and second, the amount of regular physical activity, work or exercise, that is undertaken daily.

Long-term studies on dock workers and bus crews indicated that there was a direct relationship between the absence of cardiovascular ailments and a high level of physical work and there is no doubt that a good level of physical activity, combined with a moderate, sensible diet, is the best possible preventive medicine.

But it is not just to prevent ourselves dropping dead that we want a well-controlled diet. Our main aim, more likely, is the desire to enjoy our food. On the assumption that we are starting with a good appetite – and if we are exercising efficiently we almost certainly will be – we shall not have to rely on dishes prepared solely because they are tempting. From the necessary and nourishing ingredients we need to maintain health there is plenty of tasty, enjoyable food available.

We are also likely to rely on our diet to prevent us getting fat. The genetic make-up of some people gives them a far harder battle against obesity than some of their more fortunate fellows who burn up food more quickly. But obesity is avoidable, and it is an indisputable fact that if the intake of food is regulated to the output of energy, the body will not deposit too much fat.

Since most people are to some degree overweight, the progress you make with your diet will probably be measured in terms of weight reduction. If this doesn't happen, you will simply have over-assessed the amount of food you need – i.e. you will have still been eating too much. For while we are principally concerned with running as an aid to fitness, and while we acknowledge that the overweight runner is at a disadvantage, and while we shall go on to discuss how exercise can complement a sensible diet, it must be admitted that the most powerful factor in weight control is not running or work or exercise, but food intake.

Muscle, when exercised with the appropriate loadings, will increase in strength, and with an endurance exercise such as distance running the muscles will also firm up with better muscle tone and show more definition, rather than increase in bulk. Running does not replace lost fat with muscle, it improves your muscle performance while you get trimmer. Fat is never turned into muscle, the fat cells just decrease in size.

It is a sad fact that fat is much easier to avoid than to reduce, simply because once the fat cells are laid down the number of cells remains. A reduction in fat is a reduction only of the cell size. Furthermore, the number of fat cells is fixed at adolescence, which is why it is so unkind and unfair to overfeed children.

A slim youth who puts fat on in later life is in a far better position in his attempts to reduce weight than a child who has been allowed or even encouraged to get fat and then tries to remedy his obesity when he gets older. Unnecessary weight is expensive in food and the wasted physical effort involved in carting around unwanted flesh. It places an unnecessary, even dangerous, load upon the heart. It not only requires twice the energy to lift twenty pounds as it does ten pounds, but if you try to do it at the same rate it requires a greater power output, since power is the rate at which work is done. Most fat people move more slowly because their muscular strength does not match their weight. This becomes a vicious circle because the slower they move the less exercise they take, so their muscles tend to lose strength and they end up having to move more slowly still.

All those unnecessary fat cells, wherever they are, need a blood supply, so the lungs have to supply more oxygen to the blood and the heart has to pump more blood through an enlarged vascular system and the digestive system has to convert more food to nourish useless tissue. It is as silly as that.

A Question of Balance

A balanced diet is one that allows our intake of fuel to equal, as closely as possible, the fuel we expend. Nutritionists express our energy requirements in units of heat, called calories. One calorie is the amount of heat required to raise the temperature of 1 gram of water by 1 degree centigrade. This is such a small unit that all nutrition and physiology reference is expressed in units of 1000 calories (kilocalories) expressed as Calories (or Cal.) with a capital C.

To prove that diet controls weight more effectively than exercise let's take two examples. For an untrained man in his thirties a fair performance would be running just one mile in eight minutes. If that man weighed 11 stone (70kg) he would expend energy at the rate of 15 Cal. per minute, so his mile would use up 120 Cal. But if he drinks a couple of pints of beer a day, he is adding another 2500 Cals per week. Add to that just one fish-and-chip supper while watching television one evening – 600 more Calories – and he is putting away an excess total of 3100 Cal.

To get rid of those 3100 Cal. he would have to run twenty-six miles at eight-minute mile pace. This is nearly three-and-a-half hours' hard work. It just is not on, is it? Or take the case of a forty-year-old woman who is overweight. She wants to run off a small two-ounce bar of chocolate at a slow pace. That entails running for half an hour, which is hardly worth it, and furthermore, would have to be strictly additional to her normal day's routine.

Running, to sum up, is for fitness, diet is for weight control. This does not mean however, that running is not helpful in reducing weight – it is; but dieting and running should be mutually supporting activities and are most effective when combined.

Exercising while weight-reducing has an important safety factor, in that exercise uses up the glycogen in the muscles, which increases fat utilisation. Exercise, too, prevents someone on a low calorie diet from losing lean tissue. The whole idea of dieting is to achieve that balance between input and output.

Reducing weight when you are in a poor condition is not enough. Without exercise you will only become a thin person in poor condition.

We can guess the next question: 'OK, so I need a balanced diet, but what should be in it? And, more important, how much should I eat?' There is no fixed answer to this, only what might apply to that non-existent average man or woman. A good diet should, like high level training, be geared to the individual: with proper exercise your body will change; your intake should change with it.

The first step is to get some idea of the ideal weight for you. There are several ways in which this can be done.

By taking accurate skinfold measurements at various parts of the body, the percentage of body fat in the total weight can be calculated. The figure for total weight is then adjusted to give the required body fat percentage, and this final figure is your ideal weight.

Easier, if less accurate, is to take your ideal weight from a set of tables which are compiled to consider sex and height, and sometimes age and frame as well. For distance runners, a simple estimate of desired weight is provided by the formulae of Dr Stillman who got his figures from fifty top runners in the USA. His tables are not weighted for body type or age. For men he allows 110 lb (50 kg) for a height of 5 ft, and then adds 5½ lb (2.5 kg) for each additional inch. For women the base is 100 lbs (45.5 kgs) plus 5 lb (2.27 kgs) for each additional inch. These are the average weights for non-runners; from these figures he deducts 10 per cent for ideal weights for runners.

Height		Men Average weight			Men Ideal weight			Women Average weight			Women Ideal weight		
ft	in	st	lb	(kg)	st	lb	(kg)	st	lb	(kg)	st	lb	(kg)
5	0	7	12	(50)	7	1	(45)	7	2	(45.5)	6	6	(41)
5	1	8	3½	(52.5)	7	6	(47)	7	7	(47.7)	6	10½	(42.9)
5	2	8	9	(55)	7	11	(49.5)	7	12	(50.0)	7	1	(45)
5	3	9	0½	(57.5)	8	2	(52)	8	3	(52.3)	7	5½	(47.1)
5	4	9	6	(60)	8	7	(54)	8	8	(54.5)	7	10	(49)
5	5	9	11½	(62.5)	8	12	(56)	8	13	(56.8)	8	0½	(52.7)
5	6	10	2	(64.5)	9	3	(58.5)	9	4	(59.1)	8	5	(53.2)
5	7	10	8½	(67.5)	9	7½	(61)	9	9	(61.4)	8	9½	(55.5)
5	8	11	0	(70)	9	12½	(63)	10	0	(63.6)	9	0	(57.3)
5	9	11	5½	(72.5)	10	3½	(65)	10	5	(65.9)	9	4½	(59.3)
5	10	11	11	(75)	10	8½	(67.5)	10	10	(68.2)	9	9	(61.3)
5	11	12	2½	(77.5)	10	13½	(70)	11	1	(70.5)	9	13½	(63.5)
6	0	12	8	(80)	11	4½	(72)	11	6	(72.7)	10	4	(65.4)
6	1	12	13½	(82.5)	11	9½	(74)	11	11	(75.0)	10	8½	(67.5)
6	2	13	4	(84.5)	12	0½	(76.5)	12	2	(77.3)	10	13	(69.6)
6	3	13	9	(86.8)	12	5	(79)	12	7	(79.5)	11	3½	(71.6)

Energy intake

Recommended daily intake of protein, minerals and total calories

Age ranges	Energy	Protein recom- mended	Protein minimum requirement	Calcium	Iron
years	calories	g	g	mg	mg
Males					
9-11	2,500	63	36	700	13
12-14	2,800	70	46	700	14
15-17	3,000	75	50	600	15
18-34					
sedentary	2,700	68	45	500	10
moderately active	3,000	75	45	500	10
very active	3,600	90	45	500	10
35-64					
sedentary	2,600	65	43	500	10
moderately active	2,900	73	43	500	10
very active	3,600	90	43	500	10
65-74	2,350	59	39	500	10
75 and over	2,100	53	38	500	10
Females					
9-11	2,300	58	35	700	13
12-14	2,300	58	44	700	14
15-17	2,300	58	40	600	15
18-54					
most occupations	2,200	55	38	500	12
very active	2,500	63	38	500	12
55-74	2,050	51	36	500	10
75 and over	1,900	48	34	500	10
Pregnant, 2nd and 3rd trimesters	2,400	60	44	1,200	15
Lactating	2,700	68	55	1,200	15

Let us work out a simple example, to see how these tables can be used to establish a diet.

1.   You are a male, age 38 years, height 5 ft 9 in, who is moderately active in his general working day.

2.   From the Energy Intake table (page 103) we see that a moderately active man requires an intake equivalent to 2900 Cal.

3.   We will presume that you are going to run. To ensure body maintenance we will set protein at 15 per cent, fat at 20 per cent and carbohydrate at 65 per cent. This would meet the recommended requirements of a training diet.

The body converts different foods with varying degrees of efficiency, receiving roughly 4 Cal. per gram from protein, 4 Cal. per gram from carbohydrate and 9 Cal. per gram from fat.

So the first rough breakdown of your daily 2900 Cal. looks like this:

Nutrient	Percentage	Cal.	Cal. per gram	Weight of food
Protein	15	435	4	=109 grams (3.84oz)
Fat	25	725	9	=80 grams (2.82oz)
Carbohydrate	60	1740	4	=435 grams (15.34oz)
Total	100	2900		624 grams (22.0oz)

A calorie intake in excess of this for this individual would mean a steady gain in weight, or a levelling off well above his ideal weight.

Now let us suppose that he is running 5 miles every alternate evening after work, an average of 17.5 miles per week. If this were run at eight-minute mile pace he would use up 15 Cal. per minute. Therefore he would get rid of an extra 2100 Cal. (17.5 x 8 x 15) per week.

$$\frac{2100 \ (\text{Cal. Energy})}{3500 \ (1 \ \text{lb Fat})} = 0.6 \ \text{lb} \ (9.6 \ \text{oz}) = 272 \ \text{g}$$

This food equivalent – rather more than half a pound of butter – is then available either to contribute to his weight loss or, if his weight is at the required level, is the amount to supplement his diet.

The calorific adjustment in this case should be on fats and carbohydrates. The fat content would not need to exceed 100 grams per day in any case, but should not be lower than the example.

Honesty Works

Be honest with yourself when you are working out the calorific value of your diet, and count the effect of nibbling and the sweet tooth. The biscuit with the tea, the additional milk or cream in tea and coffee, the sugar in those six or seven cups each day simply does not vanish. Bearing in mind that one pound of fat is the equivalent of 3500 Cal., you have only to achieve a deficit of 500 Cal. per day to lose 1 lb in a week. That doesn't sound too bad, does it? One hundred grams (just under 4 oz) of butter has a value of about 790 Cal., so a mere half-ounce saved would contribute 100 Cal. towards the reduction you seek. Likewise, an ounce less cheese would save over 100 Cal., the two-ounce chocolate bar and the two-ounce bag of peanuts each have over 250 Cals. It sounds even easier put that way, and the process can be accelerated by diminishing your food intake still further. Within limits this is quite safe, providing the meals that you eat in a day contain, after preparation, at least the minimum amounts of essential vitamins and minerals. After all, fat is stored by the body as a food reserve.

(It would be unwise to push the reduction of food intake *too* far without medical advice or the help of a good dietician, because below a certain blood-sugar level the brain will not function properly. Unless you are unwise enough to go on a severe crash diet, this is unlikely to be a danger.)

Summing up, a slimming diet should contain the essential nutrients in the correct quantities, but the total energy value must be cut. And the cuts should fall on the least essential, such as the refined sugars which are considered by some to be positively harmful. Cut down on the sugars, avoid sweets, pudding, soft drinks and alcohol. Meals that are based on lean meats, fish and eggs, with fresh fruit and vegetables, are fine. Watch the amount of bread. Cheese is good, but a little goes a long way, as it is rich in fat as well as protein. And do not go on to quack diets recommending just one or two 'specials'. You need a sensible variety of foods to avoid the risk of being deficient in essential nutrients.

Finally, once you have worked out the calorie loss required to achieve the weight reduction you want, do not forget that when you start running, if you have not already started, the extra energy you expend here must figure in your calculations. Good news for the seriously overweight person who has reduced his or her weight far enough to start running: you will now have the additional calories used up in running to help you.

Once you have achieved your ideal weight, and you still want to run, then the daily diet must cater for the increased demand. And remember, working up a good sweat is not losing weight. All you are doing is losing body fluid, which is immediately replaced from drink and food.

Meals to run on

It is one thing to write down facts and state the rules, but practicalities can modify the ideal. Most training and dieting authorities advise eating more frequently in small portions, say five small meals per day in place of three large ones. The advantages include a more even energy release, and the fact that you don't feel so hungry at any one time that each meal becomes a temptation to overeat. This is fine as long as it does not mean portions that are so small as to be uneconomic or difficult to prepare.

To give an 'ideal diet' for the runner would take a book in itself. The choice of foods is so varied that as long as each day's intake has something close to the advisable proportions of protein, fat and carbohydrate the rest is up to you.

In preparing your own menus it is useful to have a guide to the calorie content of different foods as they come from the shop. A pocket guide to branded foods is helpful, as both named products and supermarket own brands are identified with the calories by ounces and grams – we would recommend the *Pocket Calorie Guide to Branded Foods* by Alexandra Sharman.

Instead of trying to map out a whole meal-by-meal regime for the fitness runner, we will instead look at one typical meal that a runner might eat, and examine the way in which he might choose it. We will also look in some detail at a typical day's menu designed for a working woman. The latter offers a balanced choice which totals only 2248 Cal., a lot less than what we would expect an active man to need; it could therefore provide useful hints for any man seeking a fast weight loss.

Dinner for an active man who runs

Age: 32 years

Weight: 11 stone (154 lb; 70 kg)

Job: Warehouse supervisor, not office-bound. On his feet all day assisting with loading. Such an active man would need 3,600 Cal. per day, even without running.

Running: Competes a little, therefore his running is at a good pace – say 6½-minute miles. He runs 4 x 7 miles during the week, with a 10-miler on Sunday at 7-min.-mile pace. Total: about 40 miles per week. Total running time: about 4½ hours.

Running at this pace requires about 860 Cal. per hour above his 3600 Cal. 4½ x 860 Cal. = 3870 Cal. which averages 553 Cal. per day.

So his total requirement is 3600 + 553 = 4153 Cal. per day.

Since he is very active he can allow the proportion of fat in his diet to increase to 30 per cent of the calorific value, which will reduce the bulk of the meals; 15 per cent or more protein will maintain body repair and 55 per cent carbohydrate will supply the remaining energy. A sample meal is as follows:

	Weight	Cal.	Protein grams	Fat grams	Carbohydrate grams
Orange juice	(large glass)	120.0	1.2	0	28.8
Roast lamb	4oz (113g)	330.8	26.0	25.2	0
Boiled peas	3oz (85g)	32.4	4.5	0	3.6
Roast potatoes	6oz (170g)	279.6	4.8	8.4	46.2
Tinned peaches	4oz (113g)	105.6	0.4	0	26.0
Custard	3oz (85g)	103.2	3.3	3.6	14.4
Calorie conversion		971.6	40.2 × 4	37.2 × 9	119.0 × 4
Total calories in meal		971.6	160.8 (14%)	334.8 (30%)	476.0 (56%)

This meal would supply nearly a quarter of the daily food requirement. Additionally it would supply most of the daily vitamin need as follows: Calcium 43 per cent, Iron 58 per cent, Thiamin 46 per cent, Riboflavin 42 per cent, all the Nicotinic acid and Vitamin C. There is no Vitamin D, but this would be met with an ounce of average margarine from other meals.

One day with a working woman

Tea and coffee drinks, of course, are mainly composed of water, but the amount of tea or coffee varies considerably. These arbitary figures have been used in the menu below: tea ⅙ oz, coffee ⅒ oz.

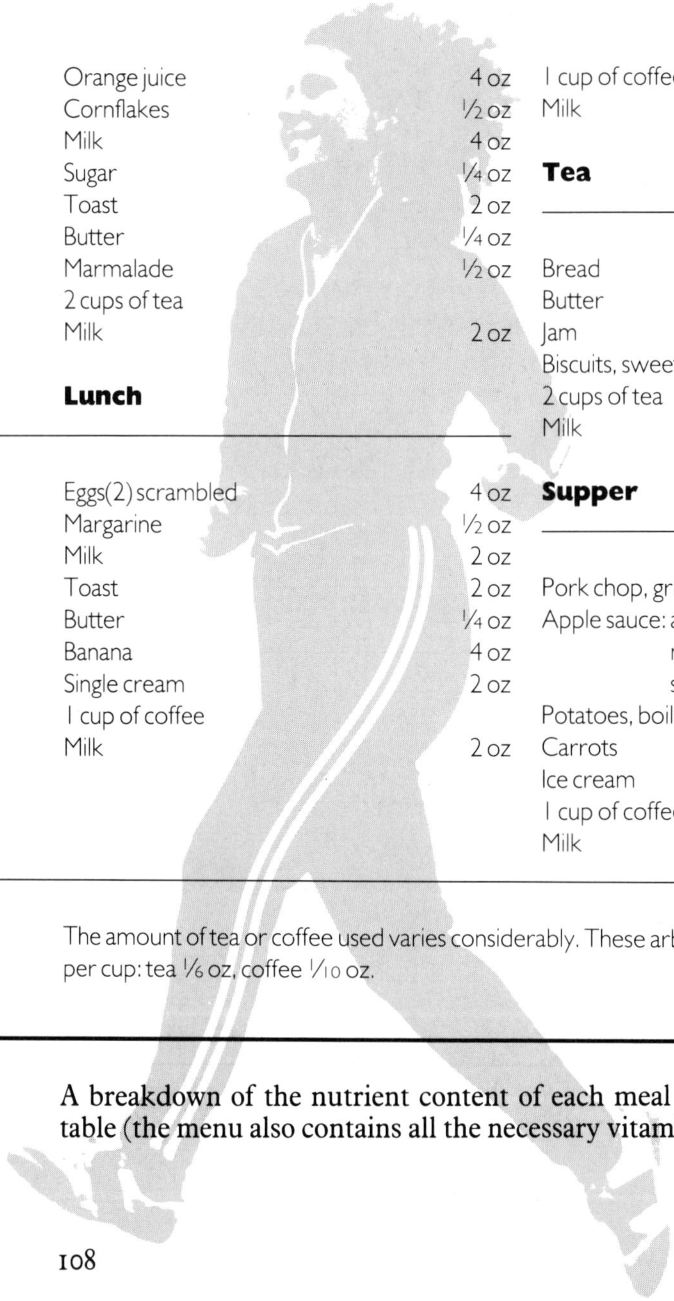

Breakfast

Orange juice	4 oz
Cornflakes	½ oz
Milk	4 oz
Sugar	¼ oz
Toast	2 oz
Butter	¼ oz
Marmalade	½ oz
2 cups of tea	
Milk	2 oz

Lunch

Eggs (2) scrambled	4 oz
Margarine	½ oz
Milk	2 oz
Toast	2 oz
Butter	¼ oz
Banana	4 oz
Single cream	2 oz
I cup of coffee	
Milk	2 oz

Snack

I cup of coffee	
Milk	2 oz

Tea

Bread	I oz
Butter	⅛ oz
Jam	½ oz
Biscuits, sweet (2)	½ oz
2 cups of tea	
Milk	2 oz

Supper

Pork chop, grilled	4 oz
Apple sauce: apple	4 oz
margarine	⅕ oz
sugar	¼ oz
Potatoes, boiled	6 oz
Carrots	4 oz
Ice cream	2 oz
I cup of coffee	
Milk	2 oz

The amount of tea or coffee used varies considerably. These arbitary figures have been used per cup: tea ⅙ oz, coffee ⅒ oz.

A breakdown of the nutrient content of each meal is shown in the following table (the menu also contains all the necessary vitamins and minerals).

Meal	Cal.	Protein grams	Fat grams	Carbo—hydrate grams
Breakfast	462	11.4	13.6	75.0
Snack	39	2.2	2.2	2.9
Lunch	729	25.0	46.1	57.5
Tea	232	5.0	8.9	35.3
Supper	786	40.2	38.6	76.6
Total dietary intake	2,248	83.8	109.4	247.3

The Snack Trap

One more quick example, just to convince those people who say that they don't eat much – only snacks:

One snack lunch: white bread, butter, cheese, lettuce, tomato, instant coffee, milk. Total weight – slightly over 10 oz (282 g). Total Calories – 643.3

One cooked lunch: Roast lamb, fried potatoes (chips), boiled peas, tinned peaches, custard. Total weight – 14½ oz (410 g). Total Calories – 646.5

The snack is giving the body almost exactly the same number of calories as the cooked meal – and any self-congratulation by the snack-eater on his abstinence is demonstrably misplaced.

Diet deficiences do not manifest themselves at once. If in any one week your intake is short of iron or vitamin C or whatever, you will not break out in spots during the following week.

While we lack an early warning system for dietary deficiencies there is also plenty of time in the following week to make up for the one week's shortfall. What we are saying is that an obsessional concern with milligrams per day of anything is neither necessary nor advisable.

Most people think of malnutrition as meaning not enough but this is only partly true. Malnutrition means bad nutrition, and too much is also bad.

Some athletes have trouble keeping their weight down even when they are in full training. Others, like Seb, have a much easier time:

I'm lucky, really, I just don't seem to be *able* to eat too much. As long as I'm sensible I just never seem to put on weight.

This is a tremendous advantage. I do try to make sure that I get the benefit of the proper ingredients for my diet – potatoes in their jackets rather than potatoes boiled away to nothing, for example, and enough salads and enough meat – but after that I can literally eat just what I want. I've never been overweight, as far as I can remember. In fact if I ever did have a problem it would probably be to maintain weight rather than lose it.

Oddly enough I find that during the track season, when I'm training hardest, I probably eat slightly *less* than when I'm doing easier work in the winter months. It's probably just that like everyone else I'm eating more in the winter to maintain body heat; and I must say that in the summer, after a long, hard track session, I physically don't *want* to eat for two or three hours.

All this makes it fairly easy for me. I usually have a cooked breakfast, a reasonably light salad lunch, and a proper cooked dinner in the evening. The evening meal is often quite late – I sometimes don't finish my training till well into the early evening, and I certainly can't eat straight after that. I do tend to nibble a bit between meals, too. I've got a sweet tooth, and I'm a sucker for chocolate biscuits.

I'm a bit more particular about drinking. I just cannot run with drink inside me – I tend to get the most awful stomach cramps. When I run first thing in the morning I may have just a quarter of a cup of tea to help the body start working, but really I'd prefer to run with nothing inside me at all. Before a race I wouldn't dream of drinking within four or four-and-a-half hours of the start. That's going to be a problem if I ever run a marathon; you really do have to drink in a race as long as that, but the idea of running with a lot of liquid swilling about inside doesn't bear thinking about.

Otherwise, though, I drink quite a lot. Not straight after a run – I don't seem to need it then – but during the rest of the day I can get through plenty of cups of tea or coffee, as well as a pint of milk at lunchtime and perhaps a pint or so of fruit juice during the course of the evening.

The one time that I might make diet concessions of any sort is when I'm racing abroad, particularly in the warmer climates. I'm careful not to eat ice-cream or fresh salads, say, or unpeeled fruit or sea food; and I stick to bottled water to drink. Some athletes have a terrible time abroad, they never seem to step off a plane without getting stomach trouble: Brendan Foster used to be a perennial victim, and poor David Moorcroft was on a strict diet of bread and jam from the moment he arrived in Athens for the European Championships last year. I've never been as unlucky as that, and I'd probably be all right whatever I ate. But it would be stupid to ruin a race just by being careless about food.'

The Alcohol Question

If it came to a straightforward case of do or don't the answer would have to be don't. Unfortunately life isn't all that simple; a lot of people enjoy a drink, and we have to make value judgments. It is the potential of alcohol that is the biggest problem. The potential for good is just about non-existent and the potential for harm is infinite.

Alcohol is a depressant and gives the illusion of relaxing the drinker. In fact it anaesthetises the nerves but not, unless drunk to excess, the muscles. What passes for acceptable social imbibing is not enough to relax muscles, and it certainly cannot remove stress symptoms.

So what does it do? Most relevant to the runner is the fact that alcohol constricts the arteries leading to the heart, it has an adverse effect at submaximal work loads by decreasing oxygen uptake, it upsets the delicate heat balance mechanism of the body, it impairs co-ordination, and it generally deludes the drinker into believing that things are better than they are. Alcohol can also destroy some essential nutrients, like the vitamin B group. Excess alcohol can also cause hypoglycaemia, and the brain cannot function properly with a low blood sugar level. And alcohol is not good for the liver, which is our glycogen storehouse.

The only pressure to take alcohol is a social one, and a romanticised one at that. It is regrettable that many of our so-called hearty sportsmen – and rugger players, for example, figure prominently among them – are obviously over-weight and not very fit. Furthermore alcohol is fattening: 1 pint of beer equals 250 Cal.

But old habits die hard, and some acquired tastes will not go away. The answer must be a compromise – less than perfect, but tolerable.

For example, Seb's compromise works like this: 'From the end of February to the end of September I drink very little alcohol. When I do, it is no more than a sipped toast at the odd reception or, equally rarely, a small glass of lemonade shandy. The replacement I use is a double Britvic orange juice with enough lemonade to fill a pint glass. For me winter drinking is an occasional half of Guinness or a lemonade shandy if I'm thirsty. I do enjoy a single glass of wine at dinner sometimes, but once serious training has commenced – no more alcohol.'

To say there are no drinking distance runners would be ridiculous, and tolerance varies with individuals, but it is our observation that intake varies inversely with your belief in your own potential. The better you believe you can be, the less you'll drink. Funnily enough, drink can be used as a good excuse for failing. 'Ah yes, I could be a lot better but I like my beer,' is a frequently heard cop-out. But if fun runners and fitness runners can still measure improvement on an occasional beer or glass of wine, then what they are drinking is all right for them.

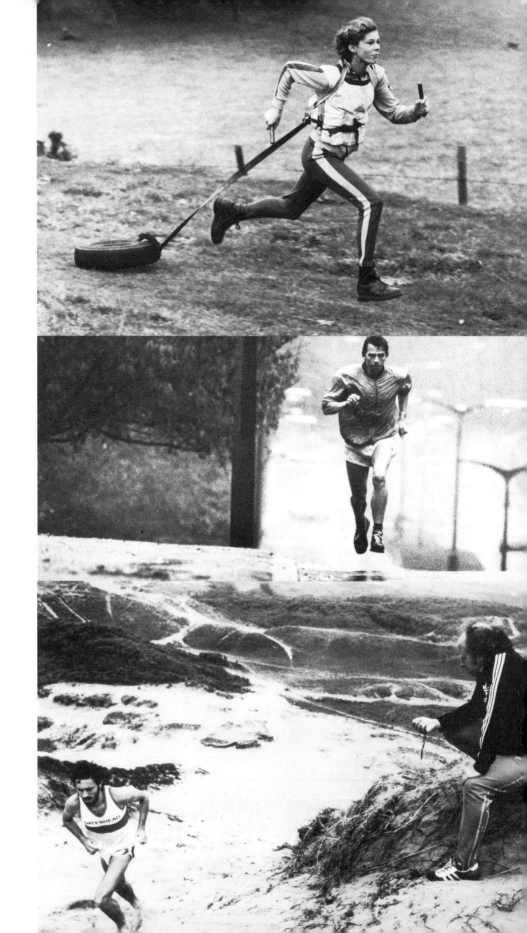

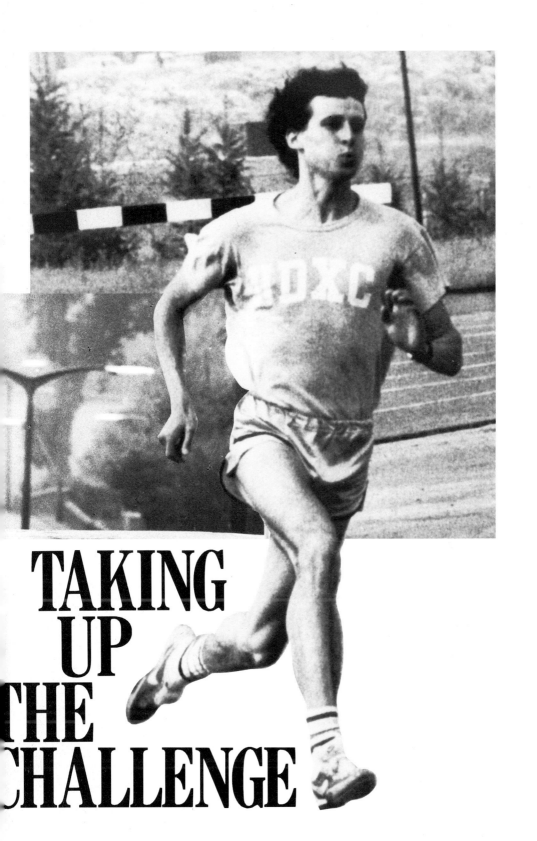

TAKING UP THE CHALLENGE

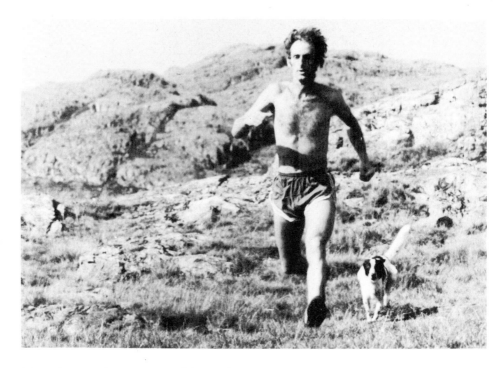

Now that you have some solid running behind you, the chances are that you will be looking ahead with fresh eyes – perhaps with ambitions that a few weeks ago you wouldn't have thought possible, perhaps with your sights now firmly on a target you set yourself years ago. Not everyone will be looking ahead to an Olympic final, but every runner will at some time or another be tempted to test his or her improved abilities on a set course or over a classic distance against the clock – and in contention with, or at least in the company of, runners of similar ability. It would be very strange if, one day, you didn't respond to the temptation.

Whenever the talk gets round to running, one question is asked more than any other: 'How much running should be done?'

Whether the aim is to run for fitness or to run for an Olympic gold medal, the reply is still the same: just enough and no more than is necessary to achieve your goal; anything more is likely to be counter-productive.

If you are aiming to be the best, then the training load will be high, but as soon as your performance levels off then you have done enough. You can examine your training schedules to see if there should be a shift of emphasis, but do not simply do more – it takes less training to maintain your condition than it does to achieve it, and while it takes 80 per cent of your maximum to apply a stimulus strong enough to bring about an improvement, it takes only a 60 per cent loading to maintain that level.

The principle is equally true with running for fitness. Once you have achieved the level you want, cut back a little and do only enough to stay fit. If you decide to compete, then you change your routine to sharpen up, but only enough to reach your new target.

And fun running is the simplest of all. First you get fit enough to run freely without strain, and then you run for fun. If you want more fun, then you run some more, and this becomes its own training. But as soon as the amount of running becomes a chore, or you start suffering undue aches and pains, you will just naturally reduce the load.

There is a general rule which says you should finish your runs feeling well worked but mentally fresh, and certainly not physically exhausted. For nearly all situations outside racing this is very true, but for the ambitious there are times when exceptions have to be made in training.

The following conversation will illustrate the point:

Peter: 'He's a nice looking runner, he has the right build and style and strength. He really should be a lot better than he is.'

Seb: 'Yes I know, Dad, but he's turned eighteen and he hasn't yet learned how to hurt himself. And I don't think he ever will.'

What Seb was saying was cruel but true: all of us can keep going that bit longer than we think, if only we are prepared to find out. Part of the art of coaching is to have a nose for the right level of development, and the right moment for your charge to test himself in this way. Runners with ambition will have to go through this more than once and not leave it only to race days.

This brings in another factor in determining what is enough. Enough is what the whole man, not just the body, will accept. The work load may be within the limit set by your body but if you mentally reject that amount of training, then it becomes too much. The sad fact is that if you cannot mentally accept what you are doing, your body will ultimately reject it as well, and you will not extract from the exercise the physical benefits you should.

Keeping the Record Straight

A training diary is well worth while. If you hate writing even a single line it may be a tedious job, but it's going to be a lot easier than the training stints you're going to be setting yourself, and the end product will be both interesting and valuable.

It doesn't have to be anything elaborate – an ordinary scribbling diary or exercise book will do. And all you have to record is the day, the mileage you run, your time for the distance, the weather, the state of your health that day, and your feelings or impressions during and after the run.

What is the point? For some of you it may be no more than a personal journal, which will be pleasant to look through and reminisce over in the years to come; but it could be much more useful than that. It will help you to check your overall adherence to your training plan. It will allow you to identify actions or events which prove to suit your training – or not to suit it. It may enable you to relate any improvement, or any injury, to some specific facet of your training. And in time it will indicate expected recovery time from any setback you may suffer – colds, flu, minor injuries and the effects of any lay-off period.

We still refer to one or more of the 'historic' build-ups when we are planning for a big event. There is no reason why you, in your own way, shouldn't benefit in the same way.

A Choice of Targets

Everyone will have their own targets, and there is no point in trying to give detailed training schedules to them all. So we are going to look at a number of runners with widely varying ambitions, and chart their progress towards those goals. We will guide our novice fitness runner towards a local fun-run type of race; our more confident fitness runner to a season of modest road racing or cross-country; our established fitness runner, who we assume will have been running steadily for a few years, towards a first-time marathon – and we'll see how an accomplished athlete prepares for a top-class international middle-distance championship. None of these may fit your own requirements precisely, but one of them, we are sure, will adapt readily to what you are looking for.

The Three-mile Fun Run

The local community centre has a member who is a regular club runner, and they have persuaded him to put on a short road race as part of their Fitness Week.

You have already been running for fitness and pleasure and feel a little glow of satisfaction at your progress and now, quite suddenly, you want to know. You want to know if you are as good as you think you are and as good as you feel. You have posted your entry form and now you find that you have barely a month to go to the race. 'What should I be doing now?' you ask. That's the easy bit – but . . .

You know that your nine-year-old son will settle for nothing less than a Dave Moorcroft runaway victory and, worse still, he hates the kid next door, whose healthy dad jumps the front garden gate every morning. And of course his dad has also entered – a happy piece of news your own lad couldn't wait to tell you.

So now the question 'What should I be doing?' (like emigrating?) takes on a new urgency.

Now, how long have you got? A month? Oh well, hard luck, you should have bought our book two months ago. Never mind, we will see what we can do. Three things before you start:

Rule 1: Play it cool – don't even tell your son what you're at. Act nonchalantly and don't let the enemy know what you are doing.

Rule 2: Don't panic – think.

Rule 3: Start from the bottom up – let's look at your feet.

Question: Are the shoes you are running in now going to be all right in four weeks' time? Never turn out in a new pair of shoes, that's a real trouble risk. The modern shoes with nylon tops and waffle soles are easy to get used to, but get them now: that way they will be OK to race in after a month. If you are going to need a repair before race day, get it done *now*. And have put aside a *tried* pair of clean socks.

Examine your feet carefully for any actual or potential trouble spots, like toenails that are growing in at the corners, corns on top or between your toes, blisters or hot spots. Once you have checked over your feet, try to keep them in condition all the time.

You are going to *race* over a three-mile course, not merely run it. What is comfortable when you are proceeding at your own pace quickly becomes exhausting if it's done too quickly, so start concentrating on pace judgment now.

Even for a beginner certain basic rules apply. If you are going to race 3 miles, train for at least 4. You will need the strength and confidence of knowing that you can last 4 hard miles. Now break down the required 3-mile time into minutes per mile. For example if your goal is 3 miles in 19½ minutes then your pace is at 6½ minutes per mile.

From here on your training splits three ways. The first will be steady over-distance running for good all-round stamina, say a run of 6–8 miles.

The second way is running a mile at race pace or better, having a short recovery, say 2–3 minutes, and then continuing for another mile with another short recovery of 2–3 minutes and then complete the third mile. Each mile should be run at least race pace.

The third line of attack will be to run 1 mile at race pace and continue at the same pace until you start to slow significantly. You will extend this type of running until you are able to run for 4 miles at your 3-mile race pace. Your month's schedule can now be planned. (A note about planning: if you have a regular hobby evening or a family activity like swimming every Tuesday evening, or your wife has a regular evening class and you are looking after the home, make that day your rest day. Then plan the days round that rest day. This avoids family disruption and guilt feelings on all sides).

Just to start somewhere we will assume that Wednesday is to be your rest day, and the race is planned for the Sunday four weeks from now.

Week 1

Monday
Run 6 miles steady at your comfortable pace
Tuesday
1 mile in 6½ mins. Jog home (J.H.) if you are training within a mile or two of your home
Wednesday
Rest
Thursday
1 mile in 6½ min. Rest 3 min. Run 1 mile in 6½ min
Friday
6 miles steady (as Monday)
Saturday
1½ miles in 9¾ min (J.H.)
Sunday
6 miles steady

Week 2

Monday
3 × 1 mile at 6½-min pace, with a 3-min rest between each mile (J.H.)
Tuesday
6 miles steady
Wednesday
Rest
Thursday
2 miles in 13 min (J.H.)
Friday
6 miles steady
Saturday
4 × 1 mile at 6½-min pace, with a 2-min rest between each mile (J.H.)
Sunday
6 miles steady

Week 3

Monday
2½ miles in 16¼ min (J.H.)
Tuesday
6 miles steady
Wednesday
Rest
Thursday
4 × 1 mile at 6½-min pace, with 1½-min rest between each mile (J.H.)
Friday
8 miles steady
Saturday
3 miles in 19½ min (J.H.)
Sunday
6 miles steady

Week 4

Monday
3½ miles in 22¾ min (J.H.)
Tuesday
8 miles steady
Wednesday
Rest
Thursday
4 × 1 mile at 6½-min pace, with ½-min rest between each mile (J.H.)
Friday
3 miles easy
Saturday
Rest
Sunday
RACE

(On the rest days and whenever you can – each day if possible – do plenty of bending and stretching to avoid feelings of stiffness.)

There, that wasn't so bad, was it?

Now that you have successfully completed your first competitive run you will have the desire and confidence to continue racing.

You will also have had enough running to start using, cautiously, the interval training we described in Chapter Four. This should improve your oxygen uptake and yield an improvement in your road running endurance and speed.

To begin with we would suggest sessions of 10 (working up to 20) x 100 metres in 18 sec, with 40 sec walk or jog recovery. Start doing this twice a week and then, after a month, increase the distance to 10 (working up to 20) x 200 metres in 38–40 sec with 60 sec recovery.

A Season on the Road

After a bit more training, and a few successful races to test your confidence and prove that you are, indeed, getting stronger, you may decide that you would like to try road racing in a limited way.

This time, though, you have made your decision well in advance – full of the joys of fitness running and celebrating Christmas, you decide to enter a number of road events later in the coming year.

Because you will be able to spend months rather than weeks on your build-up you will be in a position to introduce some more specialised and specific elements into your training. Sessions of interval training, speed endurance and fartlek will all have their place.

The events you will probably be considering are the increasingly popular 10 kilometre (6¼ mile) road races. If you are under thirty a first-time target of 40 minutes on a slightly undulating course is realistic. For the trim and fit forty-year-old the expectation is somewhat lower; a time around 46–48 minutes is a fair performance.

The following schedules, starting in January, should produce the right results six or seven months later. The four weeks after Christmas are taken up with carefully consolidating the new weekly mileage, and from then on you will train on a schedule of overall increasing mileage. The weeks that contain one or two of the fartlek, interval or speed endurance sessions will contain a lower mileage, both because they can be quite hard training sessions, and because they take up more time for fewer miles. Also, in terms of mileage it is helpful to run alternate hard and easy weeks.

This schedule should not be too hard for a runner under thirty. The 48-minute forty-year-old may feel he has to add a half a minute per mile to his earlier training pace, but he should try, without straining, to get closer to the under-thirties schedule towards the end.

The mileage chart is drawn to cover seven periods, each of four weeks, and each week should contain one rest day. This day is not an active rest day (if it's a Sunday, for example, it is not for long walks, cycle rides or a lot of swimming), it is for relaxation. It's not an absolutely fixed day but it should be well spaced at as close to weekly intervals as possible.

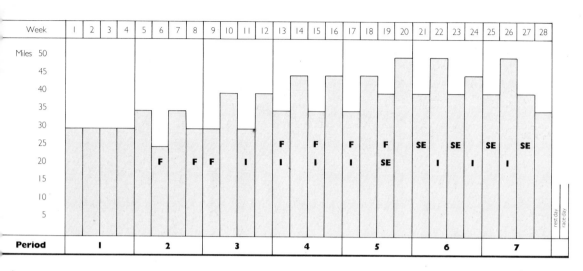

F indicates Fartlek session   **I** indicates Interval session   **SE** indicates Speed Endurance session

(Always warm up properly before these three sessions – say 2 miles – and 'jog down' 1 mile afterwards.)

For your *interval training*, take your best time for 200 metres and increase this by 20 per cent (e.g. best 200 metres is 28 sec, interval training pace is 28 + 5.6 sec = 33.6, say 34–35 sec per 200 metres). The recovery period between runs should be about three times the duration of the run (about 1½ min) and should be walked or jogged.

Your *speed endurance* runs should be around 800 metres to 1000 metres. Cyclometers and the trips on car speedos usually read off in tenths of a mile, so if you are using one of these to check a distance, then settle for the five tenths and six tenths marks on the clock. These are 880 yards and 1056 yards respectively. The pace for these runs should be based upon your best time for the distance plus 25 per cent. (This pace is one suggested only for a runner at this stage of improvement; it is not correct for faster track athletes.) The recovery should be twice the running time (e.g. best half mile time of 2 min 25 sec + 36.25 sec = 3 min 1.25 sec – say 3 min). Therefore run for 3 minutes and walk/jog recovery for 6 minutes.

Period I

Weeks 1-4
6 daily runs each of 5 miles steady running,
7min 30sec per mile pace for 4 weeks

Period II

Week 5
as above but daily average of 6 miles
Week 6
5 days of 4 miles at 7min per mile pace; 1 day
of 5 miles of fartlek
Week 7
as week 5
Week 8
5 days of 4-5 miles; 1 hour of fartlek

Period III

Week 9
as week 8
Week 10
6 days of 6-7 miles at 7min to 7min 30sec per
mile pace
Week 11
5 days of 5 miles at 7min per mile pace
Week 12
as week 10

Period IV

Week 13
4 days of 7 miles (7min pace); 1-day intervals;
1 day fartlek (1 hour)
Week 14
5 days of 5 miles (7min pace); 1 day of 10 miles
(7min 30sec pace)
Week 15
as week 13
Week 16
as week 14

Period V

Week 17
as week 13
Week 18
as week 14
Week 19
4 days of 7 miles (7min 30sec pace); 1 day
fartlek (1 hour); 1 day speed endurance (4 ×
800m)
Week 20
5 days (6,8,6,8,7 miles at 7-7min 30sec pace);
1 day 10 miles at (7min 30sec pace)

Period VI

Week 21
5 days of 7 miles (7min pace); 1 day speed
endurance (5 × 800m)
Week 22
4 days of 8 miles (7min pace); 1 day 12 miles
(7min 30sec pace)
Week 23
as week 21
Week 24
5 days of 8 miles (7min pace); 1 day intervals

Period VII

Week 25
as week 21
Week 26
as week 22
Week 27
as week 21
Week 28
5 days (9,8,7,6,5 miles) 9,8,7 miles at 7min -7min
30sec pace; 6 & 5 miles at 6min 30sec-7min
pace

Take a complete rest the day before a race. If you are under thirty, depending upon your general condition, you might very well crack the target times, but at the end of this schedule running 40 to 45 miles per week will allow you to race over distances of 3 to 6 miles every three weeks from August to October inclusive. Don't forget to do plenty of suppleness exercises.

Do not mix the fartlek or interval sessions with the steady runs, keep them for separate days – a steady run on one day, fartlek or intervals on another.

A Winter in the Mud

Training for a cross-country season will not be as specific as that for a series of road races, but the following suggestions will help any runner with a background of stamina and fitness running who wants to have a go over the country.

You will need plenty of mixed road work, fast runs over 4–6 miles for sustained pace, and plenty of steady runs over 10 miles or more for stamina. Repetition speed endurance sessions with runs over 800, 1000 and 1200 metres should also be included in your training.

If you cannot find a circuit in a hilly park or a bit of open country of, say, 2-mile laps, then you will have to find the features you want separately and practise on them in turn. Training on hills in town can be hard and useful but never quite the same – your footing is much firmer and safer in town, and the hard surfaces won't develop the ankle strength that lets you run over rough ground without worry.

Learning how to pick the best parts of a course where it is easier or safer to overtake other runners comes only with experience. Learn to gauge when the little bit of path or road can be safely negotiated with spikes, or to know at a glance when you are going to need the 15mm spikes for a grip, or whether ripples or waffles are going to be the better bet. If you do wear spikes, a heel wedge will be kinder on your calves and achilles tendons.

It is easier to perform reasonably over 10km on the road than it is at this distance over the country, particularly if you are training on a restricted mileage. The very best cross-country runner would need an average of 60–65 good miles per week at least to race well over the country, although it is doubtful if a 9-mile 'National' could be won even on this mileage.

The Lure of the Marathon

Welcome to another 'I want to know' case – the man who wants to say 'I have run the marathon'. It could very well be someone just like you.

You have seen the mass marathons on television and you know that just finishing is, for you, not enough. There are times returned in these events which preclude the possibility that the finishers actually ran the whole distance. They might have walked, crawled or swum it, but they never ran it. Out of respect for the sport and for yourself, and bearing in mind your age and the demands of your job, you have come up with a time of four hours as your target.

This is the best time that you can realistically expect. The decision to attempt the marathon is not one that is taken lightly, and you have delayed the moment of final commitment until you have only four months left before the race. Luckily for you this makes it an end-of-season event, when the autumn weather should be ideal.

Your background is fairly typical. You took up jogging a couple of years ago rather sporadically, but all last year you made a serious effort to train, and in fact got up to an average of 30 miles a week. You have a decent job where you are paid for your knowledge and ability rather than your time, and your colleagues are sympathetic to your endeavour – in fact you have got them to sponsor you per mile for charity. For someone who is not an established athlete and is strictly a fitness and fun runner, your background is ideal for success, particularly as you are not coming home whacked from contract bricklaying or concreting. What you have to do is to get in enough distance running before the day, check your diet, and pay attention to those particular aspects of running that are problems only in marathons.

Let's take mileage first. Our good friend Trevor Wright, a Sheffield athlete of great talent and experience, says that he thinks that 70–75 miles a week is quite enough mileage to run a good marathon. This may seem low to some runners aiming for the top. We will always agree that training schedules should be individually prescribed but Trevor won a silver medal in the European Championship in his first marathon in 1971 and recently ran a 2 hour 12 minute marathon. His record in cross-country and at 10,000 metres on the track is also a fine one, and he won the King of the Road title a few years back.

Now although much can be done by those at the top on 75 miles a week, it is still a lot of miles to be found, and for runners not as fast as Trevor Wright, even more time is required for the same mileage.

Furthermore, to go mad suddenly on increasing mileage at this stage is inviting the athlete to break down. The total mileage wants lifting, but very carefully and steadily – and we do not propose to set our first-time man more than 50 miles in any one week.

What prospective marathon runners must do is to establish their pace judgment. Your aim is to achieve a time of four hours for the race. If you get the feel of this pace firmly established it will help you to assess by the mid-stages of the race if you are going to be able to sustain it over the latter part of the race. If not, then you must choose one of only two options open to you. First, to see how far you can go at that pace, a good piece of knowledge in itself, or second, note the mile mark at which you are still on target, and then deliberately slow down in order to complete the distance.

This decision should be made with the following in mind. Is it a 'one-off' event to satisfy the desire to say 'I ran a marathon' or is it to say 'I set out for a four hour marathon and if it eludes me this time, next time I will succeed.'? If it is the latter then you must take the first choice and stick to your pace.

We cannot advise on this choice except to say that we based Seb's athletic career on the premise that once the target is identified you go for broke. For a marathon runner, it is best taken before the race, as it significantly changes the runner's attitude – and hence his performance – on the day.

Now, back to the problem of pace and mileage in training. Four months – or about seventeen weeks – is the time beween now and the race.

The general plan is this: learn pace judgment on the shorter runs and steadily extend the longer runs to approach the racing distance. Later on some of the shorter runs will be faster than race pace and some, or part of some, of the longer runs will be at race pace.

A marathon is 26 miles 385 yards, and to run it in four hours means a pace of 9 min 9 sec per mile. In order to get your pace judgment accurate measure off parts of your training roads – five mile sections are long enough – and during your training runs make sure that you run enough of these sections between 45 min 30 sec and 46 min in order to get the feel of the pace.

Throughout your four-month build-up there will be – and there should be – a

Marathon training chart

Week	Tues	Weds	Thurs	Fri	Sat	Sun	Mon	Total
1	6	5	ss	6	5	8	ss	30
2	5	6	ss	5	6	10	ss	32
3	6	6	ss	6	6	10	ss	34
4	6	8	ss	8	6	8	ss	36
5	5	8	ss	8	5	12	ss	38
6	10	6	ss	9	7	8	ss	40
7	11	5	ss	9	7	9	ss	41
8	6	7	ss	7	6	16	ss	42
9	6	8	6	8	6	10	ss	44
10	10	7	ss	10	7	12	ss	46
11	6	8	ss	8	6	20	ss	48
12	6	10	8	10	8	8	ss	50
13	12	5	6	6	5	16	ss	50
14	6	10	6	10	6	10	ss	48
15	7	10	ss	7	ss	16	ss	40
16	5	6	ss	6	8	8	ss	33
17	6	jog 5	jog 4	ss	ss	RACE		15

Training total 667

(ss = suppleness and stretching on rest day)

lot of mileage that you will run at faster than race pace and this running will be all to your good, but do remember to refresh your memory from time to time as to what 9 min 9 sec pace is really like. This judgment will be essential on the race day, because assuming you get through this schedule, eat properly and sleep well, the first ten miles of your marathon are going to feel easy; the real danger will be getting carried away with how well you are going and trying to cover too many miles and get too many minutes to the good; this will lead to a desperately hard last five miles.

Also, on the eleventh week of the schedule, there is a twenty-mile run. Do not, even if you still feel very good, get the wild idea of finishing the full marathon distance just to know you can do it a month later. Remember, you are training for your first marathon, not for two in one month.

You will notice that, with exception of weeks 9, 12, 13 and 14, the pattern of days 'off' and 'on' is one off, two on, one off, three on. In the event of enforced lay-offs (colds, for example) return to the exact pattern as soon as possible. If you are not feeling fully fit, return to the daily pattern at a reduced pace and/or mileage, but keep to the pattern.

All over the country runners make their long runs on a Sunday. Club runners particularly use this day and we feel that for those runners who enjoy their running more when in company this will always be the day. There may be work or domestic reasons that rule out Saturday anyway, but if after a hard Sunday run you do not feel fresh enough to face work on Monday, consider moving the mileage build-up chart back one day. This would give you an old-fashioned lay-about Sunday and ensure a better Monday.

Being fresh for work is important because any carry-over of business or domestic worries into an otherwise smooth-running preparation will have an adverse effect on the training and ultimately the race. However, the great majority of runners are 'long run Sunday' people, and you should cope with this quite happily. If you do want an easy Sunday, try not to swop in and out of Saturday and Sunday as you go along. The mileage chart is drawn up to give you adequate recovery during each and every week and the last four days before your race are to give you a chance to feed up, rest and store the glycogen.

During this seventeen-week period the diet must be watched, because in some weeks there is going to be a big increase in the total mileage.

The less useless weight a runner carries around with him the better, particularly a marathon runner, and the first eight weeks of our schedule might well be used to get rid of the few excess pounds you may be carrying.

In our chapter on diet and nutrition, we noted that a man in a sedentary job needs around 2600 Cal. per day. Running at about 7 mph requires about 870 Cal. per hour, so a forty-mile-week will need an additional 5000 Cal. per week, or 714 Cal. per day. Nevertheless, by week 11 weight changes should be stabilised and from then on a careful check should be maintained on weight control.

If the extra running does increase your hunger, eat more frequently – not more. Certainly if your percentage of body fat was correct before you started on this schedule, you should be matching the increase in mileage with a balanced addition to your diet, somewhere between 100 and 125 Cal. per mile per week.

As far as your mile-chart is concerned, remember that a top athlete going for a big marathon would have a significantly different build-up for his attempt than the one suggested for you. To start with, his programme would be spread over the year, and although he might race more than one marathon, he would always keep the big one in mind and his training would always be biased towards this race.

Furthermore, his total mileage would be at least double yours, and would very likely alternate the hard months with easy ones. While there would be an overall climb in mileage as the training progressed, there would probably be a 'macro-recovery period' every other month. In other words, a hard month is followed by a full month of lower mileage to fully recover and consolidate the improvement laid down by the stress of the hard month. Inside this overall plan would still be a 'micro-recovery period' such as one day hard and one or two days easy.

But your case is a rush job of four months – and you are not an athlete conditioned to a sixty-miles-per-week base from which to start.

The plan you have provides for a small, steady increase week by week until you reach fifty miles per week which is then held for two weeks. Though people have completed, and doubtless will complete, marathons on lower mileages, we would consider this to be about the lowest total weekly distance on which some one relatively inexperienced might expect to manage four hours in reasonable comfort.

What relief from over-stressing that can be allowed inside the time scale must be achieved during the week. The longest runs are nearly all followed by a rest day; if not, they follow one.

A Tilt at the Championship

For our final example we will suppose a big track championship meeting somewhere in Europe in August or September when three races – heat, semi-final and final – will be required.

We will also suppose our athlete is someone like Seb. For this kind of athlete there is no particular build-up in his training, you cannot bring world class athletes to the 'boil' quickly, certainly not with any likelihood of consistency. For a main event of this importance the whole year's training will be organised towards this goal, although he will have run some good-class one-offs before this. It may take five or six fast races to consolidate his speed and form before he sets out to win a major event.

We can only give an outline of a training year, and then detail the last two weeks before the big event.

The athlete will have built up a solid strength and endurance base by steady distance running and by hard weight and circuit training in the gymnasium. On to this base, using a multi-tier training programme as in our sample schedule, he will build up speed endurance – the ability, in this case, to run one half-mile flat out and then one mile nearly flat out. In addition, he will not have neglected his pure sprinting speed.

For this kind of performer the last two weeks before the race is not a build-up period, this has been done already; no, this period is better considered as a count-down time.

It would require a different kind of book to chart the fine deails of 'periodising' and specific build-up for world-class runners, but the following is a generalised scheme.

September: end of season.

October: ideally a holiday by the sea, somewhere mild and warm.

November to February: train 13 days out of 14 with runs of 6–12 miles (10–20 km) plus weight training and circuit training.

March to May: start this period as above, but introduce more hill work (hard repetition running up slopes of 100–1000 metres long), while increasing the speed content of the training. This is the main period of multi-tier training. Starting around 40 miles per week in November and working up to 65–80 miles per week by March, the mileage will then decrease as the speed content of training increases.

The main distance work will be done on road and grass as steady running. Then will come some interval training, followed by sustained speed over relatively short distances – say 600–1000 metres.

Into this training will be worked sessions of sharp sprinting speed and speed sessions such as 6 x 300 metres flat out with short recoveries and 8 x 400 metres at 95 per cent effort.

June to September: this is the main racing season, and throughout this period he will have to maintain general condition and speed with only one or two easy days before any race. Weight training and circuit training are finished by the middle or end of May.

October: brings the year full circle, with the prospect of a non-working holiday where only walking and swimming interrupts relaxation. The mental refreshment is even more important than the physical relief from the hard training.

That is a very broad summary of the way a top middle-distance runner might organise his year. Peter Coe gives a more detailed insight into the rigorous schedule he and Sebastian might devise for an important season:

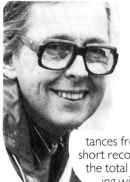

November, December, January: *5000m work.*
One short run – (9–14 km) on 5 days per week;
One long run – (16–19 km) on 1 day per week.
Additionally there will be on 2–3 days per week sessions that will be repetition running. These runs will be over distances from 100m to 1000m, all with short recoveries – usually jogging. When the total distances are low, weight training will be held twice per week, plus a circuit training session of 1 hour 30min. If the mileage is high or there are additional repetition sessions, then the circuit training may have to be omitted and only one weight session taken. One important note: always finish a session of running on an "up-tempo" note, i.e. in 95–100 per cent effort over the last 300–400 metres of a distance run.

Hill running for power: Having said that the kind of speed we want has to be sustained speed, we apply this principle to hill running when using 100m and 200m distances. These short distances are semi-sprint sessions which build up to 30–40 repetitions over the 100m and up to 10 repetitions for the 200m. The 100m slope is approximately 10 degrees, and the recovery is an immediate jog back down the hill. The 200m slope is about 7 or 8 degrees with a jog back recovery; this run is performed at about 90 per cent effort.
The long hill work is on a 1000m incline, on one single set of 6 runs with a slow run back. Our hill running is largely anaerobic and develops the ability to maintain good form when working hard. A high knee lift and a vigorous arm action has to be maintained throughout these runs.
Around April, the first time in England when the weather is suitable in our part of the country, we use a particular kind of hill running which is a coach-controlled type of fartlek training (except that there is not much play in it). It is fast and slow running around a grassy hill during which the athlete must sprint flat out between signals. The coach signals the start and finish of the sprint with a blast on a whistle. This way the runner has to respond to another's command (a track situation) and not when he feels like it. The coach chooses the flat section or the up or down part of the circuit; he varies the sprinting time from 7–15 sec and the continuous jogging recovering depending upon how long he wants the session to last. This varies between 12 and 25 minutes. This is very demanding, and is not for every runner as there is the danger of a severe "breaking down" effect.

General distance work: Most distance running will be run at 3min 20sec per kilometre pace, although occasionally during a 15 or 16km run the last 8km will be run at 3min per km pace as a check on general condition.

February, March, April, May: Multi-tier training (see schedule) plus one long run of 16–19km per week. Weight training and circuit training is still continued, but now some track sessions are shared with a 400m squad. Plus the following:

March: careful build up towards sprinting speed using 60m to 80m work and shuttle runs in a gymnasium.

April: flat out repetitions with 400m squad over 150m, 200m, and 300m (conditions permitting – keeping warm at all times).

May: when the pure sprinters take longer intervals, the 800/1500 man puts in extra repetitions; this is also the time to commence hard speed endurance sessions over 600m and 800m.

May, June: serious weight training is finished by mid-May and only general light sessions of medium repetitions on a multi-gym machine are used about once a week and the remainder of the work will be either pure sprinting, 60m–80m accelerations, or speed endurance runs of 300m–800m. By now I am supervising Seb's training more closely so that I can start to apply some of the more highly stressing sessions. Such sessions need careful observation of the runner so that they can either be shortened, or longer recovery periods be given (longer recovery may also be achieved by adjusting a work load on the subsequent days). From

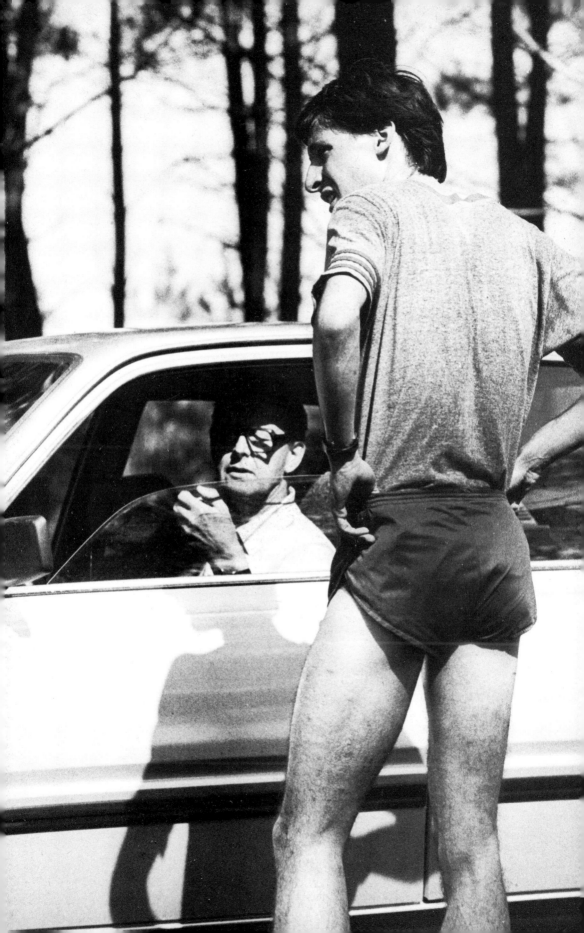

Multi-tier training

An example of a typical twelve days' work in the early part of the year for a top-class athlete

1 Sunday	4 × 1600m or 3 × 2000m	5000m Pace
2 Monday	Fartlek	
3 Tuesday	8 × 800	3000m Pace
4 Wednesday	Road	
5 Thursday	16 × 200m	1500m/1 Mile Pace
6 Friday	Rest if race If not racing – Fartlek	
7 Saturday	Race or Time Trial	
8 Sunday	4 × 400	800m Pace
9 Monday	Road Run	
10 Tuesday	1 × 300, 2 × 200, 4 × 100, 8 × 60 400m Pace	
11 Wednesday	Fartlek	
12 Thursday	Race – or choose pace for next race. (e.g., if next race is 800m, train at 1500m pace; if 400m, train at 800m pace; if 1500m train at 5000m pace).	

This is not the multi-tier training as advocated by Frank Horwill, but one modified to Seb's requirements. We believe Horwill's principles to be very sound, but every athlete should have his or her own schedules.

now on, and right through the racing season, no hard and fast schedules can be given as I keep his work under continual review, taking the actual performances in training as a guide to what part of his progress needs advancing or holding back.

(One safe generalisation is that three or four times a week there will be an easy morning run of 6.5km to 8km at 3min 20sec to 3min 30sec per kilometre pace).

There are occasions when we need a time trial to check the level of performance, either generally or in a particular area. These have to be handled with great care, and the coach must have an intimate knowledge of the athlete before he can draw a proper conclusion from the result. For example, Seb performs much better when racing than when training – the opposite can be true for many runners.

Non-running training

Weight Training: Two thirds of the work is repetition lifting in sets of six. One third will be pyramid work to reach a maximum lift. It is all-round weight work: squats, split squats, bench press and curling. Overhead lifting is limited because of the risk to the back. Slim middle-distance runners must seek to perfect their technique if they are to avoid injury.

Circuit Training: as in running, the variables are intensity, duration and frequency which progress simultaneously with the general training. Circuit training is a good time to develop dynamic strength, and bounding exercises, particularly box-jumping, are ideal for developing power. A session of less than one and a half hours is unlikely to allow sufficient variety of exercises or enough time at each station. The great Ron Clarke always said that a runner could not be too strong around the middle, and long repetitions of sit-ups should be included.

Flexibility Exercises: These should be done in any spare time and not restricted to training sessions only. The world-class athlete must be mentally prepared to take

every opportunity to protect himself from casual injury. After prolonged study he should get up from his desk carefully, be sure he is warm and bend and stretch carefully. The flexibility exercises for a hurdler are a perfect safeguard.'

However, the last two weeks might be as follows, *counting down* from day 14 to day 1.

Days 14 – 8: might be spent with an easy run of 4–5 miles each morning, with an 8-mile run at a fair pace (5min 40sec per mile) on *Day 9.* Afternoons would be speed training on the track with sets of repetition runs at distances from 80m to 400m. One of these days, perhaps *Day 8*, could be the day of travel.

Day 7: 4 miles easy in the morning and, say, two sets of 3 x 400m in the afternoon.

Day 6: 4 miles easy in the morning and speed drills in the afternoon.

Day 5: At any time during day, an easy jog of 20–30 minutes, and only flexibility exercises.

Day 4: (Heat) Jog in the morning – race in the afternoon or evening.

Day 3: (Semi-final) Jog in the morning – race in the afternoon or evening.

Day 2: Total rest, or a little jog and stretch.

Day 1: (Final) Jog in the morning – Race in the evening.

Throughout the whole period, sound sleep is essential for mental and physical recovery.

Running for one's country in international events at home and abroad, in addition to competing in some of the big European meetings, involves lost time in travel that can be ill afforded. And absence from work or study, which has to be accounted for, adds to the total stress of competition. The ordinary trials and tribulations of work and family life take on an extra dimension for the class athlete. It is very difficult to perform consistently at this level, a point worth remembering when you read reports which cast all their judgments in terms of success or failure.'

For most runners, this sort of training schedule would be frightening. How does Seb face the prospects of the hard training months each year?

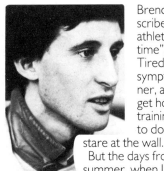

Brendan Foster once described the life of a top-class athlete as "feeling tired all the time", and I thoroughly agree. Tiredness is the commonest symptom of stress for any runner, and there are times that I get home from a hard evening training session when all I want to do is slump into a chair and stare at the wall.

But the days from late spring to mid-summer, when I'm working my body as hard as I can, are something of a challenge, too. If the training programme is going well, and I'm meeting my targets, and Peter is satisfied with my progress, the training can be exhilarating, however hard it is. I can wake up in the morning, and it's grey outside and it's starting to rain, and I know I've got to run six fast 800 metre repetitions and that my head's going to be buzzing at the end of them and that I'm going to be shattered by the evening; but I'd far rather do that than face the ordeal of walking round a department store to get the shopping.

I'm very much an "evening man" when it comes to the hard training. I far prefer the sessions in the afternoon or early evening, and I certainly wouldn't want them before 10.30 or 11 in the morning – I'm hardly alive before then. Ideally, I'd always prefer to race in the evening, too; the best time for me is

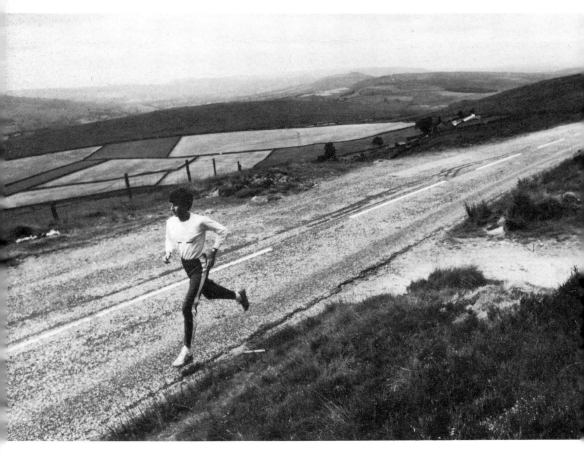

between 8 o'clock and 10 o'clock.

It isn't all hard work, day in and day out. I'm lucky in that I can compartmentalise my life to some extent. Many of my friends are not athletes, and those that are don't want to talk about running all the time. So I can switch off mentally from pace charts and lap times for most of the day. This, I'm sure, helps me concentrate better when I really have to – at the end of a hard session when I'm forcing myself to maintain style and pace and momentum even if my instincts are telling me to stop. I always seem to be able to keep in the back of my mind the thought that if the session goes well the preparation will have been that much better and the next target will be that much easier. It's all one more stepping stone to the next achievement.

Sometimes, even in the hardest sessions, there is time to take stock and adapt the training so that it works even better – that makes the toil even more satisfying. I remember a session in Italy last spring when Peter had planned a tough series of forty consecutive 200 metre repetitions at 30 seconds each with short recoveries between them. I had done about twenty of them, and I found that I had been running them faster than we had planned, about 27 seconds each, so Peter cut the total to thirty: we agreed that I had done the required work, things were going well, and an extra ten would prove nothing, only make me more tired. That seemed to me a good example of athlete and coach working well together even when training was at its most exacting. It's often just as vital for a coach to ease up an athlete during these hard months as it is to speed him up.

The best part of these heavy training months are the races themselves – they really do come as a relief. It's never good to feel completely divorced from competition, and it's like a breath of fresh air to break the monotony, wind down for a day, have a race and sharpen up the mind. That's why I've always been keen to have a few indoor races each winter. A good race proves things are going well, and the occasional bad race can always help to highlight some weakness that may have been missed. And frankly, racing is a darned sight easier than training.'

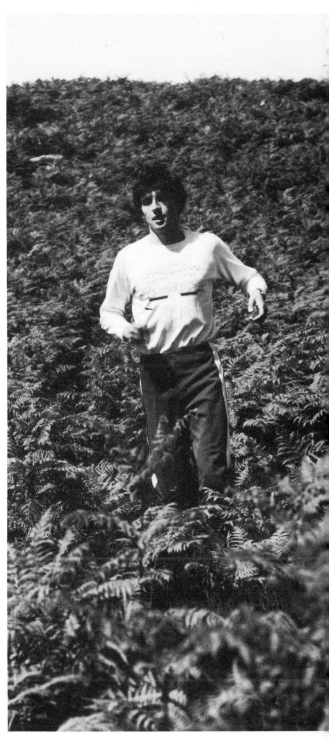

Pace Chart

In training, as well as in racing, pace judgment and pace maintenance are crucial. The accompanying chart indicates accumulated steady-pace times

Miles 1	2	3	4	5	6	8
mins secs					hrs mins secs	
4 40	9 20	14 00	18 40	23 20	28 00	37 20
4 50	9 40	14 30	19 20	24 10	29 00	38 40
5 00	10 00	15 00	20 00	25 00	30 00	40 00
5 10	10 20	15 30	20 40	25 50	31 00	41 20
5 20	10 40	16 00	21 20	26 40	32 00	42 40
5 30	11 00	16 30	22 00	27 30	33 00	44 00
5 40	11 20	17 00	22 40	28 20	34 00	45 20
5 50	11 40	17 30	23 20	29 10	35 00	46 40
6 00	12 00	18 00	24 00	30 00	36 00	48 00
6 10	12 20	18 30	24 40	30 50	37 00	49 20
6 20	12 40	19 00	25 20	31 40	38 00	50 40
6 30	13 00	19 30	26 00	32 30	39 00	52 00
6 40	13 20	20 00	26 40	33 20	40 00	53 20
6 50	13 40	20 30	27 20	34 10	41 00	54 40
7 00	14 00	21 00	28 00	35 00	42 00	56 00
7 10	14 20	21 30	28 40	35 50	43 00	57 20
7 20	14 40	22 00	29 20	36 40	44 00	58 40
7 30	15 00	22 30	30 00	37 30	45 00	1 00 00
7 40	15 20	23 00	30 40	38 20	46 00	1 01 20
7 50	15 40	23 30	31 20	39 10	47 00	1 02 40
8 00	16 00	24 00	32 00	40 00	48 00	1 04 00
8 10	16 20	24 30	32 40	40 50	49 00	1 05 20
8 20	16 40	25 00	33 20	41 40	50 00	1 06 40
8 30	17 00	25 30	34 00	42 30	51 00	1 08 00
8 40	17 20	26 00	34 40	43 20	52 00	1 09 20
8 50	17 40	26 30	35 20	44 10	53 00	1 10 40
9 00	18 00	27 00	36 00	45 00	54 00	1 12 00
9 10	18 20	27 30	36 40	45 50	55 00	1 13 20
9 20	18 40	28 00	37 20	46 40	56 00	1 14 40
9 30	19 00	28 30	38 00	47 30	57 00	1 16 00
9 40	19 20	29 00	38 40	48 20	58 00	1 17 20
9 50	19 40	29 30	39 20	49 10	59 00	1 18 40
10 00	20 00	30 00	40 00	50 00	1 00 00	1 20 00

for distances from two miles to a full marathon, with the minutes-per-mile times in the left-hand column.

10	12	Half-Marathon 13m 193y	15	20	Marathon 26m 385y
46 40	56 00	1 01 11	1 10 00	1 33 20	2 2 21
48 20	58 00	1 03 2	1 12 30	1 36 40	2 06 44
50 00	1 00 00	1 05 33	1 15 00	1 40 00	2 11 06
51 40	1 02 00	1 07 44	1 17 30	1 43 20	2 15 28
53 20	1 04 00	1 09 55	1 20 00	1 46 50	2 19 50
55 00	1 06 00	1 12 06	1 22 30	1 50 00	2 24 12
56 40	1 08 00	1 14 17	1 25 00	1 53 20	2 28 34
58 20	1 10 00	1 16 28	1 27 30	1 56 40	2 32 56
1 00 00	1 12 00	1 18 40	1 30 00	2 00 00	2 37 19
1 01 40	1 14 00	1 20 51	1 32 30	2 03 20	2 41 41
1 03 20	1 16 00	1 23 02	1 35 00	2 06 40	2 46 03
1 05 00	1 18 00	1 25 13	1 37 30	2 10 00	2 50 25
1 06 40	1 20 00	1 27 24	1 40 00	2 13 20	2 54 47
1 08 20	1 22 00	1 29 35	1 42 30	2 16 40	2 59 09
1 10 00	1 24 00	1 31 47	1 45 00	2 20 00	3 03 33
1 11 40	1 26 00	1 33 58	1 47 30	2 23 20	3 07 55
1 13 20	1 28 00	1 36 09	1 50 00	2 26 40	3 12 17
1 15 00	1 30 00	1 38 20	1 52 30	2 30 00	3 16 39
1 16 40	1 32 00	1 40 31	1 55 00	2 33 20	3 21 01
1 18 20	1 34 00	1 42 42	1 57 30	2 36 40	3 25 23
1 20 00	1 36 00	1 44 53	2 00 00	2 40 00	3 29 45
1 21 40	1 38 00	1 47 04	2 02 30	2 43 20	3 34 07
1 23 20	1 40 00	1 49 15	2 05 00	2 46 40	3 38 29
1 25 00	1 42 00	1 51 26	2 07 30	2 50 00	3 42 41
1 26 40	1 44 00	1 53 37	2 10 00	2 53 20	3 47 13
1 28 20	1 46 00	1 55 48	2 12 30	2 56 40	3 51 35
1 30 00	1 48 00	1 58 00	2 15 00	3 00 00	3 56 00
1 31 40	1 50 00	2 00 11	2 17 30	3 03 20	4 00 22
1 33 20	1 52 00	2 02 22	2 20 00	3 06 40	4 04 44
1 35 00	1 54 00	2 04 33	2 22 30	3 10 00	4 09 06
1 36 40	1 56 00	2 06 44	2 25 00	3 13 20	4 13 28
1 38 20	1 58 00	2 08 55	2 27 30	3 16 40	4 17 50
1 40 00	2 00 00	2 11 07	2 30 00	3 20 00	4 22 13

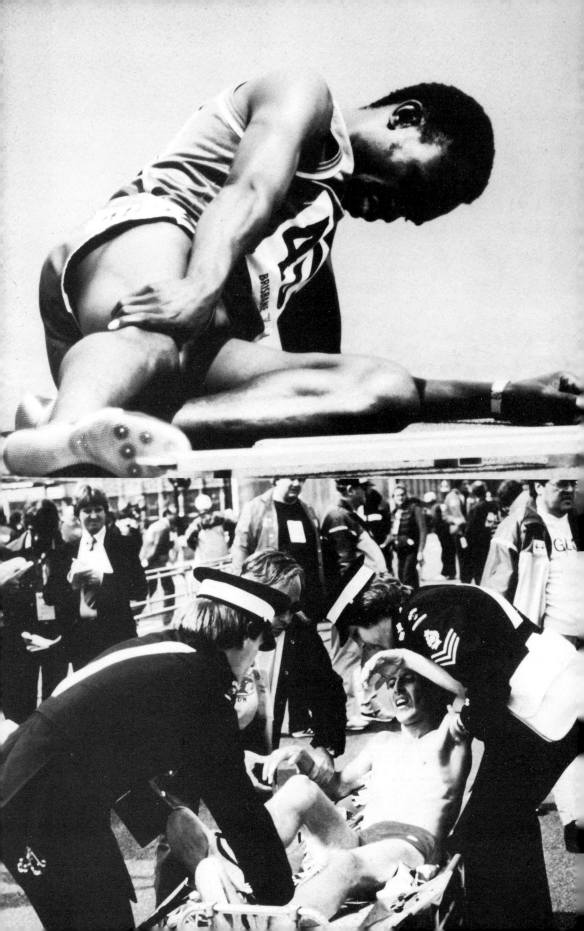

RUNNING INTO TROUBLE AND OUT AGAIN

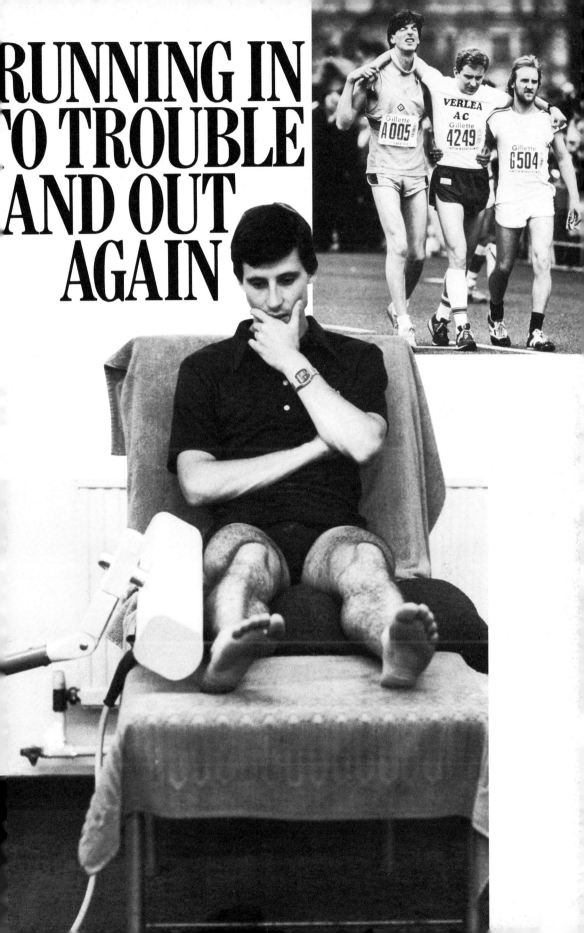

No training programme ever goes *absolutely* to plan. At whatever level you are running, you are deliberately putting extra strain on your body, and if you are competing, whatever the standard, you are putting unaccustomed pressures on your mind as well. Muscles do get strained, feet do sometimes hurt, runners catch cold just like everyone else, and, just like everyone else, they sometimes lose concentration.

An ache or a persistent niggle can hold up your training programme for a day or two; an illness or a bad injury can put you out of action for weeks, and throw a well-conceived training programme into total confusion. It is important for any runner to know what is serious and what is not, and very convenient if he has some idea of how to treat the minor things that might go wrong.

THE FEET

If your feet let you down, you really *have* had it. For no other part of the body is the saying 'prevention is better than a cure' more appropriate, and proper care of the feet will pay back a runner many, many times over.

With feet the first rule of body care particularly applies – keep them clean. Hands get washed several times a day, mainly because they are visible and

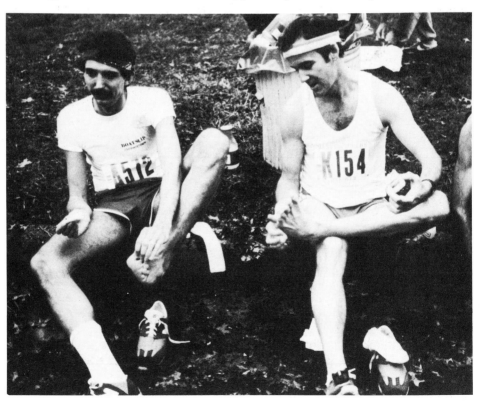

therefore attract attention. Feet, which are structural marvels, are out of sight and so ignored. Yet although they are normally covered up they can pick up a lot of dust and dirt during a day.

Don't wait for pain, examine your feet regularly. Trim toenails square, look for corns starting and the build-up of calluses. Some toughened areas of skin must be expected, and indeed do offer some protection, but if they are allowed to become too thick they create very painful pressure points and damage the soft tissue underneath. A blister under soft skin is not difficult to treat but a blister under a thickened and toughened patch can become serious, so keep down the thickness of hard skin.

Fashion shoes, male and female, are a menace. The heels are invariably too high, and have the effect of shortening the calf muscles. One American podiatrist recommends running shoes with heels as high as or even higher than everyday walking shoes, to take the strain off the back of the legs. There are not many running shoes, if any, with heels as high as contemporary male fashion would dictate. Better to use everyday shoes with low heels.

Be aware of your own shape. If you are even slightly knock-kneed you are placing an extra strain on the inside of the foot; if you are bow-legged you will have an outside-edge foot-strike with an extra twist (pronation) on landing. Being aware of these conditions can help you with shoe choice and the selection of inserts, though if you do need orthotics you should seek professional advice.

Help your feet by doing regular leg-stretching exercises. Can you comfortably touch your toes? Tightness in the calves reduces ankle flexibility, and this is often the start of tendonitis. Regular exercises to strengthen the feet provide an excellent injury prevention, especially for beginners.

After bad sprains the tendons are restored along with muscle tone, but the ligaments, which are the clever, intricate strappings that bind the foot together, are another matter. Strains weaken a foot and if great care is not taken, the foot becomes progressively more vulnerable and strains more frequently.

Exercising on a wobble board, rolling a ball or bottle around under the foot, sitting and rotating the foot to the maximum, repeated heel raises, gripping and holding with the toes, and walking around barefoot on carpet on the extreme edges (inside and outside) of the foot are all examples of what you can do to build up their strength.

Foot sores

Localised pressure that becomes too intense will form calluses, and rubbing that generates heat can produce soreness and blisters. Both problems can be alleviated by padding and taping. But general advice is difficult to give, because if padding and taping is done without expertise it can often result in relieving one problem spot and starting another. People vary in their skin response to prolonged contact with adhesive tape, too, and what might be a useful temporary help to a miler could be bad for a distance runner.

If a layer of plastic skin (now stocked by most specialist chemists) can be built up to an adequate thickness it will provide a sterile protection which does not need removing. In the time it takes to disappear it will have given some protection against all but the most severe work. But the application of the 'new skin' must not be rushed. Each thin, even layer is best dried off with a hair dryer until the required protective thickness is achieved. The effectiveness of this treatment is limited by the severity of the blistered patch.

Blisters

First of all, make sure that your shoes are a good fit, and do not run in worn-out shoes – keep them in good repair.

If you do get blisters, leave any small ones alone, but try to identify the irritation that caused it. If this is removed the blister will probably be absorbed.

If the blister is big and painful, first clean and disinfect the surrounding area thoroughly and relieve the pressure by draining. Sterilise a needle and insert it horizontally into the edge of the blister and allow the fluid to escape. Do not cut or tear the skin – leave it covering the blister. By inserting the needle this way you avoid piercing the soft tissue and causing bleeding.

After drawing the blister, again clean the area with an antiseptic and dust with a suitable foot powder. If the skin seems very delicate, cover it with a tape, but make sure that the adhesive area is not on the loosened skin; if it is, it may pull the skin away when it's removed. Leave the tape until some new skin has formed under the old.

If under hard or racing conditions you break through the thickened skin and get a raw surface which bleeds, your foot needs very careful treatment. Soccer players frequently place a full strapping of adhesive tape right round the foot and over the bare wound. The sensitive soft tissue underneath is thus protected, and since the adhesive is in contact, slipping and rubbing cannot take place.

The obvious hazard in this procedure is that soccer players, especially pros, play from game to game, but runners have to think further ahead than this. If you stick an adhesive to a bare wound any natural skin or protection that might grow is easily removed with the tape – every time you do it.

If you cannot or will not stop running, leave the wound cleaned and, as much as possible, exposed to the air or lightly covered. Then, when you run, lightly cover it with a special non-stick dressing and with broad tape cover the whole area to keep the dressing in place.

Some people advise you to relieve the pressure by sticking pads of chiropodist's felt into your shoes, suitably cut away, or by placing packing along the sides of the shoes. If your shoes are a proper fit this will be difficult, and if it is easy your shoes may be a bad fit, which probably triggered the blister in the first place. When you have run on a burst blister and released fluid, which will probably have contained blood, remember when cleaning the foot with antiseptic that the now dirty insole of your shoe will also want cleaning.

Finally, whether on track, road or field, and especially if you have run without socks, do not at the end of a run immediately pull off your shoes and walk around for relief. You may have unnoticed scratches on your skin, which could pick up an unpleasant infection.

Athletes Foot

This infection of the foot, usually between the toes, is caused by a microscopic fungus. There are many kinds of application to help cure it though the most effective are those which are most specific to the type of fungus causing the complaint. Even your doctor may have to use trial and error to find the best remedy. There is an antifungal, Griseofulvin, available in tablet form, which can aid in curing forms resistant to local treatment; it is available only on prescription.

Dhobie itch is the same complaint but on a different site, the groin. These ailments should be treated promptly and taken seriously. Go straight to your doctor. Generally, the best prevention is to keep scrupulously clean and dry in these areas. Take care that chafing does not open the skin.

DOUBTS, ACHES AND NIGGLES

Some of the troubles that beset runners are minor – magnified, perhaps, in the runner's mind by the effect they are having on his training, and causing him worry at a time when he doesn't want it. But a few can be 'run through', and with care will disappear without long-term treatment. While it is important to recover from an injury, it is also important to discover the cause, otherwise it will very likely recur on resuming running.

Stress

However much we hear about suspect knees and dodgy achilles tendons, the most common cause of disability for a runner is purely and simply stress, and it remains the most usual reason of all for bad or under-par performance.

Professor Hans Selye's theory is that we all have a fixed stress reserve. There is a reserve tank which is filled with an anti-stress agent, and no matter what the cause of the stress, mental or physical, we draw on the same tank to meet these demands. The logical conclusion from this is that if you are feeling low from overwork, examination worries or personal problems, these worries will be drawing from your anti-stress tank. If the level gets low, a series of heavy training sessions might drain the tank, and you would then begin to show one or more of the typical stress symptoms.

While a combination of various stresses may get you run down quickly, any one factor, if strong enough, will ultimately have the same effect. This does not contradict the view that a good run in the fresh air and in congenial surroundings is refreshing. It is indeed very good therapy and is a great relief from work stress.

The problem is only the old enemy – excess. When stress becomes excessive, something has to give and you must consider yourself as a whole.

First, check your general health and consider everything from your diet to an infection from a cold, a tooth abcess or a small cut. Check whether your resting pulse rate has increased. Are you sleeping well or are you keeping late hours? Have you gone on to shift work, or begun swotting for examinations? They all count. A sudden and heavy increase in your training load, even if it does not bring on injury, will certainly be stressful.

Any of the following could figure among the symptoms of stress: an unexpected weight loss, the symptoms of a recurring or long-lasting common cold such as a runny nose or sore throat and a nervous sneezing. And don't write off backache merely as driving or bad posture; this too is a sign that you could simply be run down. All these symptoms would almost certainly be accompanied by a diminished performance.

A classic symptom, one that Seb has shown once or twice over the years, is a swelling of the lymph glands, particularly in the groin. Be careful. If swollen glands persist after your training has eased off, and you still feel poorly, consider the possibility of glandular fever (*mononucleosis*) which is thought by some to be stress-induced and which, according to observations in the USA is commonly found among the fittest athletes.

Seb has experienced certain stress symptoms when the training has been going well; the training itself was not excessive, but he was also revising hard for his degree finals. The training was cut back, but the symptoms did not disappear until the exams were over. The bounce back was almost immediate, and only a short while later he broke his first world record, the 800 metres, in Oslo. In simple physical terms, that degree of recovery was just not on.

The subject of stress is very well covered in the chapter 'When Things Go Wrong' in *The Complete Middle Distance Runner*, that excellent book by Watts, Wilson and Horwill.

Of course, not every discomfort you feel is going to be the result of stress. If you suffer from an allergy, like hay fever, you may also be sensitive to bright sunlight. When you first start training and racing on a very bright day, early in the year, you can easily experience a runny nose, sneezing or sore eyes. If these pass off within a day or two they are not stress symptoms – if diagnosis was easy we would all be physicians. Everyone should learn what they can about themselves, not in submission to obsessive hypochondria, but simply to observe what does or does not suit them and, if possible, why.

Stiffness

Muscles well used in endurance work, or enlarged with strength training, tend to shorten, which in turn decreases the range of movement – the flexibility – in the joint. Unless this condition is continually relieved with the proper mobility exercises there is every likelihood that you will suffer from frequent bouts of stiffness.

The veins have a system of non-return valves to prevent blood from pooling in the lower limbs. The rhythmic contraction of the muscles alternatively squeezes and releases the veins in the muscles and because of the non-return valves the returning blood is urged towards the heart.

During hard work there is an increase of body fluid diffused throughout the muscle tissue which needs to be reabsorbed and flushed away by the returning blood. A sudden cessation of work stops this auxiliary pumping action and can leave some of the by-products of muscular work still in the tissue. This causes stiffness. So another precaution is properly tapering off at the finish of a training session. Prolonged or persistently uncomfortable stiffness can be relieved by massage.

Massage principally assists the return flow of blood and lymph by its rhythmic action. The pressure stroke on the muscle is always towards the heart. Massage also relaxes the muscle and dilates the surface blood vessels, which helps to restore a feeling of comfort and well-being. The application of heat, too, either by radiant heat or warm baths, also dilates the blood vessels, and can be very relaxing and soothing.

A variation on this heat treatment, which is often used specifically on the lower leg for tendonitis, is the alternate application of heat and cold. This promotes a significant increase in circulation, and it is believed to give relief through the vigorous flushing out effect by the blood. This hot and cold method seems to be more effective with younger people.

Take care when using rubifacients – any of the 'heat creams', for example. These creams dilate the blood vessels locally, and the increased blood supply brings warmth to the area and gives a sense of comfort and relief. But read the instructions carefully, especially about the degree of rubbing in or massage. It is best to make a test application to a small area of skin and look at the reaction. Seb finds the reaction to certain creams very fierce, sometimes accompanied by swelling.

With generalised stiffness – as long as it has not been brought on by injury – it is always best to maintain as wide a range of movement as you can without aggravating the soreness, and a good old soak in a hot bath is fine. Some soreness in muscles, though, is caused by tears in the fibres. The severity of these minute tears will determine to what extent you can carry on training.

The Stitch

The exact nature of the stitch is uncertain but it can be a sign of not being fit enough for the job in hand. When, on two occasions some years ago now, Seb had a bad stitch, they came on in cross-country races early in the year. They both came after very fast starts, and pointed to lack of training for that intensity of running.

If the stitch is slight, it is possible to run slowly through the discomfort and continue the race, by easing up and inclining the body towards the pain. But if it is severe and continuing, you must stop. A prolonged muscle spasm leaves you with a painful bruised feeling which can last for several days. That said, it is much better to be fit enough for the race than to learn how to run through the stitch.

Cramp

The exact cause of cramp associated with running is very uncertain.

Cramp is the everyday word for a painful muscle spasm. When the attack is induced by excessive sweating or heat stroke from exertion in hot conditions it is often due to a lack of salt, for which the only cure or prevention is an adequate salt intake. Other cramps can be caused by an interruption of the blood supply such as a diversion of the blood from the stomach to working muscles particularly if the exertion is too close to a heavy meal.

The simplest remedy for these painful muscle contractions is, wherever possible, to stretch the affected muscle. This may need someone's assistance, because some 'locked' muscles, such as those in the thigh or the calf are very powerful indeed.

Can Massage Help?

The position of massage in sport is not a simple one. While it has specific physiological functions, it often has a psychological one too. Massage can be compared with the excessive and incorrect warm-up routines that are adopted by some athletes; the only good they do is to serve as a mental prop, one that makes them feel more secure because they have always done it. In fact, massage incorrectly timed or incorrectly applied can do a lot more harm than the wrong kind of warm-up.

If you do require massage, choose a masseur with all the care with which you would choose a physiotherapist or a sports-medicine physician or surgeon.

The immediate effects of massage can be quite different. They range from a feeling of well-being to one of feeling badly used. To appreciate the latter you would need to have experienced the deep massage that is practised more frequently in some parts of Europe, where you feel the next day almost as if you have been beaten up, only to feel marvellously fresh and fit two days later. This does not mean that any massage that is painful is a good one. Generally it should promote pleasant feelings in the limbs. So it follows that the effects from such a range of feelings could be damaging if wrongly applied. Although the principles are relatively simple, correct diagnosis and correct application take years of intelligent experience.

Massage is used in the treatment of muscle stiffness, including cramps and spasms, deep bruising and inflammation. This is effected by stretching tissue, stimulating the circulation and dispersing fluid, and is carried out by stroking, kneading and striking.

Anyone going for massage should take care that their skin is as clean as possible around the area to be treated in order to avoid skin infections. The lubricant to avoid skin burn will be selected by the masseur.

It cannot be too strongly stressed that massage is much more specialised than just a rub down. The proper dispersal of fluids needs great skill, as does the 'freeing' of tissue after scarring or where a small nerve may be trapped, and the masseurs must know what they are doing.

However, where muscles have stiffened after prolonged exertion and relief is needed, or where ordinary flexibility exercises are either painful or are not working effectively, then proper massage can be very helpful.

As a safety measure before explosive exertions, too, massage has its place, providing the muscles are not overstimulated: overstimulation has the effect of a depressant – exactly the opposite result from the one you are seeking.

ILLNESS AND INJURY

Minor aches and pains, stitches and stiffness can, almost literally, be taken in your stride. A more important decision must be taken by the runner, though, when things have clearly become more serious than that. In times of illness or genuine injury, the runner's response could affect the rest of his running year – or the rest of his career.

The Three Rules of Injury

1. Treat all injuries as serious. This could prevent minor injuries becoming major ones, and serious injuries becoming very serious ones with the need for long lay-offs and drastic cures.
2. If in doubt – *don't*.
3. Begin treatment immediately – a good defence against the possibility of the acute becoming chronic.

Together, these rules are in line with our philosophy of balanced restraint as a guard against an excess either of enthusiasm or, on the other hand, of rationalised sloth. (The latter should be noted by anyone tempted to misinterpret rule two as meaning 'Don't train if you don't feel like it'; training, like diet, has to be maintained to be effective – if you're tempted to give in, just think of the effort that has gone before and ask if you really want to throw it all away.

Illness

Illnesses should be regarded as injuries, and our second rule on injuries holds good here – 'If in doubt – don't'. In our experience, running through an infection does not work. In fact, you don't run through it, because you will feel even worse for trying and eventually you will have to stop as the aches in the joints become even more painful.

Runners who take general care of themselves, maintaining a good diet and regular running in all weathers, will be healthier than those who do not exercise. And unless they are performing at a high level where stress-induced illnesses are more likely, they will be generally more resistant to the common ailments than the rest of the population. So if you are down or going down with something or other the chances are it is not slight, so treat it with respect. Colds, bronchitis, sore throats, any respiratory infections are not helped by rapid breathing through the mouth. Similarly with stomach upsets or any abdominal pain – heavy exertion will not cure them.

Injury

It is always dangerous to oversimplify, particularly for beginners, but it is fairly safe to say that the pain that wears off as you run is not likely to be as serious as the pain that comes on when you run, and the pain you feel continually is certainly the most serious.

For the purposes of this section we will define an athletic injury as one which (a) prevents running, (b) causes any degree of pain while running, and (c) leaves a pain that has been brought on by running. These are principally injuries to the legs, though this leaves a grey area of pain in other areas or organs, the origin of which may not be running even if the onset does occur during running.

Running injuries are mainly those of over-use. Although brought on when running or by running, they are structural injuries, and frequently the result of inherent structural weakness. The injuries of distance men are usually from prolonged repetitions of movements through the same range, seeking out the weakest link in the chain.

Before looking at some common injuries, we should make it clear that it has never been our policy to run through injuries – this is no better than playing Russian roulette with your health. Also, an injury that does not respond to the simple remedies we suggested for it must be referred immediately to at least a good and sympathetic doctor. The proper place for accurate diagnosis and treatment is a sports medicine centre, or a doctor with a genuine interest in sports medicine. A good physiotherapist is invaluable if he or she has direct sports-injury experience and is not dealing mainly with the everyday infirm; the better the physios, the more closely they will be working with a good ortho-paedic doctor. In fact the good sport physiotherapist will very likely be in touch with the best doctors to deal with sportsmen.

The following table is from a *Runners World* survey in which 800 runners, nearly all of them distance men, reported injuries which made them *stop* running. The survey does not indicate whether or not more than one injury per runner was recorded, though this is very likely. These are listed in the order of the frequency with which they occurred.

Knees	17.9%	Calves	3.6%
Achilles tendons	14.0%	Heels	3.0%
Shin splints	10.6%	Hips	2.6%
Arches	6.9%	Hamstrings	2.6%
Ankles	6.4%	Thighs	1.3%
Foot fractures	3.6%	Leg fractures	1.0%

The ICE Treatment

I.C.E. are the initial letters of the principal steps taken when dealing with injuries, particularly the traumatic kind: Ice (applied to check any internal bleeding); Compression (to prevent fluid gathering round the site of the injury); Elevation (to take the load off the limb). In the absence of a refrigerated cold pack or an ice-bag, cold water compresses, or even holding the injury under a cold tap, can help. Be careful with the cold packs or ice-bags – the skin should have a protective smear (we use olive oil) to prevent skin burns or skin sticking to the frozen pack. And crush the ice before it goes into the ice-bag, so that it can conform to the limb contours more easily than can big cubes from the refrigerator.

Knees

Knee injuries are quite often the result of some biomechanical weakness. Runners who already play a sport like soccer, where the continual twisting and turning in studded boots tends to anchor the foot to the ground, must be careful. Any knee injury due to football will be found out in continuous running.

The knee has thirteen ligaments to keep it in position, but it also depends upon the strength of the thigh muscles. Strong muscles and good muscle tone generally helps with the stability of joints. *Chondromalacia patella* is the technical name given to certain kinds of painful knee. The pain occurs behind the kneecap usually accompanied by grating – if the hand is placed over the kneecap while the knee is being flexed the underlying roughness can be felt and even heard.

This is due to a breakdown of the normally very smooth and slick surfaces. The kneecap (*patella*) protects the front of the joint and increases the leverage of the quadriceps extensor muscle so that it presses into the groove at the end of the femur when the leg is straightened. Obviously if it moves to one side because of muscular weakness or structural imbalance or both, the increased friction will wear the sliding surfaces unduly. Consult an orthopaedic specialist or podiatrist and have your feet examined. Very often the correctly designed orthotic will prevent further trouble.

Cortisone injections and surgery have been tried in past years without much success, and surgery is by no means a certain cure. The treatment recommended is isometric exercise to strengthen quadriceps, ice to reduce swelling at onset, and elevation to reduce the weight load. It is one of those pains which can be caused by running on sloping surfaces, like the sides of hills or road cambers. Finding the cause is the most important thing here.

Cartilage
Cartilage is a specialised form of connective tissue which is firm but flexible and elastic. It is found mainly as spacers between joints (backbone and joints) or the rib ends where the rib cage needs flexibility for expansion. But in common usage it is nearly always used to refer to the semi-lunar discs in the knee joint. There are protective discs between the femur and the tibia, where the joint slides. These can be torn if the knee is severely twisted, and often a torn piece can become detached and lodged in the joint. The knee can become locked with pain and swelling. Immediate treatment is our old friend ICE. This injury requires surgery, but with modern techniques the operation is precise and neat, without the old long incisions.

The Collateral Ligaments
Here the pain is felt in the side of the knee, and without proper treatment the pain will continue for months or, depending on your age, even years. If the leg is kept straight, is restrained above the ankle and the knee pushed gently inwards,

any pain might indicate damage to the medial ligament, the pain being felt on the inside of the knee. If, when the procedure is reversed and the knee is eased outwards, pain is felt on the outside of the knee, this could be the lateral ligament.

Complete rest, not just from running, is indicated if you are to avoid a long-lasting disability. Small tears will clear up with immobilisation and rest, but larger tears may require surgery.

Achilles Tendon

This is the tendon connecting the calf muscles to the heel. It slides in a loose protective sheath which is slippery internally. If, through excessive rubbing, the lubrication breaks down, the sheath becomes sore and inflamed (*tendonitis*). (It can, more rarely, become inflamed through rheumatism or infection.) If the sheath becomes so inflamed that it swells, and so constricts the movement of the tendon even more, the condition becomes serious, and combined with the small lesions in the tendon it can eventually produce a total seize-up in the tendon sheath. This can only be cleared away with surgery. The condition is made worse by continuing to run instead of resting; the repeated running keeps up the tiny internal tearing.

A sudden onset is best dealt with by ICE. Stop weight-bearing and apply cold compresses or an ice-bag for twenty to thirty minutes and continue with alternate hot and cold treatments. After treatment maintain some movement by ankle-rotating exercises with the leg raised. Anti-inflammatory drugs can be very helpful with tendonitis, but do not allow the condition to continue without obtaining expert advice, preferably from a sports medicine centre.

Try to prevent its onset by never wearing shoes that put pressure on your heel or the tendon. Never start running very fast sessions without first building up the speed work gradually. Do not run hard in a new pair of shoes, or even an old pair not worn for a long time. Avoid sudden changes of running surface for long runs – for instance, if most of your mileage is done on grass in the local park, do not suddenly run ten or twelve miles on a hard road, or vice versa. Get used to the different surfaces gradually. If any sign of tendonitis occurs, you can take the strain off the tendon by placing heel lifts, preferably spongy ones, in both shoes. But remember to raise both your heels equally, in the unaffected leg as well, to avoid creating an imbalance.

Shin Splints

This is sometimes just called shin soreness. Diagnosis is difficult because shin splints can mean anything to anyone so long as the front of the lower leg is sore.

True shin splints is technically *periostitis* of the tibia. This is inflammation of the fibrous coating of the bone, and when it is localised it is not easy for a non-expert to distinguish between this and a stress fracture. The painful area is mainly between the tibia and fibula. The cause of this injury is uncertain – the treatment is to stop running and get physiotherapy as soon as possible. Ultra-sonic treatment and hydrotherapy have all given relief. The do-it-yourself hot and cold treatment is helpful too.

Another form of shin splints is pain in the anterior tibia muscle, the long muscle down the outside of the shin that flexes the foot.

This, too, requires that you stop running immediately, rest for three days and use some form of strapping. Brian Lewis, sometime head track trainer at the University of Indiana, considers this injury to be so varied and complex that the successful treatment requires a variety of taping and support and a great deal of trial and error.

Diagnosis is a real difficulty with shin splints. Some old timers have recommended running through this complaint, which would be wrong even if it did turn out to be only shin splints. But as we said when discussing diagnosis, a localised soreness, which might even spread to a rather larger area, could be an incipient stress fracture. If a runner attempts to run through this pain, he will not emerge from the other side cured; he could go on to develop a full stress fracture which would require a minimum of six weeks' rest before he could start easy training again.

Shin soreness promptly dealt with will not normally last that long. Both kinds of shin splints can be brought on by sudden increases in mileage or even long drives with a foot poised over a foot pedal. Extra attention to careful stretching of the anterior tibia muscle can give relief.

Arches

Not all feet that appear flat-footed actually are. The longitudinal arch may appear to be flat on the floor, but only because the ankle is rolled inwards. A pronated foot will apply a painful twisting force to the ankle with further pain in the knee, even reaching as far as the lower back.

Although the function of an arch is to support weight, the ends of the arch must be fixed for it to do this. In the human foot the ball is connected to the heel by the *plantar fascia*. This strong ligament acts as a tie bar, but it is vulnerable to bruising at the attachments – runners with very high arches are more prone to this condition.

The rear attachment of the fascia is on the base of the heel bone (*calcaneum*), and it is here that some runners feel pain. At first it feels just like a bruise but if you ignore it the pain gets worse and the heel becomes deeply inflamed. Physiotherapy may assist recovery, and relief from soreness may be obtained by fitting soft inserts in the heels, with the centre cut out to relieve pressure under the heel (also a good treatment for bruising on this part of the foot).

Sometimes damage to muscles and other tissues gives rise to spontaneous deposits of calcium and this can happen here. If calcium is deposited it can turn into a heel spur. A similar condition can arise at the back and on top of the heel where, if it continues, the spur may cut into the achilles tendon – a painful and dangerous complaint. Surgical removal is necessary if the pain continues too long.

A bump on the back of the heel can also be a sign, too, that the bursa (see Bursae, below) has also become inflamed. After rest, the only lasting treatment for runners is to have properly fitted supports in the shoes.

Another way to relieve the plantar fascia of some of the strain is to tape the foot so that the ball of the foot and the heel are tied. This needs skilled knowledge, and is a better prevention than cure. If the cause is not attended to, the injuries will always continue.

Pain in the bones of the arches – particularly on the instep – is often the sign of osteo-arthritis, which will be accompanied by some inflammation. This is not too painful except when walking or running. Consult a physician for an anti-inflammatory drug, but osteo-arthritis is a wear-and-tear disease about which little can be done in the long-term. (See also our note on drugs, page 155.)

Ankles

Ankles are easily sprained by rolling the ankle outwards. A strain is a small tear in the muscle or tendons, a sprain is the same thing in a ligament. The injuries are not too serious if treated promptly with ICE and, if possible, an x-ray check to see that no bones are broken.

Rehabilitation has to start as soon as possible. Proper strapping, expertly applied, can restrict movement of the ankle sideways to allow the tear to heal, while allowing some controlled bending and straightening fore and aft. With luck you will be able to resume careful movement in two or three days, and training in less than a fortnight.

It is worth emphasising that prompt and proper treatment is essential, and also that unless any bone is shown to be broken, the ankle should in no circumstances be bound rigid.

One of Seb's rare impact injuries proved a perfect example of how – and how not – to confront a sudden ankle injury. During training on campus at Loughborough he was unlucky enough to thrust his foot down an old grassed-over post hole. The result was very painful and frightening and, with only a few weeks remaining before the 1978 European Championships, very worrying. Seb just sat on the grass stunned with the pain watching his ankle expand like a balloon.

The hospital's first instinct was to put his leg in a plaster. The treatment would not have been wrong – for anyone, that is, except an athlete. Luckily he was rescued in the nick of time and reached the haven of a *sports* physiotherapist who was able to reduce the swelling and strap the ankle in such a way that with additional treatment he was able to resume limited training in less than a fortnight and, in the Championships, win a medal.

This emphasises the importance of finding a sports medicine centre or a doctor interested in sports injuries, or finding an out-patients casualty department where the staff understand and are sympathetic to sportsmen's problems. Every club secretary worth his or her salt will know the nearest centre with a sports medicine facility.

Foot Fractures

These come in two forms. The first is an imbalance and over-use symptom and like stress fractures in the tibia and fibula, it needs no special treatment except rest. Small traumatic breakages, say in a toe after kicking a bed or chair leg, may only require strapping to the next toe. But by and large bones are so strong, and forceful breakage requires such violence, that a doctor should be consulted immediately, not only to supervise the correct setting, but also to check for the associated damage expected from great force. Ice and elevation are in order, but not the movement necessary for compressions: a bad break should not be manipulated before it is properly examined.

Stress Fractures

Stress fractures or hairline fractures are very fine cracks without displacement at the break. This type of fracture is often incomplete, and has not gone right through the bone, though continued use can cause a complete break. Sometimes called march fractures (from continuous heavy marching), they are not easy to diagnose since they do not show on x-ray plates for at least two weeks after onset, when some slight local thickening shows round the crack as repair progresses.

Six weeks' rest from running is the usual requirement. A dietary precaution is to take extra vitamin C to assist healing. Always take medical advice.

As a preventive, avoid running on slopes, either along sides of hills or road cambers. Do not do high speed work on unyielding surfaces, or increase your work load suddenly. Runners in their teens seem to be more prone to stress fractures, even on a good diet. However, check the diet for possible calcium deficiency at any age.

Calves

The calves are very strong sets of muscles, and with foot care and regular stretching they should not give you much trouble if you take care to avoid too much hard running on steep hills, especially in cold weather, and too much sprinting or speed work without experience or warm-up. Runners who have a fore-foot strike certainly place a heavier load on their calves, and while they are proportionately more developed in this area, running on slippery surfaces places more strain on them.

Distance running tends to harden and shorten calf muscles, which tighten the achilles tendons. This in turn means you should always do regular careful stretching exercises.

For general muscle tenseness and soreness a hot bath will bring relief, and general stretching, as well as easing up on distance running, is indicated.

If you have a real muscle pull, which is some degree of tearing to the muscle fibres, the treatment, once again, is ICE. Maintain elevation as much as possible for the first one or even two days. While resting the leg keep tensing the quad muscles and keep rotating the foot. Muscles lose tone quickly, and stiffness should be avoided.

All muscle tears mend with scar tissue. Subsequent exercise must be resumed with care because scars are not elastic like the rest of the muscle tissue.

Heels   See under Arches.

Hips

Aches around the hips are usually just strain from long mileage – more often from cross-country runs – and rest is the simple cure, together with reduced mileage. However, many people have one leg just a little shorter than the other, or run habitually on one side of the road, both of which cause the hips to tilt to accommodate the difference. A fallen arch on one foot only can have the effect of shortening that leg. Steady running with its repetitive movements will seek out any imbalances of this kind, and could well result in pain in the lower back. If you have not slipped or fallen and the onset of hip pain is gradual, consider any of the above causes. The remedy is probably foot care.

Hamstrings

These are the powerful muscles at the back of the thigh. If the tear is slight it may be difficult to locate and may only cause stiffness the next day. On the other hand, if a sharp stabbing pain or even a snap is felt, there will be quite a lot of pain at once.

Tears in muscle fibres are always accompanied by tears in blood vessels, so there will be some internal bleeding. The treatment is ICE, and the ice should be applied for twenty minutes, three or four times a day; the leg should be elevated for forty-eight hours. The compression bandage should be of the ACE type (see below under Thighs).

The rehabilitation programme should be undertaken slowly and carefully, and never rushed. Depending on the severity of the tear, a gentle stretching programme may be commenced after two days.

A mild pull can be left to your own care, but any hamstring pull accompanied by great pain or severe limping should have professional advice as soon as possible from a physiotherapist or a doctor.

Thighs

Injuries to the tops of the thighs or the groin are limiting strains mainly brought on by slippery surfaces. The adductor muscles pulling the legs in are often under sudden strain if the foot tries to slip sideways. Normally rest is a sufficient cure with gentle flexing exercise of the knees when lying down.

Do not do squats in weight training, and continue flexibility exercises only with great care.

Pulled muscles in the front of the thigh are often more severe than hamstrings, especially in the belly of the *rectus femoris*. These are more a speed merchant's complaint, and are infrequent in distance runners. The treatment, as for the hamstrings, is best effected with an ACE. This is a good compression pack consisting of a large piece of cotton lint that covers the affected area, which has had a liberal coating of analgesic cream. The whole is kept in place by overlapping Elastoplast strips, the ends of which cross on the pad and not on the leg. This is not the easiest dressing to apply yourself, and in any case, injuries of this type should have medical attention.

Leg Fractures

If the break is by force, you are going straight to hospital for treatment and setting anyway.

Leg fractures for runners are usually stress fractures in the lower leg, probably in the lower third of the fibula or even the tibia. Stress fractures do not suddenly go with a snap, and if you recognise the signs you can avoid them developing. The first warning is a localised soreness, more an ache, which starts right over the bone. At first there may be no additional pain with finger or thumb pressure but the site of the injury will soon become more sensitive.

Stop running at once, and completely rest the leg from load-bearing exercise. And don't rush it: whether the bone is cracked or you are only feeling the onset, you are going to have to stop for six weeks.

Check your shoes for extra wear and look for any imbalance. The fibula is a thinner bone and has to take more twisting than the big shin bone, and is more frequently troublesome.

All that we have said about stress fractures earlier applies here. Take care with surface changes, new shoes, old worn ones. A bad foot plant with excessive pronation is a prime source. Favouring an injury, say a blistered foot, on a long run can also bring on a hairline crack.

You may be advised to strap the leg, but our orthopaedic advisers have not considered it necessary, and on both occasions Seb has suffered a stress fracture he has made a complete recovery.

Bursae

These are pockets of fibrous tissue with a slippery lining which are there to reduce friction where tendons or ligaments pass over bones in joints. They can become inflamed from damage, say a sharp blow, or from extra pressure and the inflammation is often accompanied by fluid which causes them to swell. Unless it has been caused by infection, inflammation is usually the result of excessive friction or pressure.

The knees and heels – and sometimes elbows – are the bursae that most worry runners. It is usually best to rest these joints with some compression if there is excessive fluid present, until the inflammation subsides and the fluid is absorbed. Draining is always a risk and seldom recommended – an infection in a joint is always serious.

Bruising

Bruising is caused by damage to the tissue, which releases fluid. Often the very small blood vessels are ruptured and release blood into the surrounding tissue where it gradually decomposes and is absorbed. This process gives rise to the blue and yellow discoloration.

In severe cases the injury can be too painful to treat, but there are useful ointments which can help to reduce inflammation and swelling. This is done not by getting into the damaged tissue directly but by the active constituents being absorbed through the skin into the blood and thus reaching the site of the injuries. These ointments also contain ingredients to reduce stiffness, and they can be useful with sprains. Two such ointments have the trade names Lasonil and Movelat; they are non-greasy and come in tubes.

An occasional phenomenon of bruising is that it may show somewhere other than the site of the injury; thus a blow on the buttocks or thigh might show in the calf. If you can't remember any injury to the discoloured area, think of a knock you might have had somewhere else.

Slight bruising unaccompanied by severe pain can be ignored, and very severe bruising is usually the result of injury serious enough to warrant proper medical attention.

Beware of drugs

Drugs are often administered to alleviate as well as to cure ailments. All drugs have side effects. They have to be strong enough to work, and they will always have some effect on the delicate balance of the body's chemistry. Aspirin can make the stomach bleed; phenylbutazone, a powerful anti-inflammatory drug, will affect the blood cells – take enough and you will become anaemic. The trade-off is always between which is the lesser of the two evils – the symptoms of the complaint or the symptoms of the cure.

We cannot comment from personal experience on the use of hydrocortisone injections, but results with athletes of our acquaintance have varied from useless to disastrous.

There is a swing against the casual use of antibiotics, but these medicines are invaluable in the right circumstances. There is a let-down feeling and a fall off in performance after a course of these drugs which as yet is not fully explained, but may be due to interference with certain body enzymes.

If you can manage without drugs, we would advise you to avoid them.

GETTING BACK TO TRAINING

The time it takes to reach the old level of fitness after a lay-off is different for each person, and it will depend largely on what caused the lay-off.

The most easily avoided lay-off is the holiday. The hot sand, the extra cold beers and the lazy reluctance to swim much – they all have to be resisted. Getting back to form after this entails no more than a bit of extra work, so long as it is steadily taken up. Two weeks in the sun will need two weeks to get back to where you were.

Influenza or any virus infection is another matter. With these illnesses, and any illness accompanied by fever, the utmost caution is necessary. If you have had to have a doctor, and if the doctor has prescribed antibiotics, then your recovery period will be a little longer. There is very frequently an additional feeling of lowered energy and effectiveness – a loss of steam as it were – following a course of antibiotics. Do not try to force the recovery, nor should you ever fail to complete the course prescribed just because you suddenly feel better and want to hasten your return to full training. All you will succeed in doing is to spread strains of the infection which are resistant to the treatment. The doctors will love you for this.

In all attempts to resume training after illness the 'one step forward, two steps back' trap is easy to fall into. There is only one golden rule: the training must progress at a rate that always allows you to finish feeling well – healthily tired perhaps, but still feeling well.

Recovery after athletic injuries will depend upon the type and the amount of exercise you are able to carry out while not running. While you are waiting the necessary six weeks after diagnosing or suspecting a simple stress fracture of the fibula or tibia, aerobic work like swimming should be followed as much as possible. Weight training using a multi-gym or a bench is fine, though using a leg press would be silly. After about two weeks, gentle cycling would also be in order.

After surgery for cartilage trouble you must follow the instructions of the orthopaedic surgeon. If the treatment involved the arthroscopy technique, where only a small hole is made and the pieces are located accurately, the operation is so neat and clean that recovery will be rapid.

But as surgery is invasive, it is also irritating – so give the effects a proper chance to settle down. It is no use having an operation to clean out a seized-up and fouled-up achilles tendon, and then replacing the trouble with another by not allowing the healing to progress quietly.

However, most ailments that runners suffer from are those of over-use, and once these have cleared up with treatment and training can be resumed, all runners will want to return to full fitness as soon as possible. In hastening the return, quite obviously over-use is to be avoided, and here we have found that a modified form of interval training is very useful. Racing is running quickly, and since speed falls off faster than endurance when you are temporarily out of training, some speed work is needed on your return.

Distance training gives long sustained pounding, whereas *modest* speed with *adequate* recovery is less cumulatively stressful. Since it is estimated that only 60 per cent loading is required to maintain condition, as against at least 80 per cent to improve condition, it would seem sensible to stay as generally active as possible during a lay-off, and to stimulate the heart and the muscles with short-duration exercises. Short sessions of 10 x 150m progressing to 12 x 200m, plus short steady runs of about three miles were what we used in the middle of the summer of 1982 when Seb was recovering from stress fracture and para-tendonitis. Of course, these sessions were not flat out, or as fast as normal training, but they should be rather faster than normal running – say 15sec per 100m pace.

The need to immobilise an injury completely is seldom necessary, and you should resume and maintain flexibility in the limb as soon as possible. This not only speeds up recovery, but lessens the risk of injury when you start up again.

Once training is resumed take great care not to favour the injury. If you have badly sprained an ankle do not resume running favouring that foot because you will run unbalanced. The effect is similar to having one leg shorter than the other, the pelvis will be tilted to compensate and the spine becomes misaligned – just the circumstances to start off another injury somewhere else in the body.

If it is too painful to run on properly, it is too soon to train. If you are favouring it because you are frightened to put full weight upon it, then you must nerve yourself to run naturally.

Whether on a lazy holiday or during any lay-off, do not neglect your flexibility exercises – this will reduce the risk of picking up another injury due to stiffness. Even with ankle sprains or after achilles tendon operations, the doctors will tell you to start flexing the ankle as soon as possible.

For competitive athletes, injuries or illness and the subsequent lay-off and climb back to form are in many ways the most testing time of their careers. Apart from the usual ration of aches and strains and a stress fracture in his teens, Seb's career up to the start of 1982 had been comparatively trouble-free. There was that incident back in 1978 when he badly sprained an ankle during a training run at Loughborough, but apart from leaving him with one ankle slightly (and permanently) bigger than the other, that was soon forgotten.

What will never be forgotten is the traumatic year of 1982, a year that followed his astonishing string of broken records in 1981, and which was planned to culminate in a string of titles in the European Championships in Athens and the Commonwealth Games in Brisbane. Seb describes the year himself:

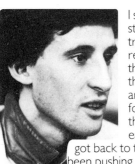

I suppose the trouble really started in January. The winter training had all been going reasonably well, and then at the end of January I had something the matter with a foot arch, and I was off for three or four weeks under a physiotherapist. I didn't run again till early March, and as soon as I got back to training I think I must have been pushing a bit too hard. Psychologically it's not very good losing a month's running in the winter, because you know that's what you're going to base your summer stuff on.

Anyway, things seemed to be going fairly well, and I ran in the Yorkshire Championships, and had two weeks' training and a 2000 metre race in Bordeaux before the start of the season proper here.

Then, three or four days after I got back from France I was out with a leg injury – it turned out to be a stress fracture at the bottom of my leg. These things take a long time to diagnose, and mine was complicated by some muscle problem in the same area. But a stress fracture it certainly was, and that meant I was out effectively from the beginning of June to the beginning of August – the one period of the year you just cannot afford to dispense with. It's a time when I'm doing all my sharpening work . . . I lost most of my hard repetitions and my speed training.

Even when I eventually got back to training I could never run more than about six miles for fear of bringing on the injury again; so far as endurance was concerned, I was in pretty bad shape.

I got back to racing after two-and-a-half to three weeks' training, and the mental relief at being back seemed to make me race above my level of fitness – I did a 1 min 44.4sec 800 metres in Zurich, and I was just coasting in the final straight. But the basic problem was simple: I didn't have enough background training, and the European Championships were on top of us.

We decided that I had to have some sort of rehearsal for Athens by running three races close together, all the time knowing that I'd be taking out endurance and speed from a very thin background of work. So I had the Zurich race, followed by the Talbot Games and a race in Cologne, and they went pretty well. And then I had that relay at Crystal Palace when the powers that be decreed that everyone who was going to Athens had to turn up and run something. It was a good run, that 4 × 800 metres when we broke the world record. I did 1 min 43.9sec, which was fast, but in retrospect it can't have done me any good. If I hadn't had that behind me I might at least have felt easier in the heats and semi-final in Athens.

When we got to the European Championships we knew we were living very much on borrowed time. Quite apart from my lack of background training I could tell from the way I was reacting to stress. I was tired, I was easily irritable, my throat was sore, my lymph glands were up – all the classic stress symptoms. I got a blister, too, which would normally have been perfectly all right, but now it seemed an extra frustration. I was mentally and physically running myself into the deck.

The heat and the semi-final of the 800 metres went satisfactorily, but I didn't find them particularly easy; they were very average times, the sort I should normally have been able to put together in one training session.

And the final was one of those occasions you just hope will never happen again. The race had gone reasonably well. I got to the final bend in front, having got rid of most of the field, then I kicked, expecting to take five or six strides out of the closest runners. Instead I only took about two-and-a-half strides. It was a dreadful feeling. I'd done it so many times in a race before, and this time it just didn't work – like sticking your foot down on the accelerator and getting no reaction. I was getting further up the straight, but I knew Hans-Peter Ferner was getting closer all the time, and as he drew level with me there was that haunting, nightmare certainty that there was nothing more, absolutely nothing, that I could give.

I felt awful, ill, after the race. Back in London at the hospital they diagnosed glandular fever. I hadn't got it now, they said, but I had certainly had it quite recently. It could have been shielded a bit in the weeks when I was laid off with the leg injury. I'd been depressed anyway, being out of action with the season slipping by, and I could have missed the symptoms.

I had a series of hospital tests and a long lay-off that autumn. Only by December was I beginning to feel anything like I felt a year before in terms of health and fitness.

When you're sidelined, frustration is the main trouble – not just missing the glory of racing and all that, but the fact that running is a daily habit – and suddenly not being able to do what you have got used to doing every day for so many years is very disturbing.

And when you're at a high level of competition, the very fact that you're not involved is doubly worrying. Everything seems to be moving away from you at an incredible pace, and there's nothing you can do about it. I try to shy away from it all. I don't want to

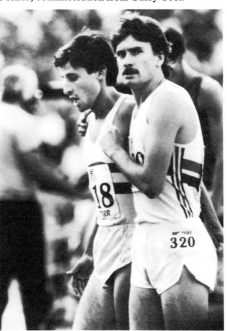

Disaster in Athens: defeat by Ferner, commiseration from Garry Cook

talk athletics, I don't even want to think athletics. All that seems to matter is getting the injury cleared up, and all I think about is the next physio session.

When you can start up again at last, the feelings are strangely mixed. It's wonderful being able to run again, and it's really exhilarating to have the challenge of getting back to racing fitness. But again there's the dreadful fear in the back of the mind that the injury could return, that you're going to end your next training session hobbling back to hospital. It takes perhaps two weeks for the fear to go. Then if you're lucky you're back to normal again.'

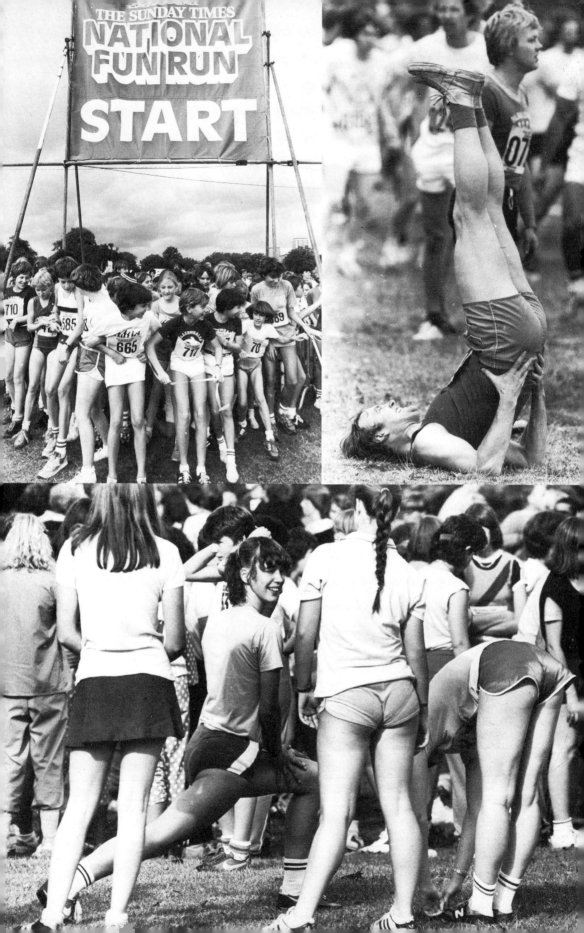

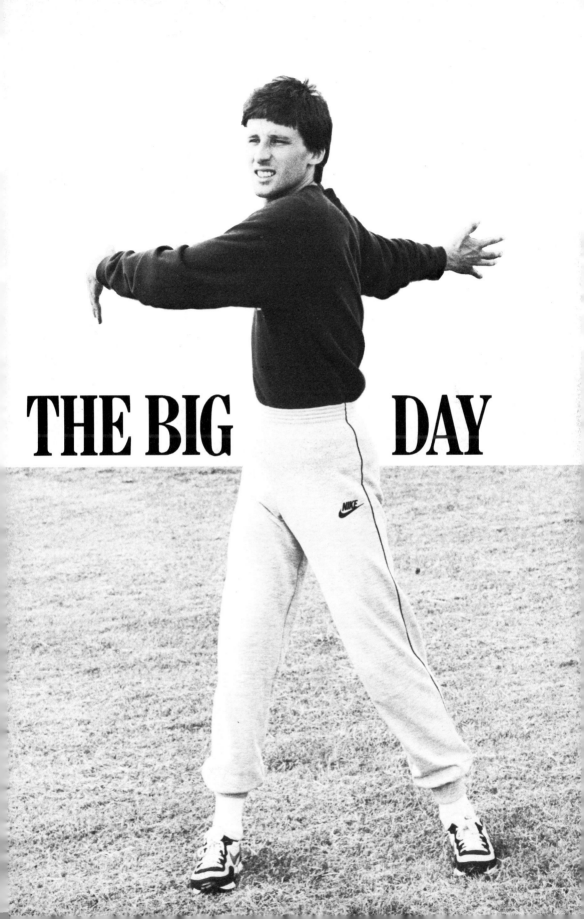

THE BIG DAY

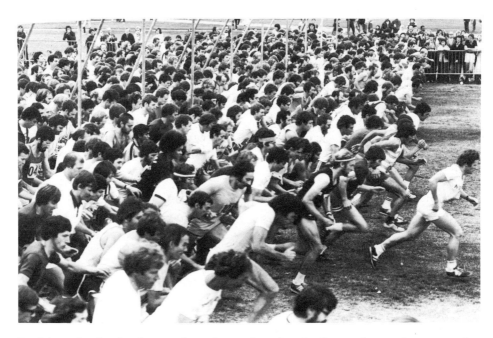

So, it's arrived – the day you have been planning for for weeks, perhaps months, or perhaps, if you have a very special talent, for the whole of your running career. It would be a tragedy if something were to go wrong to spoil the day. It might, of course, be just that someone else runs faster than you bargained for – you can't always plan for that. But a lot of pitfalls can be avoided by forethought and by careful planning; if you get these things right, you'll look back on the day with satisfaction however the race went.

You will have wound down your training in the previous few days or weeks, and with luck you will be feeling fully rested.

Get in your solid good night's sleep *two* nights before the race. If you are running on a Sunday it will be Friday night's sleep that will be the most important. On Friday night the week is over, and you can go to bed early and get up late. You will sleep well, and because the race is not tomorrow you won't toss and turn thinking about how it is going to go. On Saturday, or whatever day is the eve of the race, you can do the opposite. The edgy types should stay up a bit, or go out to see friends, so that they will be tired enough to get off to sleep as soon as they are in bed. When you're sleeping you're not worrying.

Circadian rhythms? They are not special beats from the West Indies, they are the cycles that the body passes through each day, and, with a few exceptions, they occur in everyone. The heart rate, the oxygen uptake and the secretion of various hormones all vary – for the lowest values are in the early hours after midnight. The peaks and troughs are different for women. There is evidence that some active people are sensitive to sleeping at unusual or unaccustomed times, so a couple of hours' sleep in the afternoon or early evening can upset these body rhythms and reduce the subsequent performance. So try to stick to a familiar sleep routine.

What have you forgotten?

Something else will have been concerning you on the eve of the big day, especially if you have an early start in the morning. How much are you going to take with you?

Even if this is your first event, you will have been running long enough to have acquired a lot of kit – far more than you are going to need for one race. But allowing for any contingency, from a snowstorm to a lost sock, you are still going to carry a fair amount with you. Make a list as things occur to you during the previous week, and tick it off as you pack your hold-all. Or use the checklist we have devised on page 166.

Your requirements can be divided into four categories: (1) what you wear before your run, (2) what you wear to run in, (3) what you wear or might need after the run before travelling home, and (4) the secretarial stuff, of which your running number is the most important.

Assuming you are not arriving straight from the Lord Mayor's Banquet, you will probably travel to the race in a *tracksuit*, with perhaps a *sweatshirt* underneath and, if it's cold, a *T-shirt* or a *long-sleeved thermal vest* underneath that. You may also be wearing *long johns* or thin *training trousers* under your tracksuit bottoms. You will also want to carry your *rain top* and *rainproof trousers* in case of a wet start, and probably a *hat* of some kind. Some of these can also help out if it turns really cold before the start and you find you want a long-sleeved vest or long trousers to race in. You will be wearing *trainers* or ordinary *walking shoes*.

To change into for the warm-up, and to race in, you'll carry your *vest*, *shorts*, *pants*, *socks* and *running shoes*. In cold weather you may want an *extra T-shirt* on top and a pair of *cotton gloves*. And *vaseline*, perhaps, to rub on your face and legs to prevent chafing. In summer you might want a *sweatband* or *wristbands*, or even a light *cap*.

Now remember, everything you have worn to this point might well have got either wet or sweaty even before the start. So after the race you will be searching your bag for a clean *T-shirt*, clean *pants*, a clean *sweatshirt*, clean *socks*, a *sweater*, perhaps a *windcheater*. Not to mention a *towel*, some *soap*, *foot powder* and a *comb*.

If you have taken a knock, you might be grateful for your own *first aid kit* (it's a good idea always to carry one, anyway). It should include *crepe bandage*, *safety pins*, *Elastoplast*, an *antiseptic* as well as the *vaseline*. And an *ice-pack* taken from the refrigerator before you leave and wrapped in newspaper for insulation. You can buy packs like this in sealed plastic containers – and very useful they can be.

These should suit most runners' needs. A cross-country entrant might have a variety of shoes to choose from once he has had a look at the course, and many are the runners who wished too late that they had brought a spare pair of *shoelaces*, but if you carry most of the above you are likely to be a lender in the changing room rather than a borrower.

Finally, the secretarial stuff. If you have been sent a *race number*, don't forget

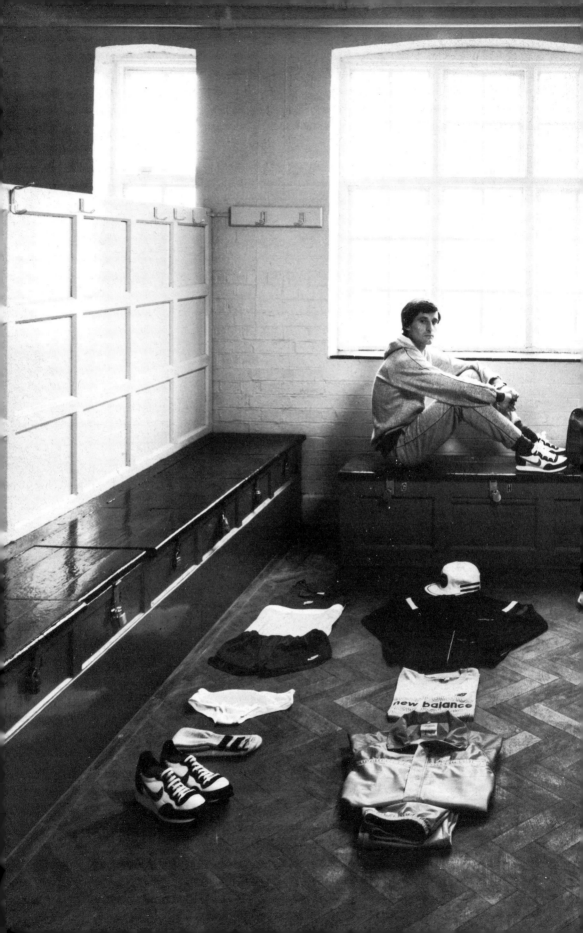

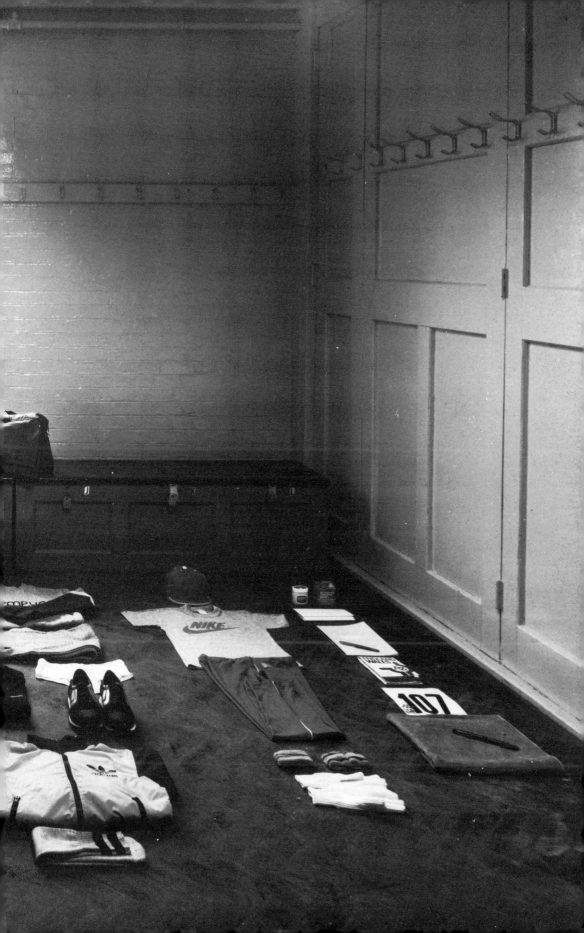

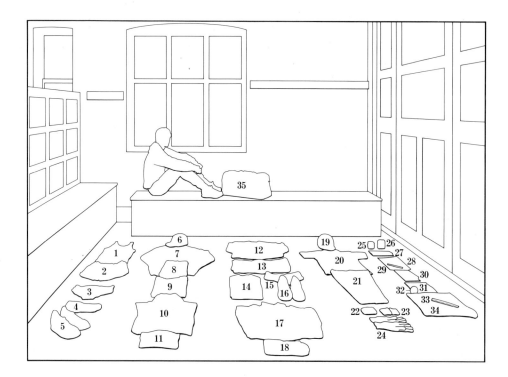

To run in
1. Vest
2. Shorts
3. Pants
4. Socks
5. Running shoes

To warm up in
6. Hat
7. Sweatshirt
8. Trousers
9. T-shirt
10. Rain top
11. Rainproof trousers

To change into after run
12. Sweatshirt
13. Trousers
14. 'V' neck sweater
15. Underpants
16. Shoes
17. Windcheater
18. Socks

Extras for running in hot or cold weather
19. Hat
20. T-shirt
21. Training trousers
22. Sweatband
23. Wristbands
24. Gloves

Miscellaneous
25. Vaseline
26. Plasters
27. Race acceptance
28. Race details
29. Pen
30. Map
31. Number
32. Safety pins
33. Comb
34. Towel
35. Hold-all

it; and in case it gets lost before the start (or during the race) memorise your number – it may mean vital points to your team, it may even be the difference between you being allowed to run or not. Bring *safety pins* to attach it to your vest. Bring some *money* for emergencies, a *pen* (not just for signing autographs – you may want to fill out a results envelope which the organisers will post to you when the final placings have been worked out). Bring the *race details* that came with your number, and a *road map* in case you get lost finding the venue. Wear your *watch*.

Getting There

Some of the most important factors determining how and when you should arrive at a race are psychological, and represent a kind of character profile.

The younger athlete who has had the same coach for a long time will certainly have been conditioned by his coach's thinking. If the coach has spotted something in his behaviour pattern that he thinks is inconsistent with a good performance he will have tried to change or eliminate it.

For example, if a runner is the nail-biting, anxious type, is he better off with the crowds with something happening to take his mind off the forthcoming competition, or is he better off out of it, where he can calm down and not get worked up by the others' feelings of expectancy and excitement? If he is away from the other competitors, does he have more time to worry about the coming trial?

At the roadside or the trackside or in the changing room there will always be those who are bragging or exaggerating to keep up their own spirits – this sort of thing can affect an impressionable newcomer.

But it is one thing to be away from the mob with a guide and confidant; it is quite another to be on your own, perhaps feeling lost and lonely.

In Seb's early running days we soon realised that running about with other youngsters was not the best preparation, and something always seemed to go wrong with all the big English Schools Championships except the last one, when Seb won the 3000 metres. This was also the one in which we arrived on our own, in our own transport and in our own time, and from this developed an unvarying pattern that we have kept to ever since.

It takes a lot of work to devise the best pattern, and the extra planning might make it a two-day rather than a one-day problem. But the results are worth it.

The anxiety you might be feeling as you arrive for your first race is nothing, of course, to the pressures on the top track stars. You will be spared the expectancy of supporters, the hopes of the whole nation, as well as the attention of newspaper reporters and television cameras.

However, you will also miss some of the small privileges that go with it, like not having to find the start or the changing rooms, or where to get a bath or where to find the numbers – the new breed of British team managers with our international athletes are a hard-working band. But for the run-of-the-mill runner these can be real irritations, and must be allowed for – in terms of time and patience.

Your first few races will seem chaotic, especially road and cross-country races and, most of all, big relays. If in doubt, arrive early – the problem of waiting for the off is not nearly as unnerving and fatiguing as trying to find the venue, change and get to the start in time with the right numbers. Travelling with a team or a coach is great fun and very supportive if you are on time, but again, if in doubt, arrive under your own steam, be sure you know exactly where the venue is and that you have very clear pre-race information and instructions.

The Cross-country Code

For cross-country meetings, a few expert tips might come in even more welcome – the varying terrain and the very informality of the sport can make it all the more confusing for a newcomer.

Unless you have run the course before, get there in plenty of time to jog round it to familiarise yourself with the layout. It will be too late to change your shoes if you have bent the spikes half way round, or selected the wrong type. If you don't know the course, study the map which should be pinned up near the start or near the changing rooms.

We have always looked for a spot with the maximum shelter to warm up in. On bad days you can get worn out trying to raise your temperature if you are too exposed to the weather.

Keep warm to the very last moment. Youngsters in school races eagerly discard coats and tracksuits and hang around for the start which can easily be delayed. Always leave your discarded gear in a waterproof bag at the finish if you don't have a clubmate looking after them all. If it starts to rain during the race you will not enjoy getting into a soggy tracksuit at the finish.

Knowing the course helps you with the start. It is fine to begin slowly and work your way through the field, the old, classic advice, but if at 300 yards from the start the course narrows to single file, by the time you are through the gap you can be so far back in the queue that you will never catch up.

Heat loss can be cruel on some days, particularly in strong, cold winds and rain. A smear of olive oil on exposed skin, light cotton gloves and long-sleeved running vests should all be considered. Experience is the best guide.

The Old Routine

Once the uncertainties of your first competitive race are over, you will readily settle into a routine for all days such as this. On occasions before a big race, Seb has evolved a sequence that hardly ever changes:

First, a good sleep for a couple of hours. Then he is woken up in time to complete the rest of the ritual, which is to shower, shave and change into freshly laundered kit. This is timed so that he can arrive at the warm-up area approximately forty-five minutes before the race. He finds that this routine reduces the pre-race tension considerably. Clearly it is good to sleep and not to worry, but it is equally bad to sleep and upset your body rhythms if you are sensitive to these changes – what suits one athlete might not suit you.

Certainly, this sequence won't even approximate to yours. But whatever it is, stick to it. The warm-up ritual you have evolved is the one that works for you, so do it as usual. The middle of the race is not the time to think 'Did I warm up enough?' If you are inexperienced, then evolve a sound routine as soon as possible – you need all the confidence you can get.

As for food before the race, don't compete on a heavy, fatty meal or with your stomach swilling around with liquid like a hot water bottle.

That switch of blood from the stomach to the muscles, which the body makes whether you want it to or not, can result in severe pain if the stomach has too much in it. The body knows it wants blood in the muscles to run; it will not know you have handicapped it with too much food eaten too late. People are different, but as a general rule allow at least two hours after a modest carbohydrate meal before you run.

Most athletes nowadays drink very little, too, in the two-and-a-half to five hours before a race – just enough to stop them feeling dry-mouthed. Though for races more than seven or eight miles on the road or across country, where dehydration might become a danger, you will find runners drinking much closer to the start.

The Vital Warm-up

The warm-up performs two functions. Primarily it is a physiological requirement before training or competition. Secondarily, it becomes a psychological requirement evolving out of the first.

The main requirement is to raise the core temperature of the body, increasing it by some 2°F (1.1°C) in order to achieve the following:

1. A reduction in internal friction: muscles contract and antagonistic muscles relax better, and therefore faster and with less risk of injury, when warm; pulled muscles are more common when an athlete is cold.

2. A dilation of the blood vessels, bringing more warmth and fuel supply to the muscles.

3. A general increase in the metabolic rate, so that haemoglobin releases oxygen more readily from the blood.

4. An increase in circulation, so that more oxygen gets to the cells.

Raising a quick sweat is not a true warm up, because although the body may be perspiring freely, and the blood, diverted to the skin for cooling purposes, may make you feel warmer, the inner temperature may not have increased sufficiently to achieve those aims. Runners do not want to, nor could they, be continually consulting rectal thermometers to ascertain their increase in core temperature; only personal experience will tell you when your body becomes freer and looser.

As in so many things, twice as much is not twice as good. In high-performance events, particularly those over shorter distances, an excessively long warm up will make inroads into the natural reserves of the body. Any warm-up routine should contain elements in which the full range of racing movement is encountered, and so you should certainly, for example, gradually work up to some fast striding.

The warm-up routine should also contain flexibility exercises, and again we emphasise that these exercises should not be done cold. They are best done not earlier than midway through your routine. And since the warm-up is, as its name indicates, to get you warm, do not stretch and risk muscle or tendon injury until you *are* warm. Your separate flexibility sessions are to enhance your range of movement so that the range which is normal for your sporting activity keeps you well short of injury.

Events like the hurdles seem to have become associated with the most elaborate flexibility routines, but all athletes would benefit by just being able to do them. If only all athletes in all sports were as flexible as schooled ballet dancers. The demands of their long, energetic roles are considerable, combining as they do running, jumping, lifting and even throwing, a kind of combined event requiring extended ranges of movement under load. Seb may be much more flexible than most middle-distance runners, his admiration for his dancing sister contains not a little envy.

The psychological aspect of the warm-up routine is also important. In competition it plays a large part in maintaining confidence and controlling nerves. Arriving late, and not having time to complete the full routine he has developed over the years, can leave an athlete worrying about not being ready to compete. And when he is doing something positive, like concentrating on his warm-up, the performer has less time to dwell upon his forthcoming trial.

Jogging, striding and stretching are the elements of a runner's warm-up, the intensity and duration of which are modified by the time of day and the weather.

Within the stricture of not taking too much out of your reserves, one might summarise by saying: the shorter the event the more intense the warm-up. Clearly the requirements of a 400 metre hurdler are not those of the marathon man, since the former has to have all systems go from the instant the gun fires.

There is a time-lag between the start of a run and the metabolism catching up with energy requirement during which, depending upon how fast the start is, a small oxygen debt will build up. In a long-distance race a slower start can be tolerated, and indeed has a sound physiological basis. But in 5000 metres and even some 10,000 metres races, the result of being too far off the pace from the start can be truly disastrous.

Besides, it takes a very brave and disciplined athlete to hold back until he is ready to increase the pace slowly and steadily until he has pulled back the gap. The problem here is that in a class race the runner may be running on his own for a long time, which is extra tough, physically and mentally.

Every athlete's warm-up routine is different. Seb's pre-race build-up goes something like this:

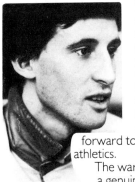

I'm usually at my most nervous when I first arrive at the stadium – particularly if I've walked there from the hotel and been part of the expectant crowd looking forward to the evening's athletics.

The warm-up for me has a genuine psychological effect. All the big stadiums have pretty good facilities now – grass areas away from the noise and the lights of the track – and once you are there you can dampen down the nerves. It's good to know, once you've started your routine, that you have somehow got into the first act of the racing evening.

It's a chance to get a glimpse of the other athletes, too. We all seem to be giving each other sideways glances, just to check who's there, perhaps. But really you are concentrating on your own warm-up, you haven't a lot of time to look at theirs. Even if you did you wouldn't learn much – they're unlikely to be actually limping, or anything like that.

I think some athletes are inclined to over-do the warm-up. It may be nervousness, perhaps, that doesn't let them stop, but I'm quite sure some runners have left their best performances in the warm-up area. You've got to remember that a warm-up is designed principally to warm you up, and if you can add to that a bit of suppleness and freedom of movement there's no need to go on flogging yourself for an hour or hour-and-a-half. Some people have almost completed full training sessions by the time they walk out onto the track.

For an 800 metre race on a reasonably warm evening I would never need more than thirty-five to forty minutes warming up, and only five or ten minutes of that would be hard work – perhaps some fast strides and some speed drills. The sequence I use has taken shape over the years. I didn't sit down and map it out, it has evolved gradually into its present shape and it works mentally and physically for me. It gets me to the start line warm, supple and mentally prepared to do what I've come to do. It goes like this:

Alternately walk and jog for five minutes or so.

Jog continuously at a slightly faster pace

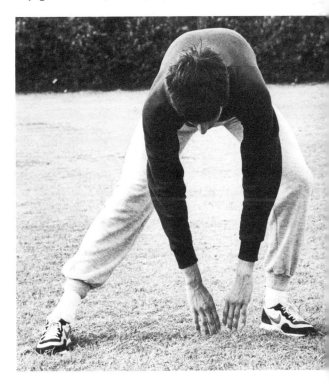

for about another five minutes, slipping in the odd high knee-lift and little burst of fast-cadence short steps, something like a sprinter's speed drill. By now I will be warm enough for stretching.

Static stretch calves and hamstrings, slowly stretching one leg at a time by leaning forward against a wall or stanchion, with the hands, and the leading leg, being ready to take the weight and control the tension, the rear leg being stretched with the heel firmly on the ground.

Loosen up the neck, shoulders and arms; combined leg and trunk stretching, by alternately placing first one straight leg and then the other, raised nearly horizontal, onto a radiator, chair or low wall, then bending the trunk forward as parallel as possible to the raised leg and placing the head on the raised knee.

Stand legs astride with hands on hips or behind the head, and bend and rotate the trunk.

Follow with a few half squats, remembering the static part – holding each position for 10–15 seconds. I would allow eight to ten minutes for the stretching exercises.

Resume jogging which, as soon as any "stretched" feeling passes off, turns into steady running. By now I am warmed up.

A set of, say, four fast strides over about 60 metres each.

Jog down for half a minute.

The whole routine is timed to finish as close to the start of the event as possible. I will stay well wrapped up throughout.'

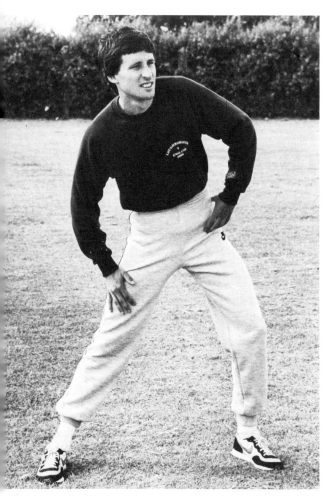
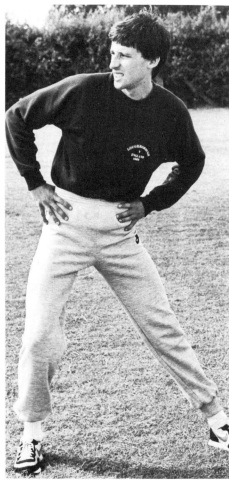

The Day of the Marathon

The day of every race is a big day – but for many runners new to the sport, the day of the marathon you have dreamed about, and towards which you have worked for months, is the big day to beat them all.

It is a day, too, that calls for more forethought and preparation than any race you might have entered during the build-up . . . because if there is one day on which you really do *not* want things to go wrong, this is the day.

The Marathon Diet

You may well have heard about glycogen-loading via a bleed-out diet. Forget it. While this diet trick can certainly help some runners, it takes a couple of tries at least to get it somewhere near right, and to ensure that you are not one of those people it does not suit.

The full bleed-out treatment involves eating a high-protein diet and hard running for a period and then, a few days before the race, switching to a high-carbohydrate diet so that the glycogen-starved body will over-compensate, and from the high-carbohydrate intake convert and store a larger-than-normal stock of glycogen.

One can easily see the effect that a hard run and a drastic diet shift might have on the learner marathoner. The easier way is to switch to high-carbohydrate meals for three days before the race – just plenty of pasta, bread and potatoes.

The Marathon Gear

What we said about foot care (Chapter Seven) is even more relevant for a marathon; and your shoes must be comfortable and protective. It may seem obvious, but we feel it is worth repeating that lightness is not everything; calculating the effort saved by lighter shoes is useless if you cannot finish the race in the super-lights you have chosen on weight alone. It may be a great shoe, but if you can feel a small stone shortly after the start think how you will feel long before the finish.

Are your shoes cool to run in? Blisters are caused by the heat from friction, and even if your shoe fits well, don't add to the heat by footwear that lacks ventilation. A marathon shoe must breathe. And the linings and inner soles must not rub, ruckle or irritate in any way.

There is nothing worse than an almost neurotic runner worrying over all the trivia instead of getting on with the running and toughening himself, but having said that, if there is a case for being ultra-careful about gear it is in the build-up period to your first marathon.

In our schedule there are no fewer than seventeen runs of ten miles or more, and this gives you plenty of time to discover the irritations that linger, and you should have encountered a sufficient variety of weather to answer such questions as: How does your skin stand up to the rain? Do you chafe easily? Is there a seam or some-such on your singlet that rubs?

Women will have some nipple protection from their bras; men who have never thought of problems in that area should be alert for it now. The continued rubbing from the wrong singlet is a problem: it is better to get a running singlet of the right cut, but otherwise use a second-skin type of adhesive cover, or even a plain adhesive strip.

Socks that may seem all right at five miles can irritate at eight miles. They then become painful at ten miles and impossible a little later. Remember that you are going to be moving your arms, legs and torso for four hours of hard work.

Head gear; you haven't forgotten that, have you? Experiment with a hat or cap if you think you will need one. Four hours' exertion in the sun is a trial to be reckoned with.

Marathon Eating and Drinking

Before the race, do not eat later than three hours before the start, and even then not a heavy protein or fat meal. As for drinking, we would suggest about a pint – not more – some half-hour before the start.

Your body's problem today is going to be the fact that it can only store enough glycogen for a modest day's living, so it is going to be looking for another fuel source when the glycogen gets scarce in the course of your marathon. That source is fat, and one suggestion, made by David Costill in *A Scientific Approach to Distance Running* is that drinking two cups of good coffee an hour before the start helps 'the fat cells liberate more free fatty acids', and has been able to extend the time to exhaustion by 19 per cent.

Costill gives one final no-no. Inside the final hour before the start, do not eat or drink anything that has much sugar in it – sweets, ice-cream, dried fruit, honey, soft drinks or even 'athletic' drinks.

During the marathon you will want to drink from time to time, and your training runs of twelve, sixteen and twenty miles should have given you a chance to establish a drinking pattern. In practice you will want about a quarter or a third of a pint every quarter of an hour or so if the day is at all warm.

You will certainly sweat, and a lot of water vapour is lost in the breath; if you lose too much water you will start to dehydrate, and dehydration can lead to overheating. There are now quite a few so-called balanced electrolytic drinks on the market which are meant to maintain the electrolytic balance (i.e. replace the various salts that are lost). However, not all the experts agree on the correctness of their composition. For example, when we lose salt through sweating, it does not leave the body in the same concentration as it exists in the body fluids. We actually lose the water faster than we lose the salt, so the salt concentration in the body is actually increasing as we run. Which calls for extremely careful

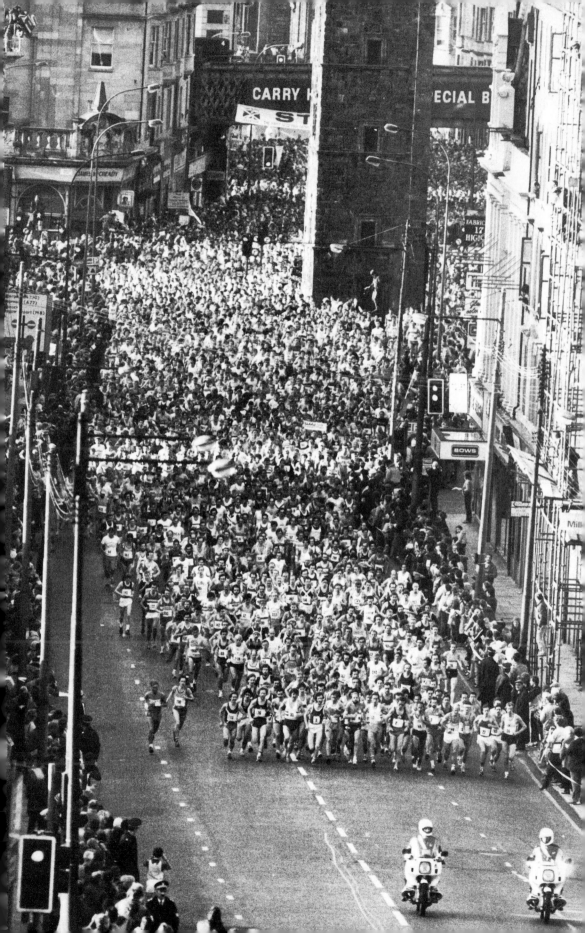

composition of salt drinks.

Until you have experimented and found something that you know improves your performance, you are probably safer with water.

The Marathon Itself

As for the race itself (and this includes any run of ten miles or more, particularly if it's a warm day), begin at slower than race pace. Hard running at the start rapidly depletes the glycogen in the muscles, and it may never get a chance to build up enough during the race.

It is wiser to run a lot slower for the first four minutes of the race, and then slowly increase speed to race pace over the next two or three minutes. This opening tactic will reduce muscle glycogen depletion and the lactate build-up that goes with it.

This starting method has only one drawback, and that is when you are running in one of the monster mass marathons when in the first six minutes of the race all sorts of oddities might decide to come past and get in the way, complete with circus props and umbrellas. But it's your day as well as theirs. Just stick to your plan and keep your cool.

The body has an elaborate heat-regulating mechanism which responds quickly to temperature changes, since it tries at all times to maintain a constant temperature. In hot weather there are two adjustments that the body makes, which are very important to runners.

It perspires so that the skin is cooled by evaporation and it also increases the flow of blood to the skin so that the blood can lose heat via the network of small capillaries and veins near the surface.

But blood diverted to the surface is blood diverted away from muscles which need all the fuel they can get. So cooling is all-important.

The key to marathon running is finding the correct pace, and in considering this problem it is helpful to appreciate two somewhat contradictory meanings of 'economy'.

The first meaning is efficiency. The most efficient pace is the pace that uses up the least energy per mile. Unfortunately this is a fast pace, which you may not be able to maintain.

The second meaning is the idea of spending (in this case energy) at a rate you can maintain, a sense of eking out your energy in order to last the distance. Unfortunately, again, this is often a slow or slower pace, and uses up more energy per mile.

While the aim is to finish the race rather than to blow up, if the pace is too slow it brings extra problems in hot and humid weather by way of excessive fluid loss. By not running so quickly you might not heat up so much, but by extending the running time under a hot sun, particularly in humid weather when sweat does not evaporate quickly, you increase the risk of dehydration and heat stroke.

Furthermore, you cannot absorb water as fast as you can lose it when running. Nearly three-quarters of your body is water and in a long run the loss of volume from the blood has to be made up from the rest of the body, and this fluid loss from the cells upsets the body's whole delicate balance.

Yes – finding your right pace is the key to the marathon.

It's All Yours

From now on you're on your own. If it's your first road race or your first time on the fells, or your first fun run or your first Olympic heat, it will be something you're not going to forget. It is your own motivation that has got you to this point – whether over the last weeks or months or years, and it's your own strength of will – as well as the quality of work that you have put into your training – that is going to get you through those next few miles or those next testing laps or the unrelenting four hours of that marathon.

If you have had the stamina to get this far in the book, we are sure you can do the rest. Good luck.

Moment of achievement: the marathon has been completed; the euphoria will come a little later

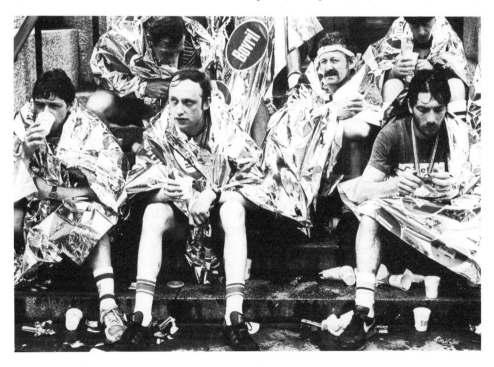

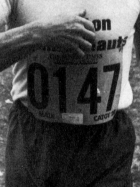

THE RUNNING MIND AND THE RUNNING BODY

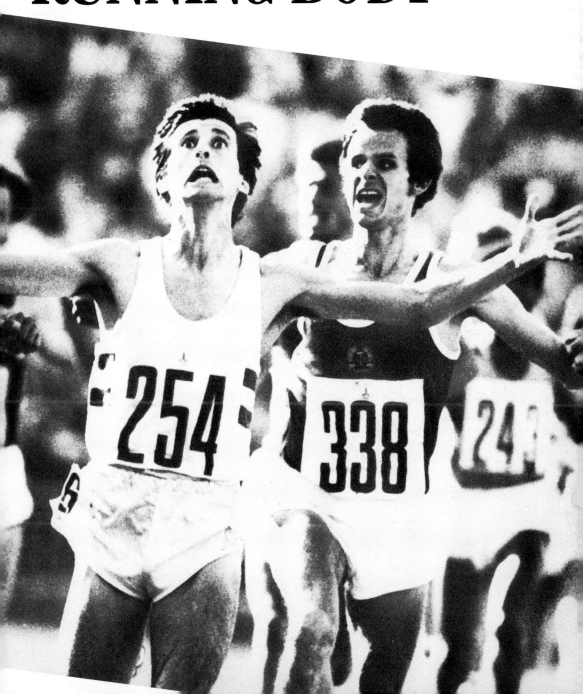

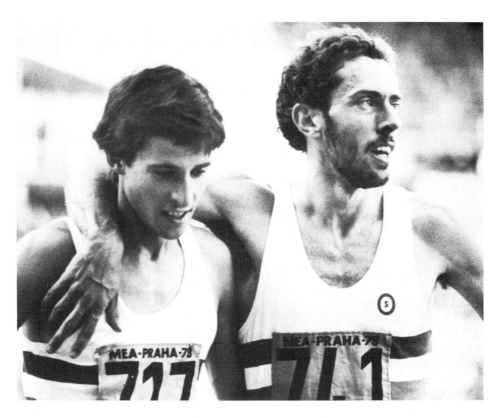

The scorn felt ten years ago by the early morning businessmen walking through Hyde Park at the sight of the sweat-soaked fitness fanatic (anybody who ran had to be a fanatic) has now changed, if not to the universal pursuit of total fitness, then at least to feelings of guilt among the sedentary, and the certainty that they are taking the trouble, in ever-increasing numbers, to count themselves among the newly converted sweat-soaked hordes.

Now you have joined them. With luck you are well on your way to a new achievement in your running career – a new distance to attempt; a new personal best time to record. Perhaps, if you are a beginner, your first competitive run is looming on the horizon: a somewhat daunting challenge if six months ago you had confined your exercise to chasing buses, but now a challenge you can face with confidence, and with a body which, as we showed in Chapter Three, is already undergoing the changes that go hand in hand with regular exercise.

Already, very soon after you began training, there will have been a strengthening of the muscles exercised, predominantly the legs but also in others in proportion to their use. Some of those significantly involved will have been those used in breathing. It is often overlooked that when running these muscles work much harder, and with a larger range of movement, than they do at rest.

The action of your heart will have improved. The heart is a non-stop muscle which more than any other depends on a plentiful supply of blood, and without developing an even greater supply it cannot in turn pump the extra that an increase in work load demands. Luckily, in order to get more blood to exercised and strengthened muscles, your fine network of capillaries has increased, including those that serve the heart.

Now a strengthened heart can pump an increased amount of blood at each stroke, and so, to do the same amount of work, it does not need to beat so quickly. In turn, a slower-beating heart has more time to fill properly so that it pumps even more per stroke. All physical activity is ultimately limited by the amount of oxygen-rich blood that can be delivered to the muscles, and this increase in the stroke-volume of your heart is basic to fitness.

Besides strengthening the muscles, your running is helping you to get rid of fat in the muscle and fat stored around the body. The reduction in useless body fat together with the greater muscle strength is increasing the power-weight ratio and the body's overall efficiency, and thereby decreasing the load on the heart.

So your lungs are becoming much healthier organs, the airways open up, and breathing is easier because there is less resistance to the passage of air, and the lungs can supply more oxygen to the blood.

The volume of blood also increases in trained runners, and you will gradually be increasing your lung capacity. Result: more oxygen uptake and more blood to circulate it. And a good supply of blood-carrying oxygen and glucose is vital to the brain – another factor in your increased well-being.

This will not all happen at once, and it would do the body no good to try to effect anything but a gradual improvement. Training not only strengthens muscles, but it necessarily strengthens ligaments, tendons and their attachments, and it is obvious that muscles and tendons should develop together: by trying to speed things up, say by using anabolic steroids, it is possible to develop the strength of muscles so quickly that severe damage is done to the tendons and the attachments to the bone which cannot stand the increased loadings. Always develop and train gradually so that the body tunes up uniformly.

Although the response to exercise lessens with age, tests on men aged between fifty-five and seventy have demonstrated significant improvement. These men had been physically inactive for at least twenty years, but after training three to five times per week in one- to two-hour sessions over an eight-week period, their maximum oxygen uptake improved 20 per cent. So it's never too late to start.

With regular exercise, the machine which is your body will be able to work much more efficiently, and thus much longer, without fatigue; and muscles that are regularly and strongly stimulated respond more readily when called upon, and do so with enhanced co-ordination.

Women's muscles and cardiovascular systems and general well-being will be affected in the same way as men's, but there really is a bonus for women who may initially be motivated to run in the hope of improving their figures. They will benefit in three ways: excess fat will be lost by means of diet and exercise; the exercise will consume the fat while preserving the lean tissue; and at the same time muscle tone will improve, posture will improve (especially if the running is accompanied by good flexibility exercises) and previously flabby muscles will improve their shape without any significant increase in size.

Round shoulders, and tummies that look fatter than they are simply because they stick out, will disappear with proper training. Almost invariably, too, an increased circulation enhances the natural complexion and the all-round enhancement of your physical condition puts back the sparkle you thought you had lost.

Not a bad selling point for the men, either.

If the idea of facing an hour's running during a week seems a bit tough on you now, it is because you do not yet know what fitness is like. Running does more than fit you for running – it sets you up for your everyday work, and for your everyday leisure.

And it isn't solely in the more obvious parts of the body that the effects are felt. The brain itself is particularly sensitive to minute chemical changes – very often in a negative sense, producing a wide range of imaginary ailments or psychosomatic illnesses. Drugs or poisons can have strange hallucinatory effects, and when deprived of small amounts of glucose or oxygen the function of the brain is impaired.

The strong healthy heart of a fit person can pump the blood containing enough oxygen and glucose to a brain that will be all the better for it. There are well-documented cases of physical gains being accompanied by emotional improvements and an increased mental alertness.

Vanity is perhaps too strong a word, but whose self-esteem would not be improved if he or she looked better? We all like to be told that we are looking fit and well and if we really know that our muscles are firm, that we have a good posture, that we are not fat and that a good circulation is helping our complexion, then we look out on the world in a much better way.

We have a nervous system of which a part carries out instructions to order, a part which once started continues functioning without being continually instructed, and another part which doesn't wait for conscious instructions at all but issues its own orders. With the central nervous system and the autonomic system so closely interwoven, and given the physiological fact that every cell in the body is connected with the others – the cells of the brain with the cells of the foot – we can be in no doubt that a holistic approach to the mind and the body must be the right one.

Mens Sana . . . ?

This attitude, we feel, is the soundest possible basis for an answer to the often-posed question: Does running have any effect on the mind? It is by no means a simple subject – a series in *Athletics Weekly* magazine by Brian Mitchell on 'Athletes' Minds' in 1982 ran to five parts, which shows there is plenty to say

– but the usual dilemma faced in attempting an answer is the old chicken-and-the-egg problem: Was it ultimately the mind that made success possible, or was it the body that allowed the mind to be successful?

It is perhaps the coach, whose job it is to train both mind and body to simultaneous performance and who can watch the results with a certain objectivity, rather than the athlete himself, who can make the most revealing contribution to the debate.

I have watched four children grow into adults sharing the same environment (house, books, music, schools), and I believe strongly that the genetic inheritance is the most important. There is no other way of accounting for the big differences not only between each of them but also within the pairs (two boys, two girls).

But I do not deny the interaction between the individual and his environment. We all have the power to modify our environment through the free choices that are open to us, and thus modify ourselves at the same time.

Today there are many clichés used on the famous to cut them down to size. They range from "If you can't stand the heat stay out of the kitchen", to "They must like it or they wouldn't do it". They may contain some of the truth, but they certainly do not tell it all.

It does take guts to continue once you have reached the top. Outside observers always seem to be hooked on the motivation problem. After a world record, an Olympic gold, or whatever else strikes them as the pinnacle of success, they all ask, "What is left now to strive for? What can motivate him now?"

There is another big problem. What is hard, and can only get harder all the time, is winning. Not the effort of maintaining the training – that's bad enough – but the knowledge that there can never be an unbroken chain of victories. Retiring undefeated looks nice in the record books, but if it is premature retirement purely to get that distinction, then it does not mean quite so much. Every class athlete knows that the last win he has just notched up brings him one race closer to defeat. One man's forty-five consecutive wins only makes the forty-sixth race more desperate.

A world record only makes defeat even more "inexcusable" in the same event at the next championship. There were two winners in the Moscow Games, of whom, after all the adulation, it can be said "only they know the true cost of their gold". Olympic titles and world records go on exacting a price long after the world thinks they are paid for. There is a common bond between champions and outlaws – both have a big price on their heads.

Carrying that pressure is every bit as tough on the athletes as the training that keeps them there. "I put up with it because I still like winning enough to endure the training. It is nice to have your body working like a 'well-oiled machine', but it is nicer not to go training in mid-winter in the early morning and the late evening with your eyes and ears frozen."

But there is a magic on the big nights which is very hard to describe, for the alchemy of the spectacular in Zurich, say, or Brussels is at the same time both brutal and subtle.

The pre-event interviews with the press and television, the media's incessant hunger for the dramatic announcement like "It's a record attempt tonight", or "I've come here to win the big one" is a maddening part of the scene one could well do without, but without which it wouldn't be the same. The siege of the autograph hunters and the genuine fans, who can make you climb fences to find rear exits from the arena, is only just bearable.

All the year you have been planning for this night. The coach has examined his athlete's progress and condition, changed the emphasis on the training, assessed the performances to date of his athlete and the other contestants and despite all the care in the preparation he accompanies his gladiator (for this is *how* it feels) to the arena knowing that at any time the unthinkable can happen. The long walk from the hotel to the stadium is almost like the walk from death row in an old Warner Brothers movie. Arrival at the warm-up area, often in the semi-darkness away from the track, brings some relief in that the action is beginning at last. The athlete has not eaten for maybe four hours or so, and the coach has starved with him – the one from practicalities, the other from nerves.

No matter how many times you have been there, it only gets harder to bear. The close bond between two people is not without pains, one of which will always be the pain of doubt. The coach is praying that there is nothing that he has not considered and the athlete is carrying the awful load, on top of all the other expectations, of not wanting to fail the coach. The longer you have been successful the greater the pressure you create. No wonder that there comes that moment when even the best have to blurt out: "What the hell am I doing here?"

Then it's through the tunnel and into the arena. The floodlights are on and, surrounded by flash guns and tracked by television cameras, the gladiator is presented to the crowd.

For him it is the Greyhound Derby, the Heavyweight Championship, the World Cup Final and Barnum & Bailey's all in one. Suddenly he is going to lay on the line thousands of hours of training and thousands of miles of running for a spin of the wheel that may only last one minute and forty odd seconds.

What is the immediate reward? The chance to lose and slip away into oblivion (but not if the world says he should have won). Or win and hope that he can get up enough strength to face the ensuing fracas which can only be likened to a coroner's court being held during a wild coronation.

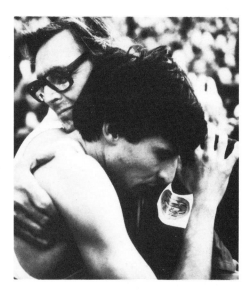

When the magic moment does come, that instant when the old "well-oiled machine" goes into overdrive and the field fades, there is only the exultation of the final drive for the line . . . unless the trackside clock is in view, when the seconds go too quickly and the tape starts to recede, prolonging the agony of the record attempt even further.

Why then do they go on? The answer surely can only be that the desire to be the best, the *numero uno*, that made them what they are in the first place, is still there.

Pride also plays a part. "I will not hang around after my best is no longer good enough – I will walk off the track and stay off." Who can argue with Seb on that?

And if anyone should ask us "Is it worth all that?" the answer is still yes.

It all comes back, it seems, to motivation. In a television interview with Seb, David Coleman once said that some runners were motivated by the opposition, "but you seem to be self-motivated. How do you do it?" Seb's reply was: "I suppose it's the motivation of just wanting to go out and run faster than I have run before, and hopefully faster than anyone else has run, and that gives me a lot of pleasure. It's sitting down before a race and feeling that at the end of the evening I may have achieved something really special."

The motivation of wanting to run faster or further than you have run before can apply to anyone. Victory is very worthwhile when it is victory over yourself, and at the end of the day the knowledge that you have had the will to force yourself to climb another few places up the finishing list can be something special to you.

So whether or not you dream of life at the top, cherish that certificate, keep that bronze medal, they are part of you. They say that you too have tried.

There were two races as a boy up Frodsham Hill and back that were Olympian in endeavour [see p. 186]. In an old photograph of the first race there is to be seen all the agony of a Calvary.

To compete means that you are submitting yourself to a test. In fact you are being examined. In a Britain which for too long has lost its way in a distortion of egalitarianism, testing, particularly of the young, has become a dirty word. We need to unlearn this attitude.

To hang on to the end, to force your way to the front and win a desperately hard fought race needs tremendous determination, and to run flat out to the end knowing that victory has gone is hardly any easier.

To compete takes courage, and courage, as distinct from foolhardiness, is an act of will.'

Ultimately, successful running is a conquest of the body by the mind.

By successful running we mean the winning of major titles by the stars *and* winning the battle to maintain the meaningful fitness schedules that the forty-plus runners have set themselves. The battle may have to be fought much harder by some than by others but then life is not always fair, and having the will to see it through and practising that will is a quality everyone can aspire to.

Every time a runner goes out for his run, that is an act of will, and every time he finishes the run he will feel himself a better man for it. The worse the weather, the greater the willpower required, and the more the will is exercised the stronger it becomes. Smugness is not a pleasant characteristic, but anyone who submits himself to a hard discipline and sticks it out has a right to be pleased with himself. The experience belongs to him – it is his bit of individuality and his bit of success – success achieved with will, with thought and with concentration.

If all this seems a bit heavy, then consider the lighter side. Pleasures simple or intellectual are not enjoyed very much when accompanied by dyspepsia, constipation and lassitude. Dragging around a poor body takes the joy out of everything from bingo to chess. Poor old Karl Marx is alleged to have said that his writing would give the bourgeoisie cause to remember his boils.

Take your pick of the old sayings – 'Blowing the cobwebs out of your mind', 'Getting some fresh air in your lungs' and the like.

From the Ancient Greeks until today, bodily health has been considered indispensable to mental health. It has been said that nothing succeeds like success, and certainly earning your own self-respect is your own success story.

At school Seb was a very modest scholar, but as soon as he found himself as a runner and started winning races his school work started improving. Even the great chess champions now know that they have to prepare for the big intellectual battle of the world title with a carefully thought-out regime of physical fitness.

So if willpower is mind-power and running can exercise the will, then surely running can improve the mind.

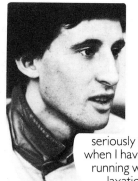

Running is much more than a convenient way of "improving the mind" and keeping the body healthy.

For me it has been my life, and I hope it will go on being my life. Running now is work and excitement and tension and a challenge, as it has been ever since I started competing seriously at the age of fourteen. But when I have retired from competition, running will be contentment and relaxation and pleasure.

When I do retire, I think the break is going to have to be a clean one. For any athlete who has competed at world-class it's very difficult to take a voluntary step down and compete at less than best. I really can't see myself two years after retirement running in my club's Christmas Handicap, or making up the numbers in a local cross-country race, or running my leg in the inter-club road relays. If the break is going to be healthy, it's got to be a break right across the board.

But running will certainly be there, and there is a lot of running that I want to do that I couldn't possibly do now. I watched the London Marathon earlier this year, when I was cheering on a friend, and the atmosphere really did affect me, it was very moving — not just the fast men at the front, but all the men and women down the field. They seemed to get such support from each other, in the easy miles early on, and in the shared pain and struggle towards the end. I'm sure I'll run a marathon one day — not to win, just to take part with everyone else.

I'll be free of programmes and schedules and stop-watches, too, when I've retired. If it's cold and raining when I get up in the morning, I can put off my run till the next day. And, in a funny way, I'll be able to take more risks. I can run across terrain that it would be mad for me to run across now — moorland paths, places like that, where the risk to legs and ankles and muscles have been too great.

I won't be inhibited in that way any more. I can just keep in shape and run and enjoy every minute of it.'

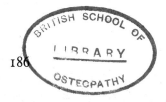
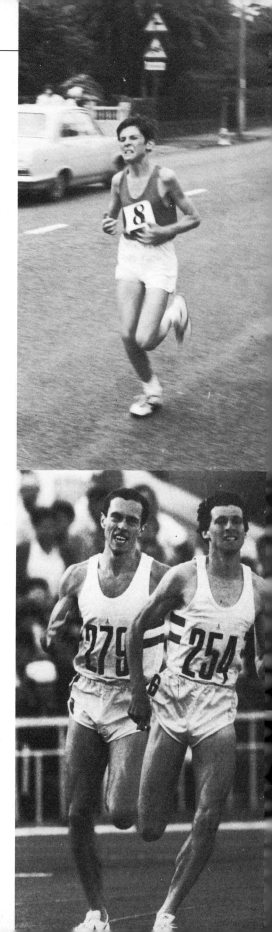

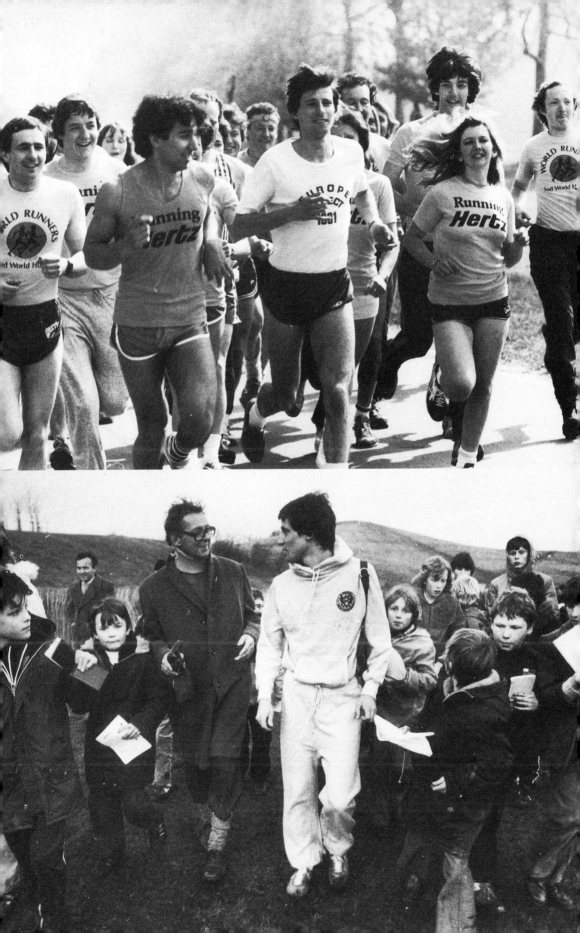

APPENDIX

Joining a Club

Not everyone will want to join a club, but they have their advantages – not only for the companionship, the coaching and the competition, but also for the fact that membership of a club is likely to allow you reduced entry fees to many events, and even get you a discount at your local sportswear shop. A letter to any of the following, accompanied by a stamped addressed envelope, will get you a list of the clubs in your area, and the address and telephone number of the secretary.

Athletics Clubs
All clubs affiliated to the Amateur Athletic Association are grouped in regions:
Southern Counties AAA and *England and Wales Women's AAA* Francis House, Francis Street, London SW1 1DL.
Midland AAA Devonshire House, High Street, Deritend, Birmingham B12 0LP.
Northern Counties AAA Studio 44, Bluecoat Chambers, Liverpool L1 BXC3.
Welsh AAA 54 Charles Street, Cardiff.
Scottish AAA and Scottish Women's AAA 16 Royal Crescent, Glasgow G3 7SL.
Northern Ireland AAA 20 Kernan Park, Portadown, Co. Armagh, N. Ireland.
Northern Ireland Women's AAA Tir na Nog, Old Calgorm Road, Ballymena, N. Ireland.
Irish Republic (Bord Luthleas na Eireann) BLE Offices, 69 Jones Road, Dublin 3.

Veterans' Athletics
Men become veterans at 40, women at 35, and there are many athletic clubs and athletic events run specially for them, as well as classes reserved for them in many open races. Members generally join the Veterans' Association for their area if they want to compete.

Parent body: *British Veterans Athletic Federation* Hon Sec Jack Haslam, 10 Higher Dunscar, Egerton, Bolton, Lancs.

Cross-Country
The area Cross-Country Association will provide a list of local clubs.

Eastern Counties Cross-Country Association. Hon Sec C. C. Bruning, 15 Karen Close, Ipswich, Suffolk IP1 4LP.

Midland Counties Cross-Country Association Hon Sec B. B. Heatley, 6 Kirkstone Crescent, Wombourne, near Wolverhampton.

Northern Cross-Country Association Hon Sec J. E. Davies, 14 Neal Avenue, Heald Green, Cheadle, Cheshire.

East Lancashire Cross-Country Association Hon Sec C. E. Haslam, 10 Higher Dunscar, Egerton, Bolton, Lancs.

West Lancashire Cross-Country Association Hon Sec Dr P. R. Thomas, 5 Newby Avenue, Rainhill, Prescot, Merseyside.

Yorkshire Cross-Country Association Hon Sec J. E. Smith, 7 Birch Avenue, Bradford, West Yorkshire BD5 8EZ.

North-Eastern Counties Cross Country Association Hon Sec M. Frazer, 11 Heslop Drive, Darlington, Co. Durham.

Southern Counties Cross-Country Association Hon Sec H. J. Hicks, 34 The Crescent, Friern Barnet, London N11 3HH.

Scottish Cross-Country Union Hon Sec J. E. Clifton, 38 Silvermowers Drive, Edinburgh EH4 5MM.

Welsh Cross-Country Association Mrs I. Lisle, 38 Nantfawr Road, Cyncoed, Cardiff.

Northern Ireland Cross-Country Association (as Northern Ireland AAA).

Orienteering

A full calendar of events, for anyone wishing to give orienteering a try, is available from:

British Orienteering Federation National Office, 41 Dale Road, Matlock, Derbyshire DE4 3LT.

You are able to try a couple of events as an 'independent', but should you wish to orienteer regularly you could be required to join a club, which would be affiliated at the same time to the area orienteering association and the national federation.

Fell Running

Members of the *Fell Runners Association* receive a full fixture list.

Membership secretary: N. F. Berry, 165 Penistone Road, Kirkburton, Huddersfield HD8 0PH.

Reading and Reference

While some of the following publications are inevitably more detailed and specialised than others, we have found them all valuable in their way over the years.

Training Theory by Frank Dick (British Amateur Athletics Board)
The Physiology of Exercise by Morehouse and Miller (C. V. Mosby)

Run, Run, Run by Fred Wilt (Track and Field News)
A Scientific Approach to Distance Running by David L. Costill (Track and Field News)
The Aerobics Way by Kenneth H. Cooper (Corgi)
The Complete Middle Distance Runner by Watts, Wilson and Horwill (Stanley Paul)
The Challenge of the Marathon by Cliff Temple (Stanley Paul)
Orienteering by Brian Porteus (Oxford University Press)
Tackle Orienteering by John Disley (Stanley Paul)
The Penguin Book of Orienteering by Roger Smith (Penguin)

Fitness, Health and Work Capacity ed. Leonard A. Larson (Macmillan)
Textbook of Work Physiology by Astrand and Rodahl (McGraw-Hill)
Strength Training for Athletes by R. J. Pickering (B.A.A.B.)
Mobility Exercises by Peter Harper (B.A.A.B.)
Fit to Exercise by Burke and Humphreys (Pelham)
Human Movement by Joseph R. Higgins (C. V. Mosby)
The Running Body (Runners World, booklet 27)

Success in Nutrition by Magnus Pyke (John Murray)
Diet in Sport by Wilf Paish (E.P. Publishing)
Teaching Nutrition and Food Sciences by Margaret Knight (Batsford)

The Athlete's Guide to Sports Medicine by Ellington Darden (Contemporary Books Inc.)
The Penguin Medical Encyclopaedia (Penguin)
Encyclopaedia of Athletics Medicine (Runners World, booklet 12)
The Sports Health Handbook by Harris, Lovesey and Oram (World's Work)
The Sunday Times New Book of Body Maintenance (Mermaid Books)

Photographic Acknowledgements:

Allsport: 7 (bottom), 8, 61, 64 (top right), 76, 92, 94 (bottom), 112 (bottom), 114, 136, 184; *Associated Press*: 186 (bottom); *Associated Newspapers*: 137 (bottom), *Glasgow Herald*: (Stuart Paterson) 112 (top and centre), (Ian Hossack) 175; *Richard Jeans*: 30 (left), *Chris Morris*: 30 (right); *Olympus Sports*: 164/165; *Record Pasta Company*: 96, 174; *Don Rose*: 64 (centre top); *Mark Shearman*: 3, 6 (right), 7 (top), 12 (top), 13, 21, 26, 45–49, 62, 64 (bottom), 79–82, 94 (top), 95, 132, 133, 137 (top), 138, 159, 161, 171, 172, 177, 180; *S&G Press Agency*: 88; *Sheffield Newspapers*: 33 (top left), 34, 67; *Sunday Times*: (Duncan Baxter) 33 (top right), (David Cairns) 38; (Derek Cattani) 32 (top right), 65 (top), (Ian Cook) 52, (Ian Dobbie) 14, (Frank Herrmann) 160 (bottom), 162, (Chris Smith) 2, 12 (bottom), 28/29, 32 (top left), 32 (bottom), 33 (bottom), 41, 64 (top left), 66, 74, 160 (top right), 178; *UPI*: 179.

INDEX